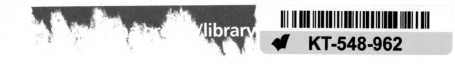
Core Paediatrics

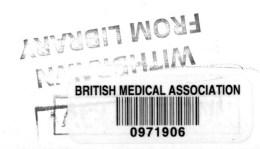

CORE PAEDIATRICS
A problem-solving approach

Steven Ryan MD, FRCPCH

Consultant Paediatrician,
Royal Liverpool Children's NHS Trust, Alder Hey, Liverpool, UK

Jackie Gregg MB ChB, FRCP, FRCPCH, DCH

Consultant Paediatrician, Community Child Health,
Royal Liverpool Children's NHS Trust, Alder Hey, Liverpool, UK

Leena Patel MB BS, MD, MRCP, FRCPCH, MHPE, MD

Senior Lecturer in Child Health, Academic Unit of Child Health,
University of Manchester and Honorary Consultant Paediatrician,
Central Manchester and Manchester Children's University Hospitals, Manchester, UK

ARNOLD

Hodder Arnold · A member of the Hodder Headline Group · London

First published in Great Britain in 2003 by
Arnold, a member of the Hodder Headline Group,
338 Euston Road, London NW1 3BH

http://www.arnoldpublishers.com

Distributed in the United States of America by
Oxford University Press Inc.,
198 Madison Avenue, New York, NY10016
Oxford is a registered trademark of Oxford University Press

Whilst the advice and information in this book are believed to be true
and accurate at the date of going to press, neither the authors nor the
publisher can accept any legal responsibility or liability for any errors or
omissions that may be made. In particular (but without limiting the
generality of the preceding disclaimer) every effort has been made to
check drug dosages; however, it is still possible that errors have been
missed. Furthermore, dosage schedules are constantly being revised
and new side-effects recognized. For these reasons the reader is
strongly urged to consult the drug companies' printed instructions
before administering any of the drugs recommended in this book.

British Library Cataloguing in Publication Data
A catalogue record for this book is available from the British Library

Library of Congress Cataloging-in-Publication Data
A catalog record for this book is available from the Library of Congress

ISBN   0 340 80971 X

1 2 3 4 5 6 7 8 9 10

Commissioning Editor: Georgina Bentliff
Development Editor: Heather Smith
Project Editor: Wendy Rooke
Production Controller: Lindsay Smith
Cover Design: Amina Dudhia

Typeset in 10/12.5 Minion by Charon Tec Pvt. Ltd, Chennai, India
Printed and bound in Italy.

What do you think about this book? Or any other Arnold title?
Please send your comments to feedback.arnold@hodder.co.uk

We dedicate this book to our families and our patients

Contents

Contents

Preface

We hope that you enjoy meeting the 40 young people whom we've come to know during the writing of this book; we also hope that through them you will achieve an understanding of the modern approach to paediatrics that is rooted in the ancient skills of history taking and examination. You will be introduced to the most common health problems in children and taken through the child's medical journey step by step. The history, examination and investigations are logically pursued for each case, and we hope to increase your understanding of why certain questions are asked and why particular examination techniques are employed. Each chapter has a section with the key knowledge that supports these clinical aspects and comes with self-tests to keep you actively learning. Background reading lists are provided as well as relevant websites. The book must be seen as an introduction. The best textbook of all is the children and their carers.

Get out onto the wards, into the community and meet them. They will tell you even more of what you need to know than the young people in this book.

Steven Ryan, Jackie Gregg and Leena Patel

Acknowledgements

We would like to thank the following people who have helped us in the production of this book:

- Staff of Royal Liverpool Children's NHS Trust and Alder Hey Hospital: Dr David Pilling, Dr Joyce Russell, Mr Roger Franks, Dr George Kokai, Professor David Lloyd, Mr Matthew Jones, Dr Linda Brookes, Mr Gary Price, Dr Hope Forsythe, Mrs Jayne Collins, Dr Amanda Bennett, Dr Audrey Oppenheim and the staff of the Medical Photography Department – Tony Hanmer, Jackie Hyland, Kenneth Maddock, Molly Mitchell, Thomas Oldfield and Raymond Hanmer.

- Staff of the Manchester Children's Hospitals and the University of Manchester: Dr Mark Bone, Professor Peter Clayton, Judith Campbell, Judith Leaver, Dr Leslie Tetlow, Helen Upright, Dr Julian Vyas and the staff of the Medical Illustration Department at North Manchester General Hospital.
- Also, Dr Sharmila Jivan and Jane Meehan.

Without their generous contributions it would not have been possible.

Steven Ryan, Jackie Gregg and Leena Patel

History and examination

Age: 7 years

STEVEN RYAN

History

As far as students are concerned, there are two purposes to the history and the examination: first, to obtain essential diagnostic information relating to the patient and, second, to learn about children and their families – what better way is there than to meet and talk to them? This is why the history taken by the student should always be comprehensive, as opposed to the focused history of a busy clinician who has little time to spare. Such an opportunity will not occur again. Take it!

In keeping with the format of this book, the processes of history taking and examination are presented as a narrative of a typical clerking (Figure 1.1):

An undergraduate medical student was interviewing 7-year-old Sam and his mother Jennie. Sam had been admitted to hospital the previous day. The student first sought permission from Sam's primary nurse that he was well enough to be examined. She then introduced herself to Jennie, explained why she was there and asked if she could take a history and perform an examination. Jennie readily agreed.

History of the presenting complaint

The student asked an open question: What is or are the main problems with Sam's health? The student then made a list of the problems.

Sam had been admitted with cough, wheeze and breathlessness the previous day. He was known to have asthma.

Self-test 1: What is a closed question and why are they generally best avoided at the beginning of histories?

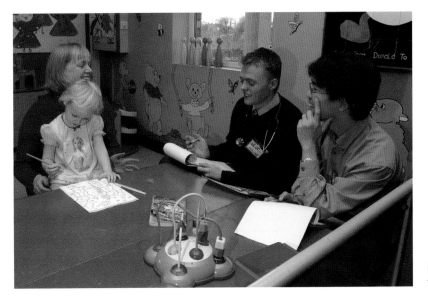

Figure 1.1 A student clerking on the paediatric ward.

Answer: One that has a limited range of answers, most typically 'yes' or 'no', e.g. 'Does Sam have wheezing at night?'. Such questions are best avoided because they can stop patients expressing their concerns and hence block a doctor's understanding of the problem. They have their place but generally later in the history to fill in any major gaps. Contrary to popular opinion, giving parents time at the beginning of a consultation to express their concerns is not a recipe for a prolonged time-wasting monologue, provided that you do not keep interrupting.

Open questions and clarification were used to flesh out the symptoms and gain an understanding of the problems in detail. As the student understood that it was important to differentiate between the acute presentation and long-term symptoms in asthma, Sam's mother was asked to look at these two aspects separately. This shows how the history can be modified in line with an understanding of the underlying problems.

The acute problem: a runny nose and fever for a day, then a steadily worsening cough over the previous night. He began wheezing in the early hours of the morning and this got worse and he became so breathless that he could not speak. He was brought to hospital by emergency ambulance.

The long-term problem: Sam has had asthma symptoms for 4 years. Currently he coughs whenever he runs and sometimes this makes him wheezy too. Whenever he gets a cold he gets a cough, which lasts about 2 weeks. He needs to use his blue (reliever) inhaler more frequently. He's worse in the winter.

After identifying the main problem/presenting complaint, 'check questions' of a more closed nature were then used to build up a more comprehensive picture of the child. These are as follows:

- **Past medical and surgical history** – details of previous illnesses, hospital admissions, general health
- **Pregnancy history** – any complications of the pregnancy; any treatment required
- **Birth history** – gestation, birthweight; mode of delivery; any difficulties in the labour or complications
- **Neonatal history** – patient's condition at birth. Did the baby go to the special care baby unit?

- Specific details about childhood exanthems (chickenpox, measles, etc.)

Sam's mother had had an uneventful pregnancy and straightforward delivery at 38 weeks' gestation. Sam weighed 3.22 kg at birth and was in good condition. He was discharged home with his mother the following day. Other than his asthma Sam was in good health. He did have eczema when he was an infant and had a right inguinal hernia repair at 1 year of age. He had had mild chickenpox aged 2.

Self-test 2: Which of the following conditions are associated with asthma?
A **Allergic rhinitis**
B **Migraine**
C **Eczema**
D **Arthritis**
E **Dental caries**

Answer: A/C.

- **Current medications:** the student listed all current regular and as-required medications including route and dose. She also noted any side effects

Sam took:
Inhaled beclomethasone (preventer) through a metered does inhaler and large volume spacer at a dose of 200 µg twice daily.

He also took inhaled salbutamol (reliever) through a metered dose inhaler and large volume spacer, at a dose of 200 µg twice daily routinely and additional doses when required.

In addition, he had received one course of oral steroid medication through the previous winter for an acute exacerbation. No side effects had been observed.

- **Allergies and side effects:** it is important to ask about allergies because they are commonly reported, but not to accept an allergy at face value because often there is none. It is also important to differentiate between allergies and other reactions. Allergies are always mediated by the immune system whereas other reactions are intolerances or pharmacological effects. Consider allergies to drugs, foods, environmental allergens (cat, dog, pollen, house-dust mite) or plasters. If an allergy is reported, it is important to detail the sequence of events accurately

Sam was on a peanut-free diet. On two occasions he had put a peanut in his mouth and within seconds his mouth had begun swelling and then his face. He was also wheezy and needed his inhalers. This sequence is consistent with immediate hypersensitivity to peanuts.

- **Dietary and nutritional history:** the standard of recording of nutritional status is generally poor in UK hospitals and this results partly from inadequate learning about principles and practice at both undergraduate and postgraduate level. By taking relevant histories in this area and basing learning around them, students can help to correct this deficit

  To obtain an outline of current diet a dietician will take a very detailed dietary history usually by asking the family to produce a 3-day food diary. This is a validated and accurate way of assessing food intake. A medical dietary history will allow at least an impression to be gained (Table 1.1)

Sam, other than being on a nut-free diet, had a good mixed diet but was not very keen on green vegetables. His

Table 1.1 Gaining an impression of a child's diet – some questions to ask

Is the child a grazer or a regular eater?
Is the diet varied or restricted?
Does the teenager eat breakfast?
Is there snacking on poor quality snack foods?
Is the child learning to eat a healthy diet with five portions of fruit or vegetables daily?
Some specific questions to ask, depending on age are:
• Breast- or bottle-fed and for how long?
• Age at starting solid food? (Too early and allergies are more common; too late and weight gain may be compromised)
• Any dietary problems? (Fussiness, grazing)
• Special dietary requirements? (Is the child already on a special diet?)

mother encouraged a healthy intake of fresh full-cream cows' milk.

- **Review of systems:** a further history should start with relevant systems. If a child has a cardiovascular problem, for example, review of the respiratory system is important. An exhaustive review using closed questions is usually not necessary – open questions are much easier for the parents. Common symptoms to find out about are shown in Table 1.2.

Sam had mild flexural eczema from time to time. He was still wetting the bed on three to four nights a week. He also had a persistently runny nose.

- **Developmental history:** for younger children think of the four domains:
  1 Fine motor and visual
  2 Hearing and language
  3 Gross motor
  4 Psychological, social and cognitive
  For older school-aged children previous problems with development will have declared themselves with the above history. Instead school progress and educational achievement should be recorded

Sam was at his local primary school and was making good progress. His teachers had no concerns about his learning. He was allowed to keep a reliever inhaler at school and this was administered before he played sport, and he could ask for it at any time. This allowed him to take a full part in sports and exercise.

- **Social history:** this needs to be asked sensitively. Open questions are useful. A history that sounds like an official interrogation may make parents feel ill at ease. Areas of clinical interest include:
  Environment – housing and surrounding area
  Schooling/nursery
  Financial circumstances – government allowances
  Transport
  Who helps and supports the family: relatives, friends, neighbours, health and social carers, voluntary workers and charities, self-help organizations
  Occupation of members of the household

Table 1.2 Review of systems

System	Occurrence	Symptom
Respiratory	Common	Cough, wheeze, breathlessness
	Occasional	Chest pain
Cardiovascular	Common	Breathlessness, cyanosis, fainting, palpitations
Gastrointestinal	Common	Constipation, diarrhoea, abdominal pain, nausea, vomiting, weight loss, rectal bleeding
	Occasional	Jaundice, distension, heartburn
Genitourinary	Common	Bedwetting, daytime wetting, frequency, dysuria, loin pain, fever, vomiting (especially in infancy)
	Occasional	Renal colic pain
Neurological including eyes	Common	Headache, vertigo, seizures
	Occasional	Loss of balance, weakness
Ear, nose and throat	Common	Earache, sore throat, snoring, colds, hearing loss, discharge
	Occasional	Vertigo, tinnitus
Locomotor system	Common	Leg pains, fracture, bow-legs, knock-knees
	Occasional	Joint swelling, pain and immobility, deformity
Skin	Common	Itchy skin – eczema, scabies, urticaria
		Red non-itchy rash – psoriasis
		Stretch marks – associated with rapid growth and obesity
Multisystem	Common	Fatigue, fever
Mental functioning	Common	Anxiety, low mood, overactive behaviour, poor concentration, poor sleep pattern, fatigue
	Occasional	Obsessional behaviour, depression
	Rare	Psychotic symptoms

Sam's family live in a local council house that they rent. There is quite a lot of damp, the ventilation is poor and there is no central heating. The area is very dusty because it is near the docks where coal is unloaded; there are chemical factories and a lot of heavy traffic nearby. Sam's mother feels that all of these factors are making Sam's problems worse and would like to move house. Neither parent smokes nor are there any pets in the household.

Sam's father is a painter and decorator working for a small local company. The family rely on public transport, so hospital appointments and visits are difficult. Sam's mother is a full-time mother and home-maker. The family moved to the area a few years ago and they have no relatives nearby. Sam's 3-year-old sister therefore usually has to come along to hospital visits too.

- **Family history:** Who is in the family? A diagram of the family tree will be helpful incorporating ages and medical history details (Figure 1.2)
  What health problems are there in the family? Especially any similar health problems to the patient

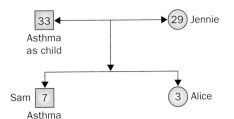

Figure 1.2 The family tree.

Are there any family health disorders that the parents are concerned about?

Sam's father had asthma as a child; he now has no problems. Would Sam also grow out of his asthma?

Self-test 3: On a family tree what are the symbols for:
Parental relationship ended?
Dead?
Twins?
Stillborn baby?

Answer: See Figure 1.3.

How to be an effective history taker

Here are some instructive tips for increasing skills in history taking. Essentially they are broad-based communication skills:

- Explain who you are and why the history is important to you
- Ask permission to take the history
- Put children and families at their ease with a little small talk appropriate for the child's age and likely interest
  - currently 3 year olds might be interested in Tweenies
  - 14-year-old boys from Liverpool might respond to talk about the city's two football teams
  - 9-year-old girls may be into the latest boy band
  - as you go round the wards, learn what children are interested in
- Talk to the child wherever possible to start with
- For older children and teenagers, allow them to be the primary historian

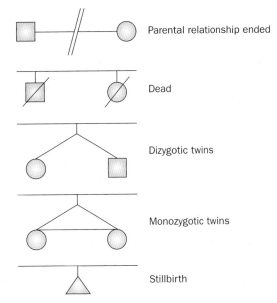

Figure 1.3 Answers to self-test 3: meaning of some symbols on the family tree.

- For younger children, engage them – get some details
- Let the parent make an opening statement
- Do not interrupt
- Listen attentively and actively
- Summarize what was said
- Check that you have understood what was said
- Leave checklists to the end
- Use open questions if possible:
  'Tell me about David's immunizations' is better than 'Is David fully immunized?'
- Be empathetic about significant difficulties and events
- Do not forget the environment:
  Is it private enough?
  Is everybody comfortable?
  Get your eye line and that of the child at the same level
  Let the child play while you take the history
- Say thank-you and ask the family if they have any questions

Examination

Below is a scheme for the general examination of a child that could be used especially for routine examination in, for example, an outpatients department or for an exam. Obviously, depending on the history, more detailed attention to a particular system may be necessary, e.g. if the child has not presented with a neurological problem, formal full neurological assessment is not required – a student will not be assessing taste in the posterior part of the tongue in a child with asthma! The nervous system is examined, but just the basics. On other occasions, more detailed assessment of a related system may be necessary, e.g. in a child with very large tonsils and a history of sleep apnoea, are there signs of pulmonary hypertension?

Self-test 4: Which is a sign of pulmonary hypertension?

A **Loud pulmonary component second heart sound**

B **Split second heart sound**

C **Pulmonary systolic ejection murmur**

D **A thrill on palpation**

E **A continuous murmur in the pulmonary area**

Answers:

A T (sign of increased pressure in pulmonary artery)

B F (atrial septal defect or ASD)

C F (pulmonary stenosis)

D F (ventricular septal defect)

E F (patent ductus arteriosus)

General examination

Observation of the child is the key to his or her physical examination. Careful observation can often give the information required or lead in the right direction (Figure 1.4).

- **Colour:**
  Record whether blue (peripheral or central)
  Is the child pale (anaemia or shock)?
  Any sign of jaundice?
- **Hydration:**
  Especially important during acute illness
  Check skin, eyes and mucous membranes – see Chapter 34
- **Nutritional status:**
  Height and weight should always be recorded and plotted on centile charts

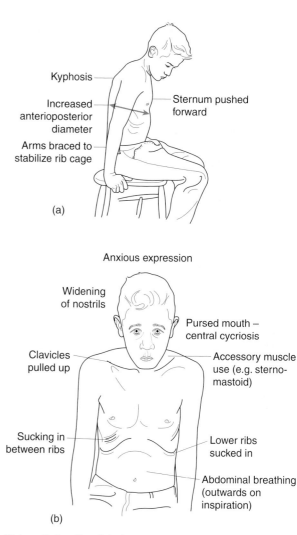

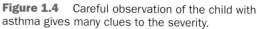

Figure 1.4   Careful observation of the child with asthma gives many clues to the severity.

Weight should be measured with light undergarments
Height should be measured:
– in bare feet
– getting the child to stand straight upright
– with heels against the base plate
– with ear hole and lower orbit in horizontal plane (Frankfurt plane)
– with feet together, knees straight
– with arms hanging loosely
– with palms facing thighs

– for children <2 years, supine length is measured instead

Assess:
– amount of subcutaneous fat
– muscle bulk
– any evidence of rickets (swollen wrists, ankles, costochondral junctions)
– conjunctival membrane for pallor of anaemia
– mouth for angular stomatitis (anaemia), smooth tongue (anaemia)
– tooth problems (decay, abnormal enamel)
– nails (pale and spoon shaped in iron deficiency)

- **Hair:** any sign of head lice?
- **Demeanour:** mood and activity
- **Relationship with carers:** a significant clue in cases of neglect and abuse
- **Hands:**
  Are nails clubbed, bitten (almost universal)?
  Skin creases (single palmar crease more common in Down's syndrome)
- **Scars:**
  Note any and enquire why present
  Note BCG scar if child old enough

Sam showed no signs of nutritional problems. His nails were not clubbed but were indeed bitten. He was not dehydrated and he was not cyanosed in air.

Respiratory

The child should be sitting up and all of the chest should be exposed. In teenage girls, their modesty may mean having to work round a partially clothed chest. The chest should be examined systematically.

- **Observation:**
  Record respiratory rate
  Note any signs of breathlessness (e.g. use of accessory muscles, indrawing of lower ribs on inspiration, abdominal breathing, mental state)
  Shape of chest:
  – hyperexpanded (increased anteroposterior or AP diameter, sternal bowing and kyphosis in air trapping with asthma and cystic fibrosis)
  Check sputum container in older children

- **Palpation:**
  Check position of trachea and apex beat to look for mediastinal shift
  Check expansion in older children with complaint
  Tactile vocal fremitus '99' in older children
- **Percussion:**
  Be gentle – only need to tap hard enough to 'feel' the noise with fingers
- **Auscultation:**
  Listen in all sectors of the lungs
  Record:
  – quality of air entry
  – ratio of time in inspiration to expiration
  – quality of breath sounds
  – any added sounds
  – vocal resonance '99'

Sam had a respiratory rate of 32 (raised) and there was mild indrawing of his lower ribs on inspiration (mildly breathless). He was able to talk comfortably. His chest was expanded in the AP plane. The trachea was central. His apex was difficult to locate because of the hyperexpansion. Percussion was generally hyperresonant, in keeping with hyperinflation. Air entry was good in all areas and expiration was prolonged. There was both an inspiratory high-pitched wheeze and an expiratory high-pitched wheeze in all areas.

Self-test 5: For each of the conditions in the left-hand column, match the most characteristic clinical finding in the right-hand column

A	Asthma	1	Increased vocal resonance
B	Croup	2	Stridor
C	Pleural effusion	3	Deviated trachea
D	Pneumothorax	4	Wheeze
E	Pneumonia	5	Dullness to percussion

Answer: A4/B2/C5/D3/E1.

Cardiovascular

This is done ideally with the child sitting:

- **Inspection:**
  As for respiratory system
  A careful check for operative scars that may be concealed in the axillae

Carefully look at the precordium for excessive activity or an abnormal shape: a bowed forward misshapen sternum may be seen in congenital heart disease

● **Palpation:**
Peripheral pulses – radial pulse acceptable in older children, brachial in infants
Note rate, rhythm and character – high volume pulse in patent ductus arteriosus
Check the femoral arterial pulse in cardiac cases (absent or weak in coarctation)
Identify apex – usually medial and inferior to the nipple
Precordium – check for thrills (a very loud murmur), heaves (an overactive ventricle)
Capillary refill time. Very important in the acute situation. Press the skin firmly for 5 seconds then release. Normal blood flow should be present within 2 seconds. Use trunk or head if child cold

● **Auscultation:**
Listen to the four main areas (under left clavicle – pulmonary; under right clavicle – aortic; base; apex); if anything abnormal heard, listen to back, neck too. In each area comment on:
Heart sounds:
– heard or not (may be hidden by loud murmur)
– volume (loud second sound in pulmonary hypertension)
– splitting of second sound (variable of fixed, e.g. the latter in an ASD)
Additional sounds: report any clicks or extra sounds
Murmurs:
– heard in systole, diastole, both or continuous
– for systolic murmurs:
same level throughout – pansystolic
crescendo–decrescendo – ejection

● **Blood pressure** – should be checked:
Use the right sized cuff – its width should be about two-thirds of the length of the upper arm. If the cuff is too small it will over-read the blood pressure and under-read it if too large

Self-test 6: For each of the findings on the left, which cardiac lesion is most likely to be responsible?

A	Pansystolic murmur at mid left sternal edge	1	Patent ductus arteriosus
B	Fixed splitting of second heart sound	2	Ventricular septal defect
C	Crescendo–decrescendo systolic murmur in neck	3	Aortic stenosis
D	Machinery continuous murmur	4	Innocent
E	A systolic murmur that disappears on extension of neck	5	Atrial septal defect

Answer: A2/B5/C3/D1/E4.

Sam had a heart rate of 120 per minute (raised) and blood pressure was 104/67 mmHg (normal). Pulse volume was normal. The heart sounds were difficult to hear because of wheezing. Capillary refill time was less than 2 seconds.

Abdomen/genitalia

The child should be lying down and you should be able to examine from knees to nipples (Figure 1.5). You do not have to keep the child this naked throughout because this may be embarrassing, especially for teenagers.

● **Observation:**
Look for scars and distension
Any signs of inguinal hernia, umbilical hernia or hydrocele?
Check the genitalia and, in boys, especially whether both testes are descended

● **Palpation:**
Initially light palpation for tenderness (look at the child's face)
Specific examination for the organs – liver, kidneys, spleen, any signs of constipation
In young infants the liver edge and spleen tip are often palpable
The spleen in infancy enlarges towards the left iliac fossa and not the right

● **Percussion:** percussion may aid definition of size of spleen and liver, and is useful in ascites

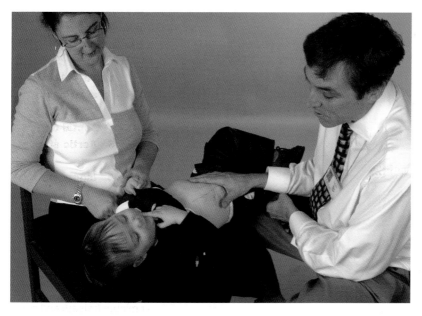

Figure 1.5 Get the child as relaxed as possible for abdominal examination. Here a toddler is examined on his mother's knee.

- **Auscultation:** useful in the acute abdomen in differentiating ileus (quiet) and obstruction (frequent and high pitched)

Sam's liver was palpable 3 cm below the costal margin in the midclavicular line. The upper edge was also displaced downwards, which was detected by percussion. This was in keeping with downward displacement by hyperinflated lungs.

Central nervous system

This is an overall basic assessment. If a neurological problem is suspected a more detailed examination is required.

- **Observation:** posture, gait and quality of movements should be observed
- **Eyes:**
  Check pupils – are they equal in size, responsive to bright light individually and consensual to accommodation? At rest the reflection from the cornea of a point source of light (the light reflex) should be equally placed in each eye
  Eye movements:
  – a full range of movement should be seen for each eye, without squint or complaint of double vision

  – the movement should be smooth without jerking (nystagmus), although a few beats observed at the very limit of lateral movement is a common finding
  Visual acuity:
  – using an age-appropriate technique – Snellen chart for older children
  – do not use the ophthalmoscope to test pupillary reaction to light because it is specially designed with low light intensity to prevent the pupil constricting!
  Chapter 25 gives details on reporting the optic fundal findings
- **Coordination and balance:**
  Check finger–nose coordination, hand patting, hopping, heel–toe walking, standing on one leg and standing still with eyes closed
  Problems may just indicate delayed maturation (many 5 year olds cannot hop effectively and rhythmic hand patting, alternating the palm and back of the hand, may be beyond many children of this age or it may mean a significant cerebellar problem)
- **Limb tone, power and reflexes:**
  As in adults, but remember to check tone across all major joints and in all directions of

movement of those joints. A general 'waggle' is not acceptable. Make power testing fun and again check all major joints. When testing reflexes, get the child as relaxed as possible and you may need to use reinforcement (e.g. gripping hands tightly together when testing knee reflexes). Routinely test biceps, triceps, supinator, knee, ankle and plantar reflexes. Remember that in the first year or so the plantar reflex is up-going

Never use the sharp end of a patellar hammer to elicit the plantar reflex in a child. It is designed for the tougher skin of adults. You will just cause pain and a withdrawal response

- **Development:**

Obviously assessed in pre-school children. Think of the four areas:
- gross motor
- fine motor and vision
- hearing and language
- personal and social

Observe, play and then formally examine where necessary – that is the order. This gives you the chance to get to know the child and for him or her to get used to you and perform to his or her optimum. Record your findings in a systematic fashion. Here is an example in a normal 8-month-old boy:

Observation	Sits without support for prolonged period, not pulling to standing
	Grasps and transfers objects but no pincer grasp yet
	Babbling but no recognizable words
	Apprehensive about examiner
Play	Crawls towards object lying on floor (commando crawl)
	Best grasp is scissors grasp not pincer grasp
	Seems interested in quiet noises outside visual range
	Increasingly playful
Examination	Cannot pick up raisin
	Turns head towards quiet high frequency rattle 1 metre (3 feet) lateral to ear
	Knows an object still exists when hidden from view (object permanence)

Ear, nose and throat

Probably the most feared part for children. Start with the ears (Figure 1.6), then the nose and the throat. Try to examine the throat without a spatula if possible. If

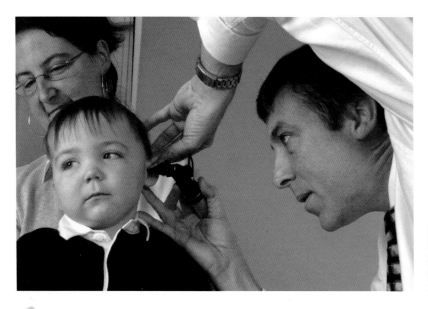

Figure 1.6 Examination of the ear. Note that the auroscope is braced against the child's head. Any head movement and the auroscope moves in synchrony.

needed, wait until the very last part of the examination. In the ears use a medium-sized speculum. Look at the eardrum and comment on:

Colour?	Grey (healthy), pink or red (infected)
Shiny or not?	Dull in disease
Retracted?	Retracted, often with fluid level visible in middle-ear disease

Any sign of a perforation?

The nasal membranes lie horizontally back from the nares. Snub the nose back and inspect in that plane. Look for normal healthy pink membranes. Abnormal membranes are red, and sometimes grey/blue in allergy and congested.

In the throat do not forget to look at the tongue, membranes, gums and teeth. What size are the tonsils? Are they scarred or pitted and do they have any exudate on them? Are they red and inflamed?

Sam's nasal membranes were rather congested, bulky and pale in places. He rubbed the end of his itchy nose several times during the examination. These findings were in keeping with allergic rhinitis, which commonly accompanies asthma.

The student summarized and presented her findings on the ward round to Sam's consultant:

Sam aged 7 was admitted with an acute exacerbation of his asthma provoked by a viral infection. He has been diagnosed with asthma for several years with exercise wheezing episodes despite preventative treatment and use of intermittent relievers. This episode is responding to treatment. He also has perennial rhinitis for which he receives no treatment. The consultant asked what the allergen responsible for perennial rhinitis was most likely to be. The student correctly answered house-dust mite faeces. He also asked what could be done to try to improve the long-term symptoms. The student answered that, as the family were not keen to increase the dose of the inhaled corticosteroids, perhaps a long-acting bronchodilator such as salmeterol could help. The consultant agreed with this management plan. Sam recovered from this episode and was discharged the next day. The salmeterol turned out to be effective and his exercise symptoms were much reduced.

Community and neonatal

A newborn with jaundice

Age: 18 days

STEVEN RYAN

Presentation

A general practitioner referred this newborn baby to the local hospital with the following referral letter:

> **Re: Sarah**
>
> Please would you see this 18-day-old white baby who has persistent jaundice. She was born at full term at the Maternity Unit at your hospital. A friend has told her mother Sally that she must stop breast-feeding and change to formula milk. I would welcome your advice as mother is now somewhat confused about what to do next. She had the routine blood screening test in the first week of life and this has been reported normal.

Self-test 1: What is the definition of prolonged jaundice in a neonate?

Answer: Jaundice present after 2 weeks of age.

Self-test 2: Which of these screening tests are currently done throughout the United Kingdom? Which of the disorders could be responsible for jaundice in the newborn period?

A Hypothyroidism

B Cystic fibrosis

C Phenylketonuria

D Galactosaemia

E Medium-chain acyl-CoA dehydrogenase

Answers:

	Screening	Can present with neonatal jaundice
A	UK	Yes
B	Some UK regions	Yes
C	UK	No
D	No (active research)	Yes
E	No (active research)	No

Initial considerations and action

There are two important but opposite principles:

- Jaundice is seen in up to two-thirds of newborn babies, and in the vast majority it is of no consequence and resolves spontaneously
- Prolonged jaundice in a neonate should always be taken seriously because it may have an important cause

However, most babies with this prolonged jaundice do not have a serious problem and it is also important to minimize parental anxiety as well as to identify important causes. Prolonged jaundice means a yellow coloration to the skin, mucous membranes and conjunctivae present after 2 weeks of age. This yellow coloration arises from increased levels of bilirubin in the blood and tissues. Two weeks is taken as a cut-off because, before this time, many babies suffer from 'physiological' jaundice. This is a natural increase in levels of bilirubin that is part of the adaptive process of changing from intrauterine to extrauterine life. By 2 weeks of age this process is usually complete. Features of physiological jaundice are:

- Full-term baby
- Jaundice appearing after day 2 and has disappeared by day 14
- Baby thriving and feeding well and active
- Urine not darkened
- Stools not pale
- Bilirubin level $<250\,\mu mol/L$

Self-test 3: What could dark urine and pale stools indicate in a jaundiced baby?

Answer: Obstructive jaundice.

History

Presenting complaint

Sally had first noted that Sarah had a yellow tinge to her skin on the third day; this yellow colour had remained until now and had slowly become more obvious. She had continued to pass urine normally, and this had remained translucent and clear. Sarah was passing about four to five sloppy green–yellow stools each day.

Feeding and nutrition

Sally was breast-feeding Sarah who appeared to be latching on to the breast well, taking about 20 minutes to complete a feed. Sarah had regained her birthweight (3.43 kg) at 10 days of age. She had posseted a small amount of milk after feeds on a few occasions.

Pregnancy and delivery

Sally's pregnancy was uneventful other than a urine infection that occurred at 28 weeks' gestation. This had been successfully treated with a 3-day course of antibiotics. Her blood group was AB rhesus positive. She had gone into labour spontaneously at 38 weeks' gestation and the first stage of labour had lasted 18 hours, the second stage 45 minutes. Sarah was born headfirst (vertex) and cried immediately. She had not been bruised and there was no history of swellings on the scalp. Other than her heel-prick blood tests for screening and vitamin K medication, Sarah did not require any medical intervention. She was discharged home after 48 hours.

Family history

Sally's partner Gus is well and, as a blood donor, he knows he has an A rhesus-positive blood group. Sarah has a 2-year-old brother Tom who is well. He too was breast-fed but did not develop jaundice. Gus and Sally are both white.

Self-test 4: What is the meaning of the following features in the history:
A Green–yellow stool and clear urine
B Passing four to five sloppy stools each day
C Mother is breast-feeding her baby
D Both parents are white

Answers:
A This is not obstructive jaundice
B This is normal for breast-fed babies
C Breast-feeding is a common cause of prolonged jaundice
D Some genetic conditions, such as glucose-6-phosphate dehydrogenase (G6PDH) deficiency, are unlikely

Differential diagnosis at this point

The details at this point have narrowed down the list of likely diagnoses quite substantially. With a jaundiced newborn baby, it is important to determine whether early onset jaundice occurred (within the first 24 hours). Early onset is likely to indicate that haemolysis has caused the jaundice. The most common causes of haemolysis are shown in Table 2.1.

In Sarah's case no jaundice is seen within the first 24 hours and the combination of parental blood groups does not indicate a risk of incompatibility. Glucose-6-phosphate dehydrogenase deficiency is associated with individuals of Mediterranean, African or Oriental origin, and with spherocytosis and elliptocytosis there is often a family history. Hence haemolysis can be discounted.

Self-test 5: What are the potential blood groups of the offspring of these parents?

Answer: A, AB or B rhesus positive or A, AB or B rhesus negative

- Onset between 48 hours and 14 days is usually physiological

In this case the onset of the jaundice after 48 hours is compatible with 'physiological' jaundice that has failed to resolve. There is no evidence of excessive blood breakdown causing the jaundice; excessive bruising, cephalohaematomas or polycythaemia can lead to excess

Table 2.1 Causes of haemolysis (early jaundice)

Types of cause	Specific causes	Tests
Blood group incompatibility	Rhesus: Sensitized rhesus-negative mother and rhesus-positive baby	Blood group and Coombs' test
	ABO incompatibility: O mother and A, B or AB baby	Blood group and haemolysins
	A mother and B or AB baby	
	B mother and A or AB baby	
Red cell enzyme deficiency	Glucose-6-phosphate dehydrogenase (G6PDH), pyruvate kinase	Red cell enzyme assay
Red cell membrane	Spherocytosis, elliptocytosis	Blood film abnormality

bilirubin production. Another cause of jaundice at this time can be infection and especially urinary tract infection. Sarah seems well from the history given, so serious infection seems unlikely but a more subtle infection, such as a urine infection, is still possible.

- Late onset and persistent jaundice can result from obstruction of bile flow. This is important to recognize before 6 weeks because surgery before this age to restore bile flow can be lifesaving

The coloured stools in this case (green–yellow) and clear-looking urine suggest that obstructive jaundice is unlikely. Obstructive jaundice results in pale stools (as bile pigment cannot reach the bowel) and dark urine (as conjugated bilirubin is excreted via the kidneys).

Examination

Sarah is examined and the following features are noted:

- Jaundiced
- No anaemia
- Well nourished (weight 3.78 kg) and well hydrated
- Handling well with normal cry, normal body tone and posture
- Liver and spleen are not enlarged – no other abdominal masses
- A green breast milk stool is seen in the nappy
- She passes clear urine

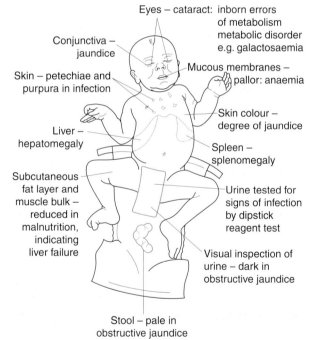

Eyes – cataract: inborn errors of metabolism metabolic disorder e.g. galactosaemia

Conjunctiva – jaundice

Mucous membranes – pallor: anaemia

Skin – petechiae and purpura in infection

Skin colour – degree of jaundice

Liver – hepatomegaly

Spleen – splenomegaly

Subcutaneous fat layer and muscle bulk – reduced in malnutrition, indicating liver failure

Urine tested for signs of infection by dipstick reagent test

Visual inspection of urine – dark in obstructive jaundice

Stool – pale in obstructive jaundice

Figure 2.1 Examination of the neonate with jaundice – what to look out for.

This examination is in keeping with 'physiological jaundice'. Sarah is outside the normal age range for this description and therefore she is referred to as having prolonged jaundice. There is no clinical evidence of anaemia, which would indicate haemolysis. She is well nourished and this suggests that her liver function is adequate. Her general health seems quite good and specifically there are no features of obstructive jaundice. The passage of green stool makes this most unlikely. The finding of a normal sized liver and spleen is also reassuring.

Enlargement of liver and spleen could indicate:

- Obstruction of biliary system
- Increased haematopoiesis as in haemolysis
- Infection with bacteria or virus
- An inborn error such as galactosaemia

Abnormalities, which can be found on examination, and their meaning are shown in Figure 2.1.

Investigations

As neonatal jaundice can be caused by a very large number of causes, the number of possible investigations that can be performed is also very large. It is therefore necessary to focus the investigations on what is likely and on those that can be used to rule out other causes. Further tests can then be undertaken depending on the results of earlier tests. The tests used will also depend on the age of the child – tests for haemolysis being principally used in the first week of life (see above).

Table 2.2 gives the baseline tests that would be undertaken in neonates with prolonged jaundice. If they give a positive result, further more detailed investigations become necessary.

Table 2.2 Investigations in prolonged jaundice

Baseline tests	Meaning	If abnormal
Total serum bilirubin	Confirms jaundice	Proceed to tests below
Serum conjugated bilirubin	Increased in obstructive jaundice	Refer for specialist assessment
Liver enzymes		
Alanine aminotransferase Aspartate transaminase	Raised with hepatocellular damage, e.g. hepatitis or obstruction	Refer for specialist assessment
Alkaline phosphatase	Raised with obstructed bile ducts	See above
Urine culture	Urinary tract infection potent cause of jaundice	Treat and investigate
Other tests		
Blood count and film	Anaemia, if persisting haemolysis, marrow suppression by virus or metabolic error	Refer for assessment specialist
Blood group and Coombs' test	Used for early jaundice and especially suspected rhesus disease	May need exchange transfusion
Red cell galactose-1-phosphate uridyl transferase (GALIPUT)	Specific test for most common form of galactosaemia	Refer to metabolic specialist – use soya milk
Abdominal ultrasonography	Detects choledochal cyst, gut malformation with obstructive jaundice	Refer to paediatric surgeon
Thyroid function tests	Hypothyroidism is a cause of persistent jaundice – usually excluded by routine neonatal screening	Refer to endocrinologist

Table 2.3 Results of investigations

Investigation	Result
Haematology	
Haemoglobin	13.1 g/dL
Normal blood film	No sign of haemolysis or abnormal red cells
Biochemistry	
Total serum bilirubin	182 µmol/L (normal range 4–20)
Conjugated bilirubin	7 µmol/L (normal range 0–10)
Alanine aminotransferase	28 international units (IU)/L (normal range 9–36)
Aspartate transaminase	28 IU/L (normal range 15–60)
Alkaline phosphatase	311 IU/L (normal range 200–1000)
Galactose-1-phosphate uridyl transferase (GALIPUT)	Normal enzyme activity
Microbiology	
Urine microscopy and culture	Some epithelial cells, no red or white cells
	No bacterial growth
Neonatal thyroid screening	Confirmed as normal

Results (Table 2.3)

These investigations exclude the presence of bile duct obstruction and rule out the presence of hepatocellular damage and hence hepatitis. Nor is there evidence of haemolysis, urinary tract infection or galactosaemia. The bilirubin level is only modestly elevated and represents no threat to Sarah's health.

Diagnosis

As a result of her continuing good health in all other respects and the negative investigations, Sarah is given a diagnosis of: **Breast milk jaundice**.

Treatment and follow-up plan

Breast milk jaundice is a benign self-limiting condition. The important principles of treatment are:

- Reassurance
- Monitoring

Table 2.4 Benefits of breast-feeding

To mother	Weight control in the long term
	Reduction in premenopausal breast cancer
To baby	Reduced respiratory tract infections (lower and upper)
	Reduced gastrointestinal infections
	Fewer allergy symptoms in early childhood
	Reduced incidence of type 1 diabetes mellitus
	Possible benefit in development

- Encouragement of continued breast-feeding (Table 2.4)

Sally was reassured that there was nothing wrong with her breast milk and that the jaundice would fade over the next week or so, and would not represent any threat to Sarah's health. The negative tests results were reviewed. To allay anxiety, follow-up was to be organized by the health visitor and general practitioner who would repeat the total bilirubin test in 2 weeks' time if the jaundice was still present. Sarah was to be reweighed and checked by the health visitor in 1 week's time. The short- and long-term health benefits of breast-feeding were reiterated (Table 2.3). Sally continued to breast-feed Sarah and, within 2 weeks, the jaundice had disappeared.

Background information

Bilirubin pathway

Haem-containing compounds are degraded to form a protoporphyrin ring and this is the precursor to bilirubin. The largest pool of haem is obviously haemoglobin, although myoglobin and cytochromes are also sources. The pathway from haem to bilirubin excretion is shown in Figure 2.2. Specific enzymatic disorders of the pathway can occur and these are also shown in Figure 2.2.

Treatments

Most babies with jaundice do not need treatment. However, very high levels of unconjugated bilirubin can pass the blood–brain barrier and damage the brain – especially the basal ganglia and acoustic nerves and nuclei. This can lead to the condition of choreoathetoid cerebral palsy and high tone deafness. The acute illness is called kernicterus and is associated with a high-pitched cry, neck stiffness and extreme irritability. Pre-term babies are at increased risk of kernicterus, as are very sick term babies with sepsis, hypoxia or acidosis. The last two processes displace bilirubin from binding sites on serum albumin and the 'free' bilirubin is highly likely to cross the blood–brain barrier.

- **Phototherapy (Figure 2.3):**
  Light radiation isomerizes bilirubin in the skin
  Can be excreted without conjugation
- **Exchange transfusion:**
  An urgent treatment when high levels of bilirubin threaten kernicterus (brain damage); blood is washed out with donor blood via an indwelling intravenous line in 5- to 10-mL aliquots – especially used for haemolytic jaundice

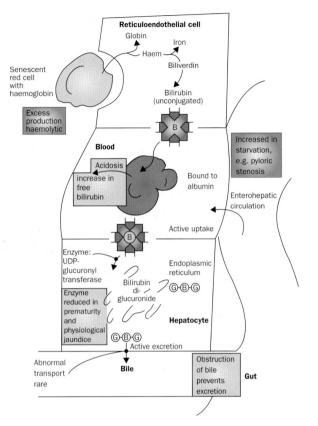

Figure 2.2 Schematic pathway of bilirubin metabolism.

- **Metalloporphyrins:**
  Specifically tin protoporphyrin and tin mesoporphyrin are used experimentally to inhibit haem oxygenase competitively (haem oxygenase is the enzyme controlling the rate-limiting step in the catabolism of haem to bilirubin), hence decreasing the production of bilirubin and lowering plasma bilirubin levels
- **Supportive treatments**
  Prevention of dehydration
  Reduction in the enterohepatic circulation of bile by feeding

How to do an exchange transfusion

An exchange transfusion usually needs to be done urgently. It's necessary to get good venous access and the most reliable site in a newborn is the

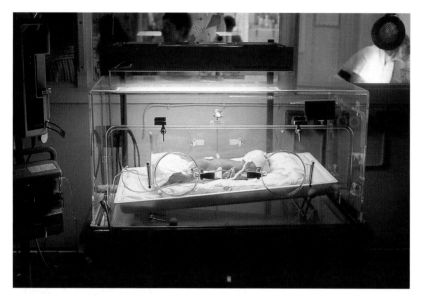

Figure 2.3 Neonate undergoing phototherapy.

umbilical vein. The umbilical stump is cut flat near the skin surface, the vein identified, and a catheter put through the vein and into the inferior vena cava. Blood is then sequentially drawn in and out until twice the baby's blood volume has been exchanged (80 mL/kg is the normal blood volume in a baby). It's important not to lose count of what's gone in and out. Even a minor discrepancy can lead to shock or overload (Figure 2.4).

Screening tests in the newborn

Wald defined screening as: 'The systematic application of a test or enquiry, to identify individuals at sufficient risk to benefit from further investigation or direct preventative action, amongst persons who have not sought medical attention on account of symptoms of that disorder.'

In the UK all newborn babies are screened for a variety of disorders both before and after birth. After birth this is by history (e.g. family history of genetic disorder; smoking in a parent, which increases risk of cot death and respiratory illness), examination (e.g. for heart murmur or dislocation of the hips) and investigation (e.g. blood test for phenylketonuria and hypothyroidism).

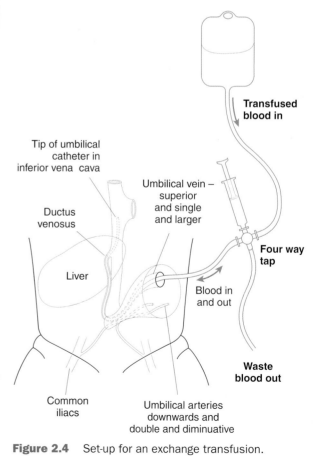

Figure 2.4 Set-up for an exchange transfusion.

Further sources of information

Articles

American Academy of Pediatrics. Provisional Committee for Quality Improvement and Subcommittee on Hyperbilirubinemia. Practice parameter: management of hyper-bilirubinemia in the healthy term newborn. *Pediatrics* 1994; **94**: 558

Dennery PA, Seidman DS, Stevenson DK. Neonatal hyperbilirubinemia. *New England Journal of Medicine* 2001; **344**: 581–90

Wald NJ. Guidance on terminology. *Journal of Medical Screening* 1994; **1**: 76

Websites

www.cs.nsw.gov.au/rpa/neonatal/html/newprot/jaund2.htm

A neonatal protocol from down-under.

www.scotland.gov.uk/library/documents6/chilpol-04p14.htm

Some basic principles from the Scottish Office.

Self test 6: Carl is 4 weeks old and presents to his general practitioner with persistent jaundice. It seemed to start when he was about a week old and has become progressively worse. He is now underweight – his mother feels he looks scrawny. She reports that his stools are like pale clay and his urine is dark. He has vomited occasionally and has had a 'snuffly nose'. His skin is rather dry. He does not appear to be anaemic.

A What are the most important features in this history?
B What is the most likely reason for these findings
C What action should the GP take?

Answers:
A The history of dark stools and pale urine
B This indicates obstructive jaundice
C Urgent referral to a paediatrician – if there is biliary atresia, an operation to restore bile flow must be conducted as soon as possible

The most common operation for this disorder is a Kasai procedure in which the small bowel is anastomosed to the porta hepatatis.

Self test 7: A 12-hour-old, full-term, white boy is noted to be jaundiced. His bilirubin level is very high and increasing rapidly.
A What is the most likely cause of the jaundice?
B What tests should be done?
C What treatment is most appropriate?

Answers:
A Haemolysis
B Full blood count, blood group and Coombs' test
C An exchange transfusion

3

Acute presentation in a neonate

A newborn with breathing difficulty and cyanosis

Age: 2 days

STEVEN RYAN

Presentation

The resident doctor is asked to go to the postnatal ward urgently by a midwife. She is caring for 2-day-old newborn baby June and her mother Susan. Over the telephone she says that, when she was caring for the child yesterday, all seemed well. Now she had been called urgently by Susan who had noted that June was a 'funny colour' and was struggling with her breathing. When the midwife looked at June she appeared blue and was having difficulty breathing.

The doctor first let the nursing staff on the special care baby unit know that there was a possible sick baby who might need to be admitted to the unit. This allowed equipment and staff to be prepared for the baby – if required. The situation sounded very urgent so an experienced neonatal nurse accompanied the doctor to the postnatal ward, taking resuscitation equipment.

Self-test 1: What are the causes of blood becoming blue in colour?

Answer: Hypoxia (the most common) and methaemoglobinaemia when ferrous iron in haem is oxidized to ferric iron

Initial considerations and action

It is important that a systematic approach is taken to the management of any sick newborn baby. Table 3.1 shows this approach.

Table 3.1 The systematic approach to dealing with a sick newborn baby

- Basic life support – assessment and action
- Does the baby need to come to the special care baby unit?
- Advanced life support
- Urgent specific medical treatment and investigations
- Review the history and examination
- Any further investigations
- Good communication with parents throughout

Self-test 2: What are the causes of persistent cyanosis in a newborn baby?

Answers:

A Congenital cardiac abnormalities:
- Pulmonary valve or arterial atresia
- Tetralogy of Fallot
- Tricuspid atresia
- Transposition of the great arteries

B Pulmonary hypertension (persistent fetal circulation – usually caused by other disorders such as sepsis or asphyxia)

C Lung disorders:
- Infection
- Malformation
- Hyaline membrane disease

Initial assessment and resuscitation

Rapid assessment of the sick neonate

The doctor arrived to find that June had been removed to the treatment room and her anxious-looking mother and father were with her. The midwife had started to give June some oxygen via a facemask. The doctor introduced himself and then, after checking that the room was warm enough, gently undressed her. He made the observations shown in Table 3.2 about June.

Table 3.2 Rapid assessment of a sick newborn baby

Airway: open

Work of breathing: laboured (see Figure 1.4)

Effectiveness of breathing:
- Air entry is heard with a stethoscope equally both sides of chest
- Looks exhausted and blue lips, tongue and skin

Circulation:
- Pulse rate is 160/minute (felt at brachial)
- Pulse volume is good

Disability:
- Pupils equal and reactive
- Responds weakly to gentle stimulation

The information in Table 3.2 indicates that June is in difficulty and appears to have a compromised respiratory system. Her exhaustion, deep central cyanosis and weak response to stimulation indicate that a respiratory arrest is imminent.

The doctor explained to Susan and her partner that June was very unwell and required urgent treatment on the special care baby unit (Figure 3.1). June was quickly pushed round to the nearby unit in her cot, accompanied by her parents. An incubator was ready for her when she arrived.

Self-test 3: Explain the ways in which an incubator keeps a baby warm.

Answers:
- **A** Stops heat loss by convection by removing drafts of air
- **B** Insulation prevents conductive heat loss
- **C** Plastic shield reduces radiant heat loss
- **D** Evaporative heat loss reduced by keeping air humid and preventing drafts

Advanced life support in the sick newborn

The doctor decided that June did need advanced life support because a brief period of time with oxygen had not improved her condition. The actions in Table 3.3 are taken.

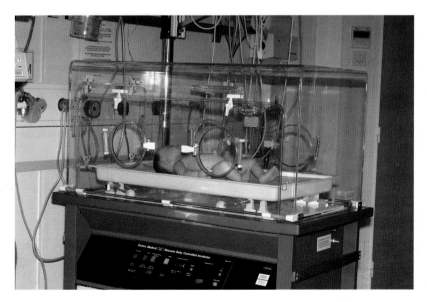

Figure 3.1 An incubator.

Table 3.3 The resuscitation

Airway: uncuffed endotracheal tube inserted after oropharyngeal suction

Work of breathing:
- Ventilated using a self-inflating bag for 5 minutes
- Pressure-cycled neonatal ventilator and circuit connected to endotracheal tube

Effectiveness: good air entry heard on both sides of chest with stethoscope

Circulation: peripheral venous access achieved with cannula – blood samples taken, then maintenance intravenous glucose solution commenced

Definitive treatment: intravenous broad-spectrum antibiotics are started as part of the resuscitation

The primary resuscitation stabilizes **a**irway, **b**reathing and **c**irculation (ABC). The rule is '**D**o not **E**ver **F**orget **G**lucose in a sick young child' (hence ABC . . . DEFG!) and this is especially true in newborns who have a high requirement for glucose and little in the way of carbohydrate reserves. In general antibiotics are administered to almost every sick neonate because infection can quickly overwhelm a neonate and the tests take some time to come back.

History

Now, after resuscitation, is the time to consider the diagnosis and its specific management. The main points of the history were the following:

Mother: Susan aged 28. Pre-pregnancy health good. Delivered one previous liveborn boy now aged 4. He has asthma requiring a preventive inhaler, only occasionally needing his reliever inhaler. Susan does not smoke and nor does her partner Geoff who also has mild asthma.

Pregnancy: This had been uneventful until 1 week previously. Membranes had ruptured 5 days before delivery and the amniotic fluid was clear. After the membranes ruptured, labour was not established for 4 days. Susan remained in hospital without a fever and her pulse rate and blood pressure remained within normal limits.

Labour and delivery: Labour lasted 13 hours altogether and the second stage just 28 minutes. It was a vertex delivery and the baby cried soon after birth and needed no active resuscitation:

- 38 weeks' gestation
- Birthweight 4.08 kg
- Length 52 cm
- Head circumference 36.2 cm
} all within normal limits
- Apgar score 9 at 1 minute, 10 at 5 minutes.

Subsequent progress: Baby had been noted to be breathing fast but without respiratory distress. This was thought to be the result of wet lungs (transient tachypnoea).

Mother had had a slight fever of 37.9°C and a moderately offensive discharge – a swab was sent and oral antibiotics started.

Interpreting the history

The are several important negative and positive points to this history:

- **Negative points:**
  Born at term: unlikely to be the result of respiratory distress syndrome (RDS) surfactant deficiency – this is usually seen in pre-term infants
  Vaginal delivery: wet lungs are more common after caesarean section and are sometimes associated with RDS in term babies
  Clear liquor: this excludes meconium aspiration syndrome – associated with asphyxia; the fetus passes stool into the amniotic fluid, which is then inhaled, causing a severe inflammatory response
  Apgar score: an Apgar score of 9 at 1 minute indicates good condition at birth – excludes birth asphyxia which can cause shock lung and be a risk factor for pulmonary hypertension of the newborn
- **Positive points:**
  Prolonged rupture of membranes: this increases the risk of ascending organisms from the vagina causing an infection
  Rapid breathing: this can be an indicator of incipient respiratory difficulty and should have prompted closer observation – it has been specifically linked with lung infection
  Maternal fever and vaginal discharge could also be

associated with ascending infection from the vagina into the uterus

The history in this patient seems to rule out a number of conditions but is supportive of a diagnosis of infection.

Examination

Principles

Once the patient has been stabilized on the ventilator and placed in the incubator, he or she is examined to:

- Look for diagnostic features
- Check on the adequacy of treatment and resuscitation

General inspection

- A good sized, well-nourished baby
- No rash observed
- External appearance normal – no dysmorphic features

Cardiovascular

- Heart rate 160/minute (normal)
- Blood pressure 54/28 (normal) using automated cuff
- Heart sounds 1 and 2 heard and normal
- Quiet systolic heart murmur heard at left sternal edge
- Cardiac apex undisplaced
- Capillary refill time less than 2 seconds (normal)

Respiratory

- On ventilator with 80 per cent inspired oxygen and inspiratory pressure of 30 cmH$_2$O (high)
- Air entry reduced with reduced chest movement but equal on both sides
- Crepitations (or crackles) heard throughout both lung fields
- Copious secretions suctioned from trachea via endotracheal tube
- Blood oxygen saturation 89 per cent by pulse oximetry
- Trachea central

Abdomen

- Soft and non-distended
- Normal bowel sounds

- Liver enlarged 3 cm below margin of ribs
- Spleen enlarged 2 cm below margin of ribs

Central nervous system

- Fontanelle soft
- Floppy tone and posture

This examination has confirmed that resuscitation and initial treatment have stabilized the situation, but also indicate that this child is very sick. The inspiratory pressure is high and the lungs are moving very little – they lack compliance. This can be demonstrated graphically by plotting the pressure within the lung generated by different volumes of air (Figure 3.2). The less compliant the lung, the greater the rise in pressure for any given volume of air.

Some dysmorphic syndromes are associated with respiratory problems (such as Pierre Robin syndrome in which the tongue of a small lower jaw 'falls back' into the pharynx through a cleft plate and obstructs the airway). The quite heart murmur is probably 'functional' and of no significance but it could just represent an underlying congenital heart defect. Table 3.4 shows the common heart defects and their presentation.

Self-test 4: Which of the conditions in Table 3.4 is most likely to be present?

Answer: Transposition of the great arteries.

This infant also has enlargement of the liver and spleen. The liver can be enlarged in heart failure, but

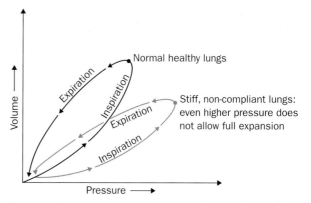

Figure 3.2 Volume–pressure graph showing decreased compliance in June's lungs.

Table 3.4 Cardiac causes of cyanosis

Cyanosis with good systemic circulation

● Transposition of the great vessels	Most common cardiac cause of cyanosis
	Starts in first few days of life
	Systemic and pulmonary circulations disconnected
● Tetralogy of Fallot	Cyanosis starts in later infancy
	Ejection systolic murmur in pulmonary area

Cyanosis with heart failure

● Hypoplastic left heart	Starts within a few days
	Severe cyanosis and very poor systemic circulation (shock)
	Liver enlargement
	Very poor volume pulses

Heart failure (lung fluid retention and reduced systemic blood flow)

● Patent ductus arteriosus	Usually in pre-term babies
	Continuous machinery murmur
	In pulmonary area
● Ventricular septal defect	Usually gradually increasing failure in first weeks
	Loud pansystolic murmur at lower-left sternal edge
● Coarctation of the aorta	May present at a few days of age
	Narrowing of the aortic arch
	Hypertension in the arms
	Low blood pressure in the legs
	Weak femoral pulses

this child has an adequate peripheral circulation now so this seems unlikely. A more probable explanation is that the liver and spleen have become enlarged in response to infection. This is also supported by the crackles heard through the lung fields and the increased respiratory secretions. The floppy tone and posture are non-specific reactions to being very unwell and unlikely to represent specific neurological problems. The possibility of a lung malformation has also been reduced by the negative examination. Congenital diaphragmatic hernia in which one lung is displaced by abdominal contents herniating through a defective, usually left-sided, diaphragm would usually be associated with reduced air entry on the affected side, a right-shifted heart apex and possibly deviation of the trachea that way too. This is not seen here. A pneumothorax would also give asymmetrical signs.

Investigations

● **Haematology:** important to check adequate haemoglobin for carrying around what oxygen there is: abnormal white cell count may indicate infection
Haemoglobin: 16.8 g/dL
White cell count: 2.3×10^6/L (with low neutrophil count)
Platelets: 66×10^6/L (low)

● **Biochemistry:** check the blood gases for oxygen tension and carbon dioxide tension – raised in respiratory failure. This may also cause a respiratory acidosis and of course shocked, sick babies may develop a metabolic acidosis
pH: 7.28 (low – normally >7.36)
P_{CO_2}: 7.7 kPa (raised – normally 4.4–5 kPa)
P_{O_2}: 7.8 kPa (slightly low – normally 9–12 kPa)

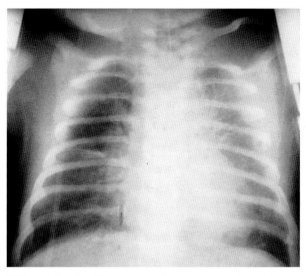

Figure 3.3 A radiograph showing pneumonia in a newborn baby. Unlike older children the infection is widely distributed through both lungs and has a homogeneous appearance.

- **Microbiology:** obviously looking for infection

Blood culture	Positive for group B streptococci
Cerebrospinal fluid (CSF) culture	Negative
Sputum culture	Negative
Maternal high vaginal swab culture	Positive for group B streptococci

- **Chest radiograph:** looking for abnormal lungs (relatively easy) or an abnormal shape to the heart, which may reflect congenital heart disease – this is much harder

The film (Figure 3.3) shows that there is bilateral homogeneous opacification within both lung fields.

Meaning of the results

These investigations show that June has a lung infection with group B β-haemolytic streptococci, with which she has become infected during her birth. The organism can be a commensal organism in the female genital tract. The low neutrophil count and the low platelet count are also seen in serious bacterial infection in neonates. Unlike older children and adults in whom lung infection is often localized (e.g. lobar pneumonia with *Streptococcus*) or patchy (viral pneumonia), a ground-glass appearance is commonly seen in neonatal pneumonia. It can be impossible to differentiate this appearance from that of hyaline membrane disease as a result of surfactant deficiency. In this case the other features of infection help make the correct diagnosis.

The blood gases and pH demonstrate a respiratory acidosis and some continuing hypoxia despite artificial ventilation. The ventilator may require adjustment.

Self-test 4: A blue neonate has these blood gas results:

pH   7.28 (low – normally >7.36)
P_{CO_2} 3.7 kPa (raised – normally 4.4–5 kPa)
P_{O_2} 4.8 kPa (low – normally 9–12 kPa)
What abnormalities are present?

Answers: Metabolic acidosis (low pH but a low P_{CO_2}) and hypoxia.

Diagnosis

Respiratory failure caused by perinatally acquired infection with group B β-haemolytic *Streptococcus*.

Treatment and progress

Direct treatment

Antibiotics: penicillin and gentamicin to which the organism is sensitive.

Supportive treatment

- Assisted ventilation until respiratory failure resolved
- Fluids and nutrition:
  - intravenous glucose solution
  - nasogastric milk feeds when tolerated
  - temperature control
  - nursed in incubator
- Support for June's mother and family

June made steady progress and made an uncomplicated recovery. She was discharged home 2 weeks later.

Background knowledge

The Apgar score

The Apgar score was originally devised by an American anaesthetist, Dr Virginia Apgar, to measure the effect of maternal anaesthetic agents on newborn babies, but it has now become a universal method for describing the health of newborn babies.

Feature	Score		
	0	1	2
Heart rate/min	0	<100	>100
Breathing	Absent	Gasping	Regular/crying
Tone	None	Floppy	Good/active
Response to suction	None	Grimace	Cough
Colour	Pale	Blue	Pink

The scores have the following meanings:

Score	Assessment	Actions
8–10	Healthy	No action
4–7	Primary apnoea	Stimulation
		Airway opening manoeuvres
		Gentle mouth suction
		May need bag and mask
		Ventilation with oxygen
1–3	Terminal apnoea	Ventilation
		Possible intubation
		Possible cardiac massage
0	Cardiac arrest	Intubation
		Ventilation
		Cardiac massage
		Adrenaline (epinephrine)
		Intravenous fluid

Cyanosis

Cyanosis occurs when the concentration of desaturated haemoglobin reaches a level at which a blue colour can be observed in the patient. This generally occurs at a level of desaturated haemoglobin concentration greater than 5 g/dL. Figure 3.4 shows the mechanisms by which cyanosis can present in a newborn baby.

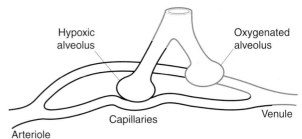

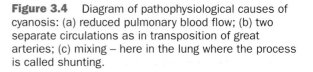

Figure 3.4 Diagram of pathophysiological causes of cyanosis: (a) reduced pulmonary blood flow; (b) two separate circulations as in transposition of great arteries; (c) mixing – here in the lung where the process is called shunting.

Other rare causes of cyanosis include methaemoglobinaemia which results from increased formation of methaemoglobin from haemoglobin. This is incapable of binding and carrying oxygen, and is formed when iron in the haem molecule is oxidized from the ferrous (Fe^{2+}) to the ferric state (Fe^{3+}). A variety of drugs and chemicals may be responsible, including nitric oxide – a vasodilator used to treat pulmonary hypertension in the newborn.

How to read a blood gas report

See Figure 3.5.

Further sources of information

Books

Behrman RE, Kliegman RM, Nelson WE, Vaughan VC (eds). *Nelson: Textbook of Paediatrics*, 14th edn. Philadelphia: WB Saunders, 1992.

Rennie JM, Robertson NRC. *Textbook of Neonatology*, 3rd edn. Edinburgh: Churchill Livingstone, 1999.

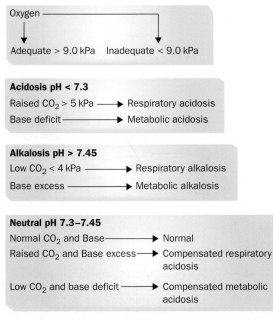

Figure 3.5 How to read a blood gas report.

Both these books are postgraduate textbooks with plenty of detail for further understanding.

Websites

www.dcmsonline.org/jax-medicine/1998journals/september98/cyanotic.htm

Approach to cyanotic heart disease in the first month of life.

www.vh.org/Providers/TeachingFiles/PAP/Neonatal ChestDiseases/NeonatalChestDisIndex.html

Neonatal Chest Disease Index.

Self-test 5: A baby boy is born after a normal pregnancy and delivery. At 2 days of age it is noted that he is cyanosed and somewhat breathless. A chest radiograph shows that the lung fields are clear and the heart is slightly large with a narrow base. When the child is put into a very high concentration of oxygen (nitrogen washout test), no improvement in oxygen saturation is observed.

A What system is likely to be responsible for the cyanosis?

B What evidence points to this system being responsible?

C What investigation would confirm the diagnosis?

D What treatments are available?

Answers:

A Cardiac

B Normal lungs on chest radiograph; abnormal shaped heart; failure of nitrogen washout test

C Echocardiography or cardiac catheter; transposition

D Temporary – reconnecting the circulation by making an artificial hole between the two atria (a balloon septostomy)
Permanent – switching the two arteries back to their original positions

Self-test 6: A baby born at 29 weeks' gestation becomes breathless within 2 hours. The pregnancy was complicated by maternal hypertension and an emergency caesarean section was undertaken. The baby is placed on a ventilator for respiratory failure. The radiograph is shown in Figure 3.6.

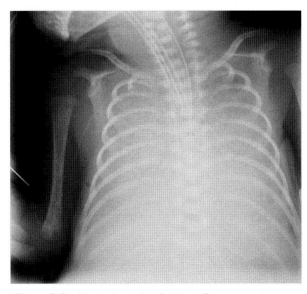

Figure 3.6   Radiograph for Self-test 6.

After the radiograph, treatment is administered directly into the lungs via the endotracheal tube.

A What does the radiograph show?

B What is the likely diagnosis?

C What was the treatment that was administered?

D What treatment could have been administered to the mother to prevent the disorder?

Answers:

A Homogeneous ground-glass appearance in both lung fields

B Hyaline membrane disease (respiratory distress syndrome)

C Surfactant replacement therapy

D Corticosteroids – enhance surfactant production by the fetus

A baby with vomiting

Age: 6 weeks

STEVEN RYAN

Presentation

A 6-week-old baby boy presents to his general practitioner. He had been vomiting for about 3 weeks and this had been getting steadily worse. He had been treated with a proprietary alginate/antacid compound with little benefit and his grandmother was becoming increasingly concerned. It was also noted, by referral to the parent-held child health record, that he had gained little weight over the last 2 weeks (Figure 4.1). The GP referred him to the local paediatrician for urgent assessment.

Initial considerations and action

Vomiting is a very common symptom in childhood and can be thought of as 'localizing', i.e. representing specific pathology in the gastrointestinal tract, or 'false localizing' where the pathology lies elsewhere. In the neonate and the young infant, this symptom is at its most common and may represent significant and sometimes life-threatening pathology. Figure 4.2 shows the range of disorders that can be responsible for vomiting.

However, even the brief amount of information available at this stage is already starting to narrow down the possibilities. First, given the age of the child, we are dealing with a persistent disorder and, as the relative frequencies of various causes are known, it is possible to construct a list of likely diagnoses. Also, at this age the child's diet should consist of milk alone and this would rule out some dietary causes such as coeliac disease (gluten-sensitive enteropathy). The possible diagnoses include those in Table 4.1.

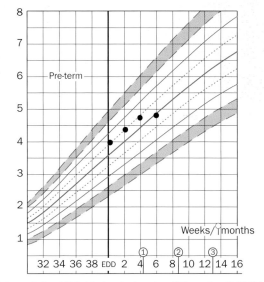

Figure 4.1 Weight chart showing little gain. © Child Growth Foundation. The chart shown here is intended for illustrative purposes only. The range of UK growth reference charts may be purchased from Harlow Printing, Maxwell Street, South Shields, NE33 4PU.

Self-test 1: In the blood of a child with adrenal deficiency caused by congenital adrenal hyperplasia, which of these is most likely?

A **Raised sodium–raised potassium**

B **Raised sodium–low potassium**

C **Low sodium–low potassium**

D **Low sodium–raised potassium**

E **Normal sodium–normal potassium**

Answer: D.

What other biochemical feature may be seen?

Answer: Hypoglycaemia

Non-localizing

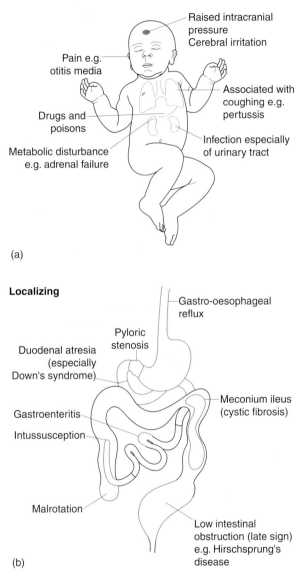

Raised intracranial pressure
Cerebral irritation

Pain e.g. otitis media

Associated with coughing e.g. pertussis

Drugs and poisons

Metabolic disturbance e.g. adrenal failure

Infection especially of urinary tract

(a)

Localizing

Gastro-oesophageal reflux

Pyloric stenosis

Duodenal atresia (especially Down's syndrome)

Gastroenteritis

Intussusception

Meconium ileus (cystic fibrosis)

Malrotation

Low intestinal obstruction (late sign) e.g. Hirschsprung's disease

(b)

Figure 4.2 Causes of vomiting in a neonate: (a) non-localizing; (b) localizing.

Table 4.1 Probable causes of vomiting in the neonate

Pathology localized to GIT	Pathology elsewhere
Gastro-oesophageal reflux	Urinary tract infection
Pyloric stenosis	Other persistent infection
Overfeeding	Metabolic disorders[a]
Milk allergy	Raised intracranial pressure or other CNS lesion[a]

[a]Uncommon but important.
CNS, central nervous system; GIT, gastrointestinal tract.

Presenting features

- Vomiting started 3 weeks ago and is getting worse
- Vomiting immediately after being fed and tends to be quite hungry again afterwards – often takes another feed; otherwise quite contented
- Once or twice the vomit has been quite forceful – 'like a fountain'
- There is no blood or bile in the vomit although it does contain clear mucus and some curds
- Simon has a whey-based infant cows' milk formula
- His stools have become firmer, greener and less frequent
- He is passing less urine and it smells quite strong

Other history

- Born at 37 weeks' gestation weighing 2.9 kg
- The pregnancy had been complicated by maternal high blood pressure
- He had no problems in the first 3 weeks, having regained his birthweight within 11 days, and weighed 3.2 kg by 3 weeks of age
- The weight recorded by the GP today was 3.22 kg
- He had been delivered normally by spontaneous labour with vertex presentation

Family history

- His mother had also had vomiting as a baby and had an operation but could not remember what it was for
- A 4 year-old sister is fit and well
- There is no family history of atopy or allergy

History

The patient turns out to be Simon aged 6 weeks and his mother and paternal grandmother accompany him. The history obtained is as follows.

Table 4.2 Interpretation of the history

Feature	Possible reasons
Vomiting getting worse	The pathological process is advancing, e.g. gastro-oesophageal reflux, urinary tract infection, raised pressure, pyloric stenosis
Vomiting immediately after feeds	Pyloric stenosis possible; can be very delayed (up to time of next feed) in gastro-oesophageal reflux
Feeding immediately after vomiting	Also a feature of pyloric stenosis
Projectile vomiting	Seen in pyloric stenosis but also seen in other conditions, although usually less persistent
No bile in the vomit	Important history that excludes intestinal obstruction below the ampulla of Vater
Change in bowel habit	Could indicate starvation – lack of milk transiting bowel or reduced milk intake as a result of decreased appetite
Reduced urine output	Could be caused by reduced milk intake or fluid losses resulting from vomiting
Poor recent weigh gain	Indicates a very significant disease process
Mother's history	Sounds as though mother has had a surgical condition causing vomiting as an infant; this could have been pyloric stenosis – children of affected mothers have a high (up to 25%) chance of being affected
Absent family history of atopy	Makes cows' milk allergy less likely as a cause

Self-test 2: What are curds and whey?

Answer: Whey is the soluble protein component of milk whereas casein is the insoluble component that forms curds when in contact with the acid and proteases of the stomach. It is no surprise therefore to see this in a child's vomit. The greater the casein content of the milk, the greater the quantity of curds seen in the vomit. Modern formula milks contain greater quantities of whey because this is felt to mimic the protein constitution of human milk best.

Interpretation of the history

Table 4.2 shows the interpretation of the history. Clearly several of the features point towards pyloric stenosis as a cause, but at this stage it is important not to rule out other causes until such a diagnosis can be confirmed.

Examination

General examination

- Wasting with reduced subcutaneous fat and muscle bulk
- Slight jaundice
- Reduced tone and lethargic
- Sunken fontanelle and eyes
- Skin turgor (elasticity) reduced
- Weight 3.22 kg; height 57 cm; head circumference 38.7 cm

Abdomen

- Soft, non-distended
- Visible peristalsis in left upper quadrant
- 'Olive' felt to right of epigastrium and projectile vomiting observed during test feed (Figure 4.3)
- No hepatosplenomegaly

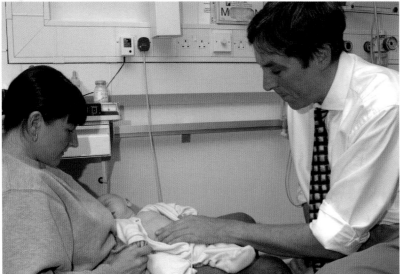

Figure 4.3   A baby having a test feed.

Central nervous system

- Soft but sunken fontanelle
- Generally reduced muscle tone
- No focal neurological abnormalities found

Cardiorespiratory system

- Heart rate 170/minute (raised)
- Blood pressure 70/45 mmHg (normal)
- Respiratory rate 36/minute (normal)
- Capillary refill time 3 seconds (slightly prolonged)

Self-test 3: What is the most likely cause of the slight jaundice?

A Haemolysis

B Increased enterohepatic circulation

C Biliary obstruction

D Liver damage

E Breast milk jaundice

Answer: B.

Interpretation of the examination

These findings show a baby 'on the edge' with severe malnutrition and features of dehydration bordering on the edge of shock. The slight jaundice could represent an increased enterohepatic circulation of bilirubin caused by a lack of milk reaching the small intestine from the stomach. The reduced tone and lethargy probably result from a combination of malnutrition and dehydration. Here the dehydration is assessed as moderate (Table 4.3).

The increased capillary refill time suggests that failing circulation and 'shock' are not far away. Fluid therapy will be required quickly to support the circulation.

Self-test 4: What diagnosis is suggested most by the findings so far?

A Gastroenteritis

B Congenital adrenal failure

C Obstruction caused by malrotation

D Pyloric stenosis

E Gastro-oesophageal reflux

Answer: D.

Investigations

A number of investigations are required to:

- Make the diagnosis
- Assess the degree of dehydration
- Assess the degree of metabolic disturbance
- Exclude other possible diagnoses
- Prepare the child for anaesthesia

Table 4.3 Assessment of dehydration in infants and children

Feature	Mild	Moderate	Severe
Percentage dehydrated	<5	5–10	>10
Circulation:			
Pulse rate	Normal	Fast	Fast
Capillary refill time	Normal	Slightly increased	Increased
Blood pressure	Normal	Normal	Reduced
Shock present	No	No	Yes
Mental state	Normal	Lethargic but rousable	Irritable
Appearance:			
Mouth	Dry	Dry	Dry
Fontanelle	Normal	Sunken	Deeply sunken
Eyes	Normal	Sunken	Deeply sunken
Skin turgor	Normal	Decreased	Like dough
Urine output	Normal	Reduced	None in 12 hours

The following investigations were done and these results were obtained:

- **Haematology:**
Haemoglobin: 19.4 g/dL (raised)
White cell count: 13.2×10^9/L (normal)

Self-test 5: Why is the haemoglobin level raised?

Answer: Haemoconcentration caused by dehydration.

- **Biochemistry:**
Sodium: 128 mmol/L (low)
Potassium: 3.2 mmol/L (low)
Chloride: 79 mmol/L (low)
Bicarbonate: 38 mmol/L (high)
Urea: 7.2 mmol/L (high)
Creatinine: 37 μmol/L (normal)
pH (capillary): 7.56 (high)
- **Microbiology:**
Urine microscopy and culture: no abnormality detected
- **Imaging:**
Ultrasonography of pylorus (Figure 4.4): the pylorus is 28 mm in length (normally <17 mm),

and the width of both walls is 5.8 mm (one wall must be >3.5 mm). This supports the diagnosis of pyloric stenosis

Interpretation of the investigations

The following are the aims of the investigations:

- **Confirmation of the diagnosis:** the diagnosis is confirmed by the imaging and, in addition, the typical biochemical features of pyloric stenosis are seen – a hyponatraemic, hypokalaemic, hypochloraemic, metabolic alkalosis
- **Assessment of the degree of dehydration:** the haemoglobin level is elevated through dehydration (haemoconcentration) and the urea level is modestly elevated. Note, however, that in severe malnutrition there is a fall in urea production and the 'true' level would have been higher than this
- **Assessment of the degree of metabolism:** there is a great deal of disturbance to electrolyte levels and to the acid–base balance. The vomit contains sodium and potassium and chloride, explaining their low levels. There is also a net loss of acid, resulting in metabolic alkalosis. This will also drive

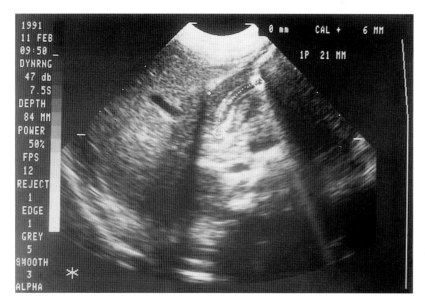

Figure 4.4 An ultrasound scan of the pylorus in pyloric stenosis.

down the potassium level because potassium ions will enter the intracellular compartment in exchange for hydrogen ions

- **Exclude other possible diagnoses:** urinary tract infection has been excluded
- **Prepare the child for anaesthesia:** the metabolic disturbance is such that anaesthesia would be a grave risk to this child. The anaesthetist will want the metabolic derangement rectified before surgery

came back to normal. He then had his dehydration and metabolic disturbance slowly corrected over the next 48 hours with an intravenous infusion of water, sodium, potassium, chloride and glucose. By this time his metabolic disturbance was totally corrected. He was then taken to the operating theatre and safely anaesthetized. He underwent a pyloromyotomy (Rammstedt's procedure). He made an uneventful recovery and was discharged home 3 days later. It turned out that his mother had also had the same condition and operation as a young infant.

Diagnosis

Pyloric stenosis with dehydration and severe metabolic disturbance.

Management and prognosis

The principles of management are:

- Support the circulation to prevent shock
- Correct dehydration
- Correct metabolic disturbance
- Stop feeds
- Operation to correct stenosis

Simon received a relatively rapid infusion of saline to support his circulation and his circulatory parameters quickly

Background information

Normal development of the gastrointestinal tract

The gut is formed from a tube that appears dorsal to the yolk sac, eventually forming the primitive foregut, midgut and hindgut by week 4 of gestation. The midgut remains attached to the yolk sac by the vitelline duct. After this the dorsal mesentery forms, allowing the gut tube to be suspended in the coelomic space. The gut tube is completely occluded by tissues at around 6 weeks and recanalizes subsequently. The gut, with its apex at the vitello-intestinal duct, then herniates into the umbilicus and rotates through 90° counter-clockwise; after this it returns to the abdomen in the normal configuration.

Table 4.4 Developmental abnormalities of the gut

Abnormality	Cause	Clinical features
Tracheo-oesophageal fistula	Failure of membrane formation between foregut and respiratory bud	Frothy oral secretions at birth, respiratory distress, abdominal distension
Oesophageal atresia	Failure of recanalization of foregut	Frothy secretions, failure to pass nasogastric tube, often associated with fistula (see above)
Duodenal and small intestinal atresia	Failure of recanalization of primitive midgut	Bile-stained vomiting, increasing distension if low intestinal obstruction
Malrotation	Gut fails to rotate counter-clockwise after embryonic herniation – obstructive bands over duodenum and narrow pedicle of midgut loop	Obstruction and volvulus of midgut – anything from recurrent abdominal distension to complete infarction of midgut
Hirschsprung's disease	Failure of migration of neural crest ganglionic cells into distal bowel	Bile-stained vomiting, abdominal distension, delayed passage of meconium (>24 hours)
Meckel's diverticulum	Remnant of vitellointestinal duct	Common (3%): usually asymptomatic, blood loss, inflammation – recurrent abdominal pain
Anorectal malformations	Failure of cloacal septation into urogenital sinus and anorectal canal	Imperforate anus, anterior anus, rectal–urogenital fistulae, genital abnormalities

At the top end, an outpouching of the ventral surface of the foregut becomes partly separated by plates growing into the midline and separating off the trachea and oesophagus. Lung buds then form. The liver, pancreas and gallbladder form buds from the duodenal foregut at 5 weeks' gestation. At the lower end the anorectal canal separates from the urogenital sinus and anal patency is established at 8 weeks. Table 4.4 shows developmental abnormalities of the gut.

How to make sense of sodium and potassium results

See Table 4.5.

Further sources of information

Books

Campbell AGM, McIntosh N (eds), *Forfar and Arneil's Textbook of Pediatrics*, 5th edn. Edinburgh: Churchill Livingstone, 1999

Larsen WJ. *Essentials of Human Embryology*. Philadelphia: Churchill Livingstone, 1998

Rennie JM, Robertson NRC. *Textbook of Neonatology*, 3rd edn. Edinburgh: Churchill Livingstone, 1999

Articles

Davenport M. Surgically correctable causes of vomiting in infancy. *British Medical Journal* 1996; **312**: 236–9

Jolley SG. Gastroesophageal reflux disease as a cause for emesis in infants. *Seminars in Pediatric Surgery* 1995; **4**(3): 176–89

Orenstein SR. Infantile reflux: different from adult reflux. *American Journal of Medicine* 1997; **103**(5A): 114S–19S

Websites

www.aafp.org/afp/20000501/2791.html

Bilious vomiting in the newborn: rapid diagnosis of intestinal obstruction

Table 4.5   How to make sense of sodium and potassium results

Electrolyte	Raised/Lowered	Abnormality	Common?	Example
Sodium	Elevated	Salt poisoning	Very uncommon	Deliberate harm
		Water loss	Uncommon	Diabetes insipidus
	Low	Gut salt loss	Common	Vomiting – pyloric stenosis, diarrhoea
		Urinary salt loss	Uncommon	Adrenal failure
		Water retention	Common	Too much intravenous fluid
				Inappropriate ADH
Potassium	Elevated	Acidosis	Common	Diabetic ketoacidosis
		Adrenal failure	Uncommon	'CAH'
	Low	Alkalosis	Uncommon	Pyloric stenosis
		Gastrointestinal losses	Common	Vomiting
		Urinary losses	Uncommon	Renal tubular disease

ADH, antidiuretic hormone; CAH, congenital adrenal hyperplasia.

www.emedicine.com/emerg/topic397.htm

E-medicine – chapter on pyloric stenosis.

Self-test 6: A 1-day-old boy who is suspected of having Down's syndrome starts to vomit at 12 hours of age. He is breast-fed. The vomit contains a deep-green pigmentation. On examination he is not dehydrated and his abdomen is soft and non-distended. A nasogastric tube is inserted into his abdomen and the appearance shown in Figure 4.5 is seen on radiograph.

A What intestinal lesions are associated with Down's syndrome?

B Which is most probable in this case and why?

C What is the green pigmentation?

D What appearance is seen on the radiograph?

E What other malformation is most commonly associated with Down's syndrome?

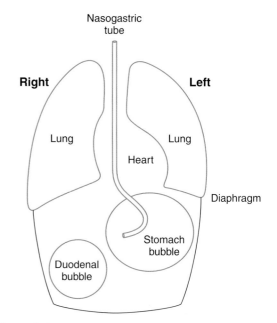

Figure 4.5   Illustration for self-test 6.

Answers:

A Duodenal atresia and Hirschsprung's disease

B Duodenal atresia – because there is no abdominal distension and the vomiting has occurred very soon after birth; it usually take a bit longer to develop in lower intestinal obstruction

C Bile – indicating an obstructive lesion that must always be taken seriously

D A 'double-bubble' – diagnostic of duodenal atresia

E Cardiac malformations – most typically atrioventricular septal defects

Self-test 7: An 8-week-old boy is seen by his general practitioner. He started vomiting after 2 weeks of age and it has persisted. He can vomit from just after his last feed until just before his next feed is due. Frequently the vomits are small 'possets'. He is gaining weight, however, and otherwise seems well. The carpets at home and his bedding are starting to smell, however.

A What is the most likely diagnosis?

B What features are against this being pyloric stenosis?

C What advice can be given to the mother to help reduce the vomiting?

D What simple treatments might be prescribed?

E What is the prognosis for this patient?

Answers:

A Gastro-oesophageal reflux (GOR – up to one in five infants have clinical GOR)

B Good weight gain; vomiting delayed up to next feed time

C Positional advice: a more upright posture tends to reduce the symptoms; this is particularly useful just after feeds

D Alginate/antacid compound such as Gaviscon Infant Sachets or feed-thickening agents

E It should remit spontaneously as a more upright posture, more solid foods and maturation of the lower oesophageal sphincter mechanism occur

Chronic disorder

Has the baby got Down's syndrome?

Age: newborn

JACKIE GREGG

Presentation

Daniel is born at term, weighing 3.1 kg, by normal vaginal delivery to 32-year-old Jayne and her husband 36-year-old Martin. The couple have a 4-year-old daughter. When the attending midwife examines Daniel, she notices that he appears somewhat dysmorphic with almond-shaped eyes and a flat occiput, and that he is rather floppy. She thinks that Daniel may have Down's syndrome and contacts the consultant paediatrician.

Initial considerations and action

Down's syndrome is the most likely diagnosis because it is the most common and most familiar of all the dysmorphic syndromes. Other dysmorphic syndromes are much rarer; however, it is now recognized that the adverse effects of alcohol and certain anticonvulsants on the fetus may be more prevalent than formerly realized. A rare possibility is that the child has inherited a number of facial features from his parents, which may make him look dysmorphic, when in fact he does not have a syndrome.

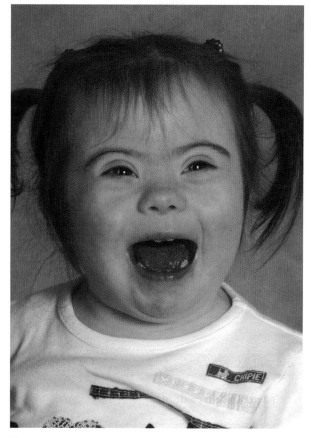

Figure 5.1   Facial features in a child with Down's syndrome.

Self-test 1: What are the typical facial features of Down's syndrome?

Answer: Upslanting palpebral fissures, epicanthic folds, Brushfield's spots on iris, flat occiput, small nose and low nasal bridge (Figure 5.1).

The consultant paediatrician asks the midwife whether the family have raised any concerns about the baby. If they had it would be important to address those as soon as possible. The midwife replies that they haven't and that

Daniel's father has gone home. He is due to return in a couple of hours by which time his wife will have transferred to the postnatal ward and had a rest. The paediatrician arranges to see Daniel's parents on the ward later.

History

The paediatrician meets Daniel's parents later and explains that he has come to carry out a medical assessment of Daniel. First he takes a brief history from Daniel's mum, Jayne. Jayne has been well throughout the pregnancy and hasn't required any medication or hospital admissions. She is healthy and doesn't have any chronic medical conditions. She doesn't smoke and has had one or two glasses of wine per week throughout her pregnancy. Jayne had had the detailed ultrasound scan of the baby at 19 weeks' gestation. She explained that she had refused the triple test in view of her religious beliefs because she 'wouldn't have had anything done about it anyway'.

Self-test 2: Which tests are available to detect Down's syndrome antenatally?

Answer: Chromosomal analysis of a sample of blood taken by chorionic villous sampling and chromosomal analysis of a sample of amniotic fluid.

Martin, too, is healthy as is their daughter. There is no relevant family history.

Examination

The paediatrician examines Daniel.

Self-test 3: As well as looking for the physical features of Down's syndrome, which medical conditions associated with Down's syndrome is it important to detect?

Answer: Congenital heart disease, duodenal atresia, congenital cataracts.

Findings

- Typical features of Down's syndrome (Figures 5.2 and 5.3)
- Centrally pink, normal pulses and blood pressure in all four limbs – no evidence of cyanotic congenital heart disease
- Grade 2 systolic murmur audible at the lower left sternal edge
- Respiratory rate 36/minute, apex beat 140/minute, liver not enlarged – no indication of heart failure which would necessitate urgent cardiological assessment
- Eyes fixing, normal red reflex – indicates normal visual responses and absence of congenital cataracts
- Bowel sounds are normal, the abdomen is not distended, Daniel has had two breast feeds and opened his bowels – no indication of bowel obstruction

Self-test 4: What is the significance of the heart murmur?

Answer: Congenital heart disease is very common in Down's syndrome – may indicate a left-to-right shunt, such as a ventricular septal defect (VSD).

Interpretation of the examination

The paediatrician is confident that Daniel has Down's syndrome. Congenital heart disease is present in almost 50 per cent of individuals with Down's syndrome, and therefore all children should have ultrasonography of the heart (echocardiography) to exclude structural abnormality. Daniel has a heart murmur and, although he is not in cardiac failure, a cardiac opinion should be arranged as a matter of priority.

Up to 5 per cent of individuals may have a structural abnormality of the gut, most commonly duodenal atresia. Daniel has opened his bowels and examination of the abdomen was normal, so he is unlikely to have any congenital malformations of the gastrointestinal tract.

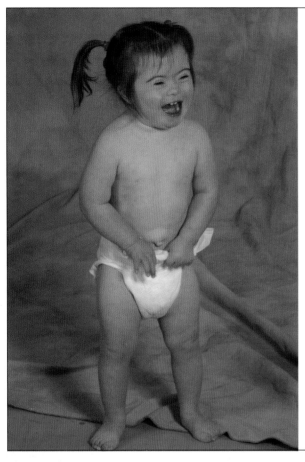

Eyes:
Upslanting palpebral fissures which tend to be narrow and short, epicanthic folds, Brushfield's spots (speckled iris), cataracts, blocked tear ducts

Craniofacial:
Flat occiput, small nose and low nasal bridge, small dysplastic ears, short neck with loose folds of skin, fine soft hair, protruding tongue. Tendency to develop microcephaly

Central nervous system:
Generally hypotonic with hyperextensible joints

Cardiovascular system:
Cardiac defects; atrioventricular septal defect (40%), ventricular septal defect (VSD) (30%), atrial septal defect (ASD) (10%), tetralogy of Fallot (6%)

Gastrointestinal tract:
Duodenal atresia, Hirschsprung's disease, constipation, gastro-oesophageal reflux, feeding difficulties.

Skin:
Tendency to:
– develop redness of cheeks and nose
– dry skin, cutis marmorata

Hands and feet:
– short stubby hands and fingers
– transverse palmar crease
– incurving little finger
– small middle phalanx of little finger
– gap between first and second toe with plantar crease

Figure 5.2 Features of Down's syndrome. (With special thanks to Libby for posing so beautifully and to her mum for offering advice on what families want to know.)

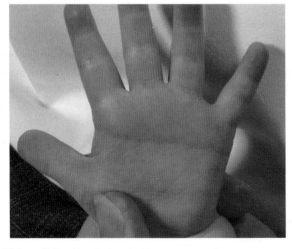

Figure 5.3 Hand showing transverse palmar crease.

Investigations

Down's syndrome can be diagnosed in pregnancy. Tests that indicate increased risk are:

- Thickening of the fat pad at the back of the neck (nuchal translucency) detected on ultrasound scan between 10 and 12 weeks' gestation
- Cardiac defect detected at the detailed ultrasound scan at 19 weeks would raise suspicion of Down's syndrome
- The 'triple' test, which involves measurement of maternal serum α-fetoprotein (AFP), unconjugated oestriol and human chorionic gonadotrophin, with adjustment for maternal age, is being used as

a screening tool to identify fetuses at increased risk of having Down's syndrome

Definitive tests

- Chromosomal analysis of a blood sample by chorionic villous sampling (CVS) at 10 weeks' gestation
- Amniocentesis at 16–19 weeks

Both of these procedures carry an increased risk of miscarriage of 1–1.5 per cent and 0.5–1 per cent, respectively.

Daniel's mother had a normal ultrasound scan at 19 weeks' gestation. She was not offered amniocentesis in view of her age and had declined the triple test. Chromosome studies on a sample of blood from Daniel will be needed to confirm the diagnosis.

Self-test 5: What is the chromosome abnormality?

Answer: Trisomy 21.

Diagnosis

Discussion with the family

The paediatrician now needs to discuss his concerns with the family and obtain their consent for chromosome studies and a cardiac opinion. 'Breaking the news' requires good communication skills, sensitivity and empathy, in addition to experience and knowledge – all doctors should receive adequate training. Parents usually remember how and what they were told in great detail and this can affect how they come to terms with the situation. It is important to remember that Daniel is a child first not a syndrome.

How to break the news

- Who? Ideally the senior doctor
- Where? Privacy is important, because there must be no interruptions
- When? Ideally, as soon as possible after the diagnosis is certain or almost certain
- How much? Most families want to know as much as possible. Be guided by the parents about the pace at which they want information. It might be necessary to do this over several consultations
- How? Both parents should be seen together, although in a medical emergency this might not be possible. Arrangements must be made to see the other parent as soon as possible. Circumstances vary and a lone parent may wish a friend or relative to be present. It is usually helpful for the mother's named midwife to be present if the parents agree. Avoid medical jargon. Encourage the parents to express their feelings freely. Allow enough time. Be honest about treatment, prognosis and any uncertainty. Use appropriate body language to convey empathy, warmth and reassurance to the family. Keep a balanced outlook – don't be too pessimistic. Be sensitive to cultural differences and use a trained translator if necessary. Assess the parents' understanding of the situation. Once the parents have heard the diagnosis, they may have no recollection of the ensuing discussion. A written summary of the discussion may be helpful. Provide written information and contact details of support services. Arrange a time for review within a few days
- Finally: document the information given and inform other professionals including the family doctor and health visitor

An issue specific to a diagnosis of Down's syndrome is the likely development of a child with Down's syndrome. Parents may have very pessimistic expectations. It is important to point out that it is impossible to predict how any individual child will develop. Parents need to be informed of the associated medical problems.

Self-test 6: Which of the following problems are associated with Down's syndrome

A Autism

B Hearing problems

C Refractive errors

D Hypopituitarism

E Bleeding disorder

Answer: A/B/C.

It may be the parents who are concerned that their child has Down's syndrome. These concerns must be taken seriously and arrangements made for a senior doctor to examine the child and discuss the concerns with the parents.

Treatment and follow-up plan

Follow-up meeting

Arrangements should be made to see the family again as soon as the results of the chromosome tests are available, which is usually within a few days. The maternity unit social worker may be helpful in giving the family information and offering practical help, and giving advice on how to tell other family members. Written information should be made available, including a contact name and number for the local and national offices of the Down's Syndrome Association. Meeting another parent of a child with Down's syndrome may be helpful for some families. An appointment should be made for the family to meet the local child development team. The community paediatrician, who will be responsible for monitoring the child's health and development, may be available to meet the family on the ward before discharge.

People react in different ways to being told that their child has a disability. Occasionally, one or other parent may 'disappear' for a day or two, perhaps even leaving their child in hospital. It is essential that professionals manage this period with the utmost sensitivity. Most parents will mourn the child they might have had, but at the same time adjust to living with their 'different' child. Bereavement analysis proposes four stages for adjustment:

1 Shock – psychological confusion and feelings of grief or numbness
2 Reaction – feelings of anger and denial may alternate with sadness and anxiety

3 Adaptation – parents seek out ways of helping the child
4 Orientation – parents begin actively to plan ahead

In reality, parents are likely to slip in and out of these stages at different times. However, they provide a useful framework within which both parents and professionals can work.

Daniel's treatment plan includes:

● Cardiac assessment
● Advice on atlantoaxial subluxation
● Genetic advice

Cardiac defects are important because they are the main factor that determines life expectancy. Many children will be symptomatic soon after birth and require urgent assessment by a paediatric cardiologist. Early detection is important to prevent secondary complications and to give appropriate advice on antibiotic prophylaxis. Other defects may not be detected clinically in the neonatal period and therefore all children should have a cardiology assessment within the first few weeks of life.

People with Down's syndrome have a small risk for acute or chronic neurological problems caused by cervical spine instability – atlantoaxial subluxation. There is no screening procedure that can predict those at risk. Parents should be advised to seek urgent medical attention if there is an unexplained change in gait or sphincter control. Children should not be barred from sports because there is no evidence that this increases the risk any more than for the general population. Advice should be given on appropriate restraint in cars.

It is important that the family receives genetic counselling and understands the risks of recurrence in relation to maternal age and the chromosome results. Advice from a clinical geneticist may be necessary in more complex cases.

Outpatient follow-up

Daniel will require regular follow-up to address the following issues:

● General health and growth monitoring
● Developmental surveillance

- Audiological assessment
- Vision assessment

Self-test 7: What degree of learning difficulties do individuals with Down's syndrome have?

Answer: Usually severe learning difficulties, but the degree is variable.

General health and growth

Short stature is a recognized physical characteristic of most people with Down's syndrome and specific growth charts are available. Some conditions leading to poor growth, such as congenital heart disease, sleep-related upper airway obstruction, poor intake as a result of feeding problems and hypothyroidism, occur more frequently in Down's syndrome. Regular checks on general health and growth should aid early identification of pathological causes of growth retardation. Thyroid disorder does not affect only growth: it also affects development. Diagnosis of thyroid disease clinically is difficult and regular biochemical testing is indicated. There is an increased incidence of respiratory infections, leukaemia and epilepsy.

Development

Children with Down's syndrome usually have learning difficulties, which most often are severe, although the degree is variable. As with any child it is impossible to predict ultimate intellectual functioning. In the first few years, cognitive development may approach the normal range, although there is usually delay in motor skills. Some children may not sit until 12 months and may not walk until well into the third year of life. A developmental physiotherapy programme is helpful from about 6 months of age to promote motor development. Learning problems become more evident after the age of 3–4 years. Children with Down's syndrome tend to have additional delay in language development compared with their other skills. There may be a need to use a simple signing system such as Makaton while the expressive language is developing, to reduce frustration.

Children with Down's syndrome are often said to be musical and of a placid and friendly personality. This is not always the case and behavioural problems may

develop. Although rare, social impairment, hyperactivity and autism can occur in children with Down's syndrome. It is therefore important that the child development team monitors all children with Down's syndrome. The team usually consists of the community paediatrician, physiotherapist, occupational therapist, and speech and language therapist with input from a clinical psychologist. Such teams have close links with the social work team for children with disabilities and the preschool education team, which usually includes an educational psychologist, a preschool teacher and a Portage worker. Together they can ensure that parents receive appropriate advice and support in how best to promote their child's development and eventually to find the most appropriate educational provision. Most children with Down's syndrome attend mainstream schools, usually with additional support.

Hearing

Most children with the syndrome have mild-to-moderate hearing loss, which is usually a conductive loss caused by secretary otitis media. Many children require grommets and some require hearing aids for a period of time. Regular surveillance is important in view of the association of hearing loss with impaired language development. In addition to middle-ear disease, children are prone to developing large adenoids and tonsils and chronic rhinitis, and often require an ear, nose and throat (ENT) opinion leading to surgery.

Vision

All newborns should be checked for congenital cataracts and visual behaviour should be closely monitored in the first year of life. There is a high incidence of refractive error and squint, and children should be referred for ophthalmological and orthoptic assessment in the second year of life.

Prognosis

Congenital heart disease and an increased risk of infections reduce life expectancy. There is a high incidence of presenile dementia as a result of Alzheimer's disease, particularly in the over-50s. However, it is estimated that approximately half will survive into their late 50s and early 60s in good health. Girls may menstruate and can be fertile whereas males are infertile.

Background information

Epidemiology

The word 'syndrome' means to 'run together' and the word 'dysmorphic' means 'abnormally formed'. Thus a dysmorphic syndrome refers to a collection of abnormalities of bodily structures that are found to cluster together more often than would be expected by chance. The cause may be a chromosome disorder, a defective single gene, exposure to an adverse intrauterine event, such as an infection or toxin, or a biochemical disorder (the last very rarely). Around 2000 syndromes have already been identified.

Down's syndrome is the most common autosomal trisomy and the most common genetic cause of severe learning difficulties. It occurs in all races. The incidence is about 1 in 650 of all live births. The risk is also related to maternal age; it rises from less than 1 in 1000 in young mothers, to more than 1 in 100 in women aged over 40. Although the risk of having a baby with Down's syndrome is higher for older women, a large majority have had their babies before they are 30 and therefore most babies with Down's syndrome are born to women in this age group (Table 5.1).

Cytogenetics

There are 46 chromosomes in the nucleus of each body cell, of which 22 are matching pairs with matching genes and are called autosomes. The remaining pair, the sex chromosomes, are alike in the female, labelled XX, but in the male there is only one X chromosome and a smaller chromosome, Y. In the ovum or sperm, there are only 23 chromosomes and this ensures that at fertilization the normal human chromosomal complement is reconstituted.

Down's syndrome is caused by an additional chromosome, chromosome 21, i.e. trisomy 21, which may result from non-disjunction, translocation or mosaicism (Figure 5.4).

Non-disjunction occurs in 94 per cent of cases and is usually caused by an error at meiosis, the likelihood of which increases with maternal age. The pair of chromosomes 21 fails to separate, so that one gamete has two chromosomes 21 and the other none. Fertilization of the former results in trisomy 21. Ten per cent of non-disjunctions are paternally derived, but this appears to be unrelated to age. The risk of recurrence is 1 in 100 for mothers less than 40 years and is twice the age-specific risk above 40.

Translocation occurs in 5 per cent and is the result of a chromosome 21 being attached to another chromosome, usually number 14, and more rarely 15, 22 or 21.

Table 5.1 Age-related risk of Down's syndrome

Maternal age (years)	Incidence
20–25	1/2000
25–30	1/1200
30–35	1/900
35–40	1/350
40–44	1/100
>44	1/37

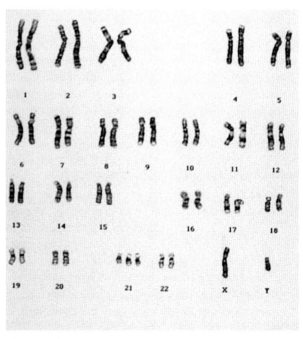

Figure 5.4 Karyotype with an extra chromosome 21.

It is unrelated to maternal age. The risk of recurrence is 10–15 per cent if the mother is the translocation carrier and 2.5 per cent if the father is the carrier. This has implications for the whole family who should be screened. If a parent carries the rare 21/21 translocation, all the children will have Down's syndrome.

Mosaicism occurs in 1 per cent. Some of the cells are normal and some have trisomy 21. This usually arises after the formation of zygote, by non-disjunction at mitosis.

Further sources of information

Books

Wiedemann H-R, Kunze J. *Clinical Syndromes*, 3rd edn. London: Times Mirror International, 1997

Cunningham C. *Down's Syndrome, An Introduction for Parents*. London: Souvenir Press (E&A) Ltd, 1988

Guidelines

Paediatric practice guidelines. *Right From the Start*. PPG/96/02. London: British Paediatric Association, 1996

Website

www.info@downs-syndrome.org.uk

Down's Syndrome Association.

Self-test 8: Seven-year old Louise, who has Down's syndrome, attends clinic for her annual medical assessment. Her mum has some concerns that she seems tired all the time, although sleeping well. She eats well and has a good diet, but has become constipated. Comments from school are that Louise's progress has been poorer than the teachers would have expected.

A What are the important features in the history?

B What might you find on examination?

C What investigation would you organize?

D What is the likely diagnosis?

Answers:

A Tiredness, but sleeping well, constipation, poor school progress

B Slowing of growth, dry skin, thin dry hair

C Thyroid function tests

D Hypothyroidism

Presentation

Carole is a health visitor working in an urban setting in the Midlands. She has been monitoring the health of an infant girl Molly since she was 2 weeks of age. She is now 9 months old. Of particular concern is the fact that Molly's weight gain has been very poor, especially over the last 3 months (Figure 6.1). Despite the advice she has given Molly's mother, there does not appear to have been an improvement. Carole discusses her concerns with Molly's general practitioner. They agree that Molly's growth is suboptimal and decide to initiate a programme of investigation to determine the problem, but first of all they review what they already know.

Self-test 1: Which is the best definition of failure to thrive?

A Weight remaining below the 0.4th centile for weight from birth to 9 months
B Crossing down two centile lines on the 9th centile chart
C Sustained rate of weight gain below the 5 per cent confidence interval for that expected
D Poor weight gain with associated clinical symptoms
E Body mass index (BMI) in the bottom quartile

Answer: C, although B is simpler and used in health screening.

Initial considerations and action

- Definition of failure to thrive
- 'Organic' versus 'non-organic' failure to thrive

- An infant with a low weight centile is not necessarily failing to thrive

Poor weight gain in infancy is termed 'failure to thrive'. It is important to note that this is not a diagnosis but a 'symptom'. It is defined, in general, by the observation of a rate of weight gain significantly below that which is usually expected. A more precise definition is a reduction by 2 or more centile lines on the weight and height charts.

- Centile fall >2 lines: mild-to-moderate failure to thrive
- Centile fall >3 lines: severe failure to thrive

Other definitions that are used include a single measurement of weight below the second centile or a reduction in weight gain velocity below the 5th centile of a specific infant weight gain velocity chart. Such specific charts are quite complex and not routinely used, but they are the 'gold standard' definition. These definitions are not evidence based. No one has calculated their sensitivity and specificity when detecting pathology and during subsequently improving growth. They are all essentially screening procedures, which allow health professionals within the community to identify children who have an increased likelihood of disease.

A simple model of failure to thrive suggests that there are two main groups of causes:

- Organic
- Non-organic

A child with organic failure to thrive (Figure 6.2) has a clear-cut pathology that is responsible for this. When this pathology is identified and treated, the child

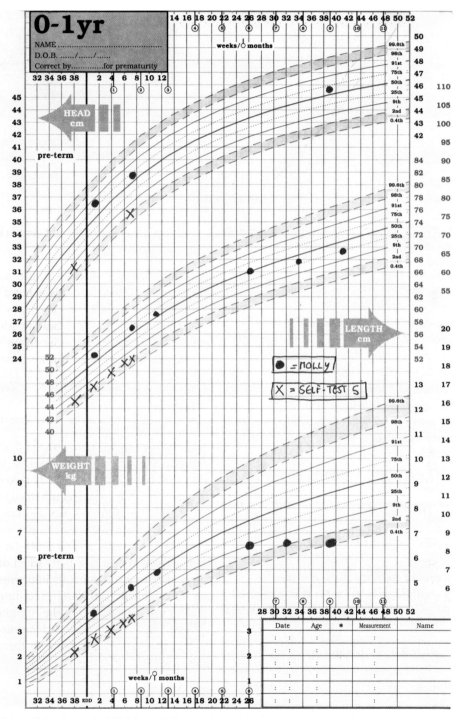

Figure 6.1 Molly's weight chart. © Child Growth Foundation. The chart shown here is intended for illustrative purposes only. The range of UK growth reference charts may be purchased from Harlow Printing, Maxwell Street, South Shields, NE33 4PU.

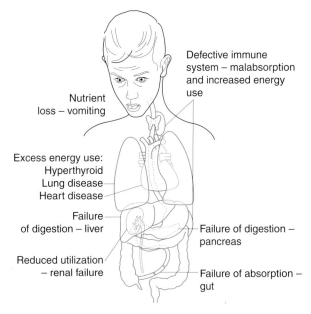

Defective immune system – malabsorption and increased energy use

Nutrient loss – vomiting

Excess energy use:
Hyperthyroid
Lung disease
Heart disease

Failure of digestion – liver

Reduced utilization – renal failure

Failure of digestion – pancreas

Failure of absorption – gut

Figure 6.2 Diagram of organic causes of failure to thrive.

will thrive. An example would be cystic fibrosis. When this is confirmed with a positive sweat test result (see below), the child will receive appropriate treatment (pancreatic enzyme supplementation) and weight gain will be improved. It is not that simple, however. Some of the diseases that are associated with failure to thrive can be associated with impaired food intake, e.g. chronic chest infection in cystic fibrosis may cause anorexia. The factors associated with non-organic failure to thrive (see below) are also seen in children with chronic illnesses and their families. Some of the factors such as stress and poverty are more likely to be seen in such families – that's what chronic illnesses can do.

In a child with non-organic failure to thrive no such disease can be detected by clinical assessment or by investigation. Ninety-five per cent or more of children with failure to thrive are within this category. The final pathway in this situation is reduced food intake. Important factors include:

- Socioeconomic deprivation
- Recurrent viral infections
- Abuse and neglect
- Inappropriate food selection

- Poor parental education
- Difficult or disorganized feeding behaviour
- Parental mental health problems

Self-test 2: Give examples of poor parental education that might lead to failure to thrive.

Answer: Selection of inappropriate foods, failure to understand and hear advice from professionals (e.g. weaning age, what to drink), failure to read food instructions, poor contact with health services; more likely to be socioeconomically disadvantaged.

Many of these factors interact with and influence each other and commonly non-organic failure to thrive is a complex disorder and, as you can imagine, the solution is usually not simple.

By the time of the birth some children's short stature and accompanying low weight centile are established and permanent. In addition some children naturally grow down the centile lines as an adjustment is made from 'uterine weight' to 'genetic weight' (see 'Management and prognosis' for more information).

History

The health visitor and the GP now review the history in the light of these factors.

First, the growth parameters recorded in the parent-held child health record are reviewed – see Figure 6.1. This is done to confirm that there is 'failure to thrive' and to determine its time course, because this can give important diagnostic information.

Features of organic disease

A careful history of gastrointestinal function is obtained, as this is especially relevant to this situation:

Feeding	This infant does not like feeding. It always seems a battle. She is able to take drinks from the bottle and can swallow mashed up solid food without coughing or choking

Vomiting	Molly has vomited with intercurrent illnesses and posseted (small frequent vomits) up to the age of 4 months
Stools	Molly has her bowels open two to three times per day and it is rather sloppy – her mother describes the consistency as like porridge. Stools are not especially offensive
Abdominal pain	There is nothing to suggest that Molly has abdominal pain, although she is felt to be a fussy child
Immune system	Although she has had her fair share of coughs and colds, Molly has not suffered from any severe infections
Respiratory system	As above, only occasional coughs and no wheezing. Persistent respiratory symptoms can represent such chronic disorders as cystic fibrosis and also immune deficiencies, which often present with recurrent or persistent chest infections. There is no evidence of chronic problems with the upper respiratory tract
Cardiovascular system	No relevant symptoms (breathlessness, cyanosis) are noted

Molly's birth history and her mother's pregnancy history are obtained:

- Born at 41 weeks' gestation weighing 3.8 kg, head circumference 36 cm
- A straightforward delivery with an Apgar score of 9 at 1 minute; no resuscitation was needed
- Breast-feeding was attempted but was not successful, so formula milk was substituted at 6 days of age
- The pregnancy was uncomplicated and maternal weight gain and fetal growth were recorded as satisfactory – despite mother smoking 10–15 cigarettes a day

Features of non-organic failure to thrive

The health visitor considers each of the categories listed above.

Socioeconomic deprivation

- The family are not well-off financially:
  - mother is 19 years old and Molly has a 2-year-old sibling called James – he is well and thriving
  - Molly's mother is single and Molly's father has never taken parental responsibility – he is unemployed, 23 and lives with his parents
  - the family live on income support and benefits – a limited income
  - they reside in a one bedroom, local-council rented flat; the flat is in a poor condition
  - there is little family support for Molly's mother – she is very isolated
  - Molly's mother smokes – this places an additional financial burden on the family

Recurrent viral infections

- Molly has had a number of infections, from which she has always recovered, but she has had a poor appetite for a least a week with them

Abuse and neglect

- Molly is always clean and well cared for. There have never been any signs of injury

Inappropriate food selection

- This does seem to be a problem. In the inner-urban environment, on a low income and reliant on public transport, the variety and quality of food the family obtains are poor
- There is little fresh fruit and vegetables and an over-reliance on processed foods, fast foods from local outlets and snack foods. Gluten-containing foods have been used from around 4 months of age despite the health visitor recommending that they should not be
- Also fresh cows' milk was introduced at the age of 7 months despite the health visitor recommending that it should be delayed until 1 year of age

Poor parental education

- Mary, Molly's mother, left school at 16 and had been a poor attender for the whole of the previous year

Difficult or disorganized feeding behaviour

Although Molly was initially a good feeder on milk, she was always fussy on solids and feeding had become a battle – she spat out solids frequently and liked the taste of very few foods. She was reluctant to let her mother feed her. Her brother James was a distraction at meal times, regularly seeking attention and disrupting feeding. Molly's attention to feeding was interrupted and it was difficult to get her started again.

Parental mental health problems

Mary admitted to feeling lonely, isolated and harassed. She did not appear to be clinically depressed, but was at risk of depression according to the general practitioner.

Specific nutritional information

Mary was asked to keep a feeding diary for 2 days for Molly, and this was passed on to the community dietician who provided the following report:

Nutrient	Intake (percentage of reference nutrient intake or RNI)
Energy	83
Protein	85
Iron	57
Calcium	92
Vitamin C	67
Vitamin D	78

Comment: generally poor intake of most nutrients related to poor solid food intake. Especially poor iron intake related to intake of fresh cows' milk. Also suboptimal intake of vitamins

---

Self-test 3: Which of the following descriptions is inappropriate for healthy daily intake in a 9-month-old child?
A Vitamin A: 350 mg
B Vitamin D: 400 IU
C Protein: 70 g
D Energy: 900 kcal
E Vitamin C: 25 mg

Answer: C – it should be about 12–15 g; 70 g is the usual adult intake.

Interpretation of the history

Poor intake of important nutrients – energy, protein, iron and some vitamins – suggests that this is the probable reason that Molly is not gaining adequate weight. Many factors related to non-organic failure to thrive are present. Some symptoms (loose stools) could be related to underlying disease. It is important to examine Molly for features of organic disease.

Examination

Accurate measurements

The current growth parameters are seen on the chart along with previous measurements (see Figure 6.1, p. 47).

How to weigh and measure an infant

Head circumference

Place the measure around the largest occipitofrontal circumference that you can find. Take and note the measurement. Take off the measure and then repeat twice. Note the largest measure – this is the occipitofrontal circumference

Weight

Weigh the child naked. The room has to be warm. Wait until the child is still and the needle or digital readout settles. Electronic scales do this automatically – usually beeping when the result is available.

Length

Under 2 years of age, the supine height is recorded. The infant should be naked. One person stabilizes the child's head at the top and holds it steady in the neutral position. The base plate is then moved up to touch the infant's heels. Try to keep the child as relaxed as possible. If he or she is upset, he or she flexes and the length will be under-read.

Nutritional assessment

- Hair: healthy
- Skin: rather pale, with pale conjunctivae, skin dry
- Eyes: bright, not sunken
- Mouth: smooth tongue, sore at corners of mouth
- Nails: healthy
- Subcutaneous fat: reduced
- Muscle bulk and tone: reduced bulk noted in biceps but good muscle tone

Self-test 4: Which of the following is the most likely cause for a smooth tongue and sore corners of the mouth?

A **Iron deficiency**

B **Vitamin B$_{12}$ deficiency**

C **Folic acid deficiency**

D **Vitamin C deficiency**

E **Milk allergy**

Answer: A.

Search for organic disease

No sign of a genetic abnormality or dysmorphic features	
Cardiovascular system and respiratory system	Healthy and in particular no breathlessness, cyanosis, heart murmurs or abnormal chest shape
Abdomen, perineum and genitalia	Abdomen somewhat protuberant but soft with normal bowel sounds No hepatosplenomegaly
Central nervous system (CNS)	Soft fontanelle, normal tone and posture, no evidence of a squint
Ears, nose and throat	Left ear drum retracted and dull – fluid level seen behind it Nose and throat look healthy

- Development assessment — Sitting from 7 months; now pulling to standing, vocalizing well but no recognizable words yet Able to grasp and transfer objects, wary of strangers Passed distraction hearing test 1 month ago

Interpretation of the examination

The examination confirms the presence of failure to thrive and there is evidence of malnutrition with reduced nutrient stores in subcutaneous fat and muscle. Despite this, there is no evidence of CNS compromise. Development seems to be within normal limits. The smooth tongue (atrophic glossitis), angular stomatitis and pale conjunctivae could all indicate iron deficiency. The protuberant abdomen may be significant. This could represent malnutrition but could also indicate a bowel abnormality. Iron deficiency is a common nutritional disorder in older infants and toddlers and it can be caused by:

- Dietary iron deficiency
- Iron malabsorption
- Intestinal blood loss

There is enough concern here to consider the possibility of organic disease. Molly is seen at the day-case unit at the children's health department where investigations are performed.

Investigations

Haematology

Haemoglobin	8.3 g/dL (low)
Blood film	Red cells are small (microcytic) and pale (hypochromic)
Serum ferritin	6.8 mg/dL (normal >16 mg/dL)
Anti-endomysial antibody titre	Strongly positive

Microbiology

Urine No abnormalities on microscopy and bacterial culture negative

Stool No ova, cysts and parasites seen on microscopy but undigested fat droplets seen

Interpretation of the results

The presence of a microcytic/hypochromic anaemia confirms the clinical impression of anaemia and shows that it is iron deficiency anaemia. The presence of anti-endomysial antibodies and undigested fat in the stool makes gluten-sensitive enteropathy (coeliac disease) very likely.

Molly was subsequently referred to a paediatric gastroenterologist who did an upper gastrointestinal endoscopy. A biopsy was taken (Figure 6.3) and the following report was issued:

'There is subtotal villous atrophy affecting the jejunal mucosa together with hypertrophy of the crypts. The tissue layer beneath the mucosa is heavily infiltrated with inflammatory cells. There is no evidence of the presence of *Giardia lamblia*. The appearances are consistent with coeliac disease.'

Diagnosis

Coeliac disease (gluten-sensitive enteropathy) with social difficulties also noted.

Management and prognosis

The paediatric gastroenterologist and dietician placed Molly on a gluten-free diet. Her stools became firmer, her appetite improved and she gained weight well. She also received iron and vitamin supplements, and her dietary intake of protein and energy was also increased while she was catching up. It is planned for her to remain on a life-long gluten-free diet (no wheat, barley or oats). Her mother and brother were also screened for the condition and found not to have it.

The health visitor arranged for a regular nursery place-ment for Molly's brother, which helped her mother greatly. As the family received income support, a social worker arranged for extra income to cover the increased cost of food for Molly. The community dietician also gave advice on healthy eating for the whole family.

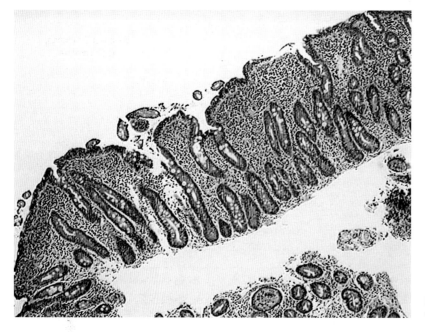

Figure 6.3 Microscopic findings on jejunal biopsy in coeliac disease.

Background information

Catch-up and -down growth and the Shire–Shetland cross

One confounding factor in assessing infant growth is the transition from intrauterine programming to genetic programming. Crosses between Shire horses and Shetland ponies result in the information in Table 6.1.

This experiment shows an important principle. Uterine capacity and nutrient production determine size at birth. Only around 20 per cent of the variability in final adult size is determined by this time. Subsequent infant growth is towards that genetically programmed. By age 2 years in humans, 80 per cent of the variation of adult height is determined.

Hence, some children are growing up and down centile charts depending on the difference between these two influences and some such children may be labelled 'failing to thrive'. There are some clues that suggest catch-down growth:

- Smooth growth down the centiles in all parameters
- Genetically small parent or parents
- Larger than expected birth size for the mother
- A healthy baby apparently feeding well

It can be difficult to differentiate these children and those with true failure to thrive. So detailed assessment and monitoring are undertaken.

In general, therefore, larger babies on average tend to grow down the lines and smaller ones tend to grow up them. This effect can be described as 'regression to the mean'.

Table 6.1 The Shire–Shetland experiment as a model of early infant growth

Parents	Size at birth	Subsequent growth
Shire mother	Shire	Grow-down centiles
Shetland mother	Shetland	Grow-up centiles

Reference nutrient intakes

In the UK, the most authoritative advice on nutrient intakes is provided by the Panel on Dietary Reference Values (see Department of Health in References). For each nutrient the Panel has produced dietary reference values. These are taken from the normal reference curves for the nutrient requirement across the UK population. The curve is shown in Figure 6.4. The reference intakes are:

- **Estimated average requirement (EAR):** the mean amount required
- **Reference nutrient intake (RNI):** 2 standard deviations above this value (likely to be adequate for all individuals)
- **Lower reference nutrient intake (LRNI):** 2 standard deviations below this value (lowest intake that will meet needs of some individuals)

For example, for iron the reference values at 7–9 months of age are:

- **EAR:** 4.2 mg/day
- **LRNI:** 6.0 mg/day
- **RNI:** 7.8 mg/day

Molly's intake was 4.4 mg/day.

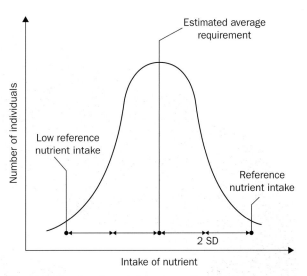

Figure 6.4 Graph explaining how the 'recommended' nutritional intake is calculated.

Iron deficiency

The normal full-term infant is born with a haemoglobin level of around 16 g/dL, falling to around 11 g/dL at 10 weeks. This is a result of the rapid onset of erythropoiesis during the second month. This tends to deplete iron stores during the second 3 months, so that up to one-third of infants will develop features of iron deficiency by the end of this period.

- **Birth:**
  - iron stores replete
  - red cell production reduced (new high-oxygen environment suppresses erythropoietin)
- **Six weeks old:**
  - red cell production increases
  - dietary iron now needed
- **Four to six months:** iron stores diminishing
- **Six months plus:**
  - haemoglobin synthesis requires 30 per cent of dietary iron
  - risk of iron deficiency if iron intake marginal

The following dietary factors are associated with iron deficiency:

- Delayed weaning on to solid foods
- Use of fresh cows' milk before 1 year
- High dietary phosphate content
- Tannates (e.g. in tea)
- Bran
- Lack of citric acid (aids iron absorption)
- Low protein intake
- Low vitamin C intake

Organic causes of failure to thrive

Although uncommon there are organic causes of failure to thrive. Table 6.2 is a list of some of the more common causes and their features and diagnostic tests.

Coeliac disease (gluten-sensitive enteropathy)

Prevalence
- As high as 1 in 300 in western Ireland
- It is a common cause of malabsorption

Table 6.2 Organic causes of failure to thrive

Cause	Features	Tests
Cystic fibrosis	Recurrent or persistent chest infections Diarrhoea or steatorrhoea	Sweat sodium and chloride increased Mutation at CFTR protein locus
Immunological deficiency	Persistent, severe or unusual infections	General immunoglobulin levels White cell count and differential and lymphocyte subsets
Urinary tract infection	Poor appetite, vomiting, fussiness Diarrhoea, offensive urine	Urine microscopy and culture
Gastro-oesophageal reflux	Persistent vomiting	Oesophageal pH probe, barium swallow, endoscopy
Coeliac disease	Irritability, diarrhoea, anaemia	Anti-endomysial antibodies, jejunal biopsy
Hypothyroidism	Developmental delay, hoarse voice, umbilical hernia (unusual – usually detected by neonatal screening)	Thyroid function tests
Genetic condition	Dysmorphic features, developmental delay	Depends on suspected condition but may include chromosomal analysis or DNA analysis

CFTR, cystic fibrosis transmembrane conductance regulator.

- The incidence is increased in immunoglobulin A (IgA) deficiency and type 1 diabetes mellitus

Pathogenesis

Permanent intolerance (hypersensitivity) to ingested gluten (wheat, oats, barley, rye) causes complete villous atrophy, with crypt hyperplasia of proximal small intestinal mucosa. Patients develop IgG antibodies. A number of immunological abnormalities are likely to mediate the mucosal damage.

Presentation

Characteristic presentation is after 6 months of age (between 9 and 18 months), when gluten products are introduced into the diet, in a previously well child. Infants and toddlers usually present with symptoms within weeks or months of the introduction of gluten:

- **Common:**
  - chronic diarrhoea (large, soft, pale, greasy and foul smelling)
  - abdominal distension
  - abdominal pain
  - poor appetite
  - poor weight gain/failure to thrive
- **Older children:**
  - short stature
  - delayed puberty
  - pallor (iron deficiency anaemia)
  - behavioural problems

- **Other:**
  - rectal prolapse
  - constipation
  - puffiness (oedema)
  - mouth ulcers
  - rickets

Investigations

- **Anti-endomysial IgA antibodies:**
  - a reliable (high specificity) and non-invasive screening test except when coeliac disease is associated with IgA deficiency
  - elevated level before and normal level after a gluten-free diet confirms the diagnosis
  - useful in monitoring compliance with gluten-free diet
- **Anti-gliadin and anti-reticulin antibodies:** elevated but less reliable
- **Jejunal biopsy:** shows complete flattening of villi and deepening of the crypts (Figure 6.5)

Management

- **Gluten-free diet lifelong:** symptoms, anti-endomysial antibody positivity and villous atrophy disappear within 6 months
- **Other family members:** should be investigated if symptomatic and screened with anti-endomysial antibodies if asymptomatic

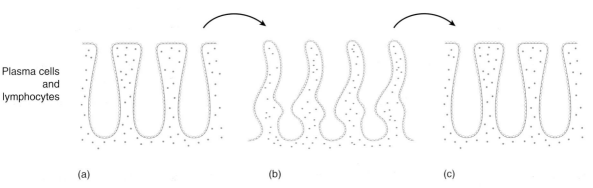

Plasma cells and lymphocytes

(a) (b) (c)

Figure 6.5   The proximal small intestinal mucosa in coeliac disease. (a) at diagnosis on diet containing gluten; (b) on gluten-free diet; and (c) after re-challenge with gluten. In (a), there is increased shedding of enterocytes leading to villus atrophy, which in turn leads to a reduced absorptive surface area; there is also elongation of the crypts of Lieberkühn and infiltration of the lamina propria. In (b) there are normal villi and crypts with a villus height:crypt length ratio of >1. In (c) there is a relapse.

Further sources of information

Books

Department of Health. *Dietary Reference Values for Food Energy and Nutrients for the United Kingdom.* Report on Health and Social Subjects. London: HMSO, 1991

McLaren DS, Burman D, Belton NR, Williams AF. *Textbook of Paediatric Nutrition.* Edinburgh: Churchill Livingstone, 1991

Articles

Wright CM. Identification and management of failure to thrive: a community perspective. *Archives of Disease in Childhood* 2000; **82**: 5–9

Wright CM, Callum J, Birks E, Jarvis S. Effect of community based management in failure to thrive: randomised controlled trial. *British Medical Journal* 1998; **317**: 571–4

Websites

www.nlm.nih.gov/medlineplus/ency/article/000991.htm

Review of failure to thrive.

www.medinfo.co.uk/conditions/coeliac.html

Coeliac disease.

www.ridgeway-surgery.demon.co.uk/pregnant/healthvi.htm

Role of the health visitor.

Self-test 5: The growth chart of a 9-week-old baby girl is shown (see Figure 6.1). She was born at 38 weeks' gestation weighing 2.2 kg. No dysmorphic features are seen and clinical examination reveals no abnormalities. She has now been referred as 'failure to thrive'. She has had persistent small vomits and occasional large vomits – especially if she is laid down after a feed. She seems to be taking appropriate amounts of feed.
Questions:
A Is she failing to thrive?
B What is the likely cause of the vomiting?
C What is the most likely pattern of her future growth?

Answers:
A No
B Gastro-oesophageal reflux
C To remain on her present centiles

An infant with delayed development

Age: 2½ years

JACKIE GREGG

Presentation

Referral letter from GP to developmental paediatrician:

Please see two and a half-year-old Paul whose parents have become increasingly concerned over the last 6–12 months that his development is delayed. The health visitor has observed Paul at home. She noted that he has been slow to achieve all his developmental milestones and that his language and play are delayed.

Initial considerations and action

Developmental delay is a rather meaningless term because it can be used to describe a child with mild and fairly minimal delay to one with profound difficulties. It may also imply to families that the child will 'catch up'. However, it is a useful term in the early stages of assessment.

Learning disability is the term commonly used to describe the individual with significant developmental delay. It is divided into gradations of intellectual ability; however, the medical classification differs from the educational one. Most developmental paediatricians working closely with their educational colleagues favour the educational classification because it causes less confusion to parents:

- Severe learning disability (SLD): IQ < 50
- Mild (may also be termed 'moderate') learning disability (MLD): IQ 50–70

- Specific learning disability: deficit in one or more areas, e.g. dyslexia, dyscalculia

Note that the term 'mental retardation' is now rarely used and people with developmental problems find the term 'learning disability' more acceptable.

The age at which a child with delay in his or her development presents will depend on the severity of the delay, the presence of recognizable specific disorders, the parents' knowledge of normal child development and the quality of paediatric services. Children with mild or more specific learning difficulties may not present until well into school age. Paul's parents, his GP and health visitor are concerned and therefore it is likely that his delay is significant. The paediatrician arranges to see Paul in his clinic in the Child Development Centre (CDC).

Assessment of Paul needs to address:

- The magnitude of the delay
- A diagnosis and/or cause (if possible)
- Recommendations for intervention
- The need for involvement of other agencies

Diagnosis is very important for both parents and professionals:

- It gives information on the likely functional ability and prognosis
- It can give pointers to the most appropriate treatment approaches
- It can help with genetic counselling/recurrence risk
- It can help families understand their child and more readily come to terms with their problems
- It can help open more doors to services

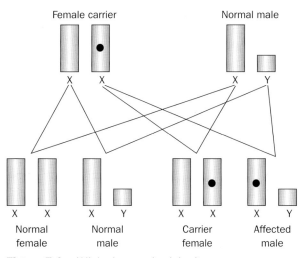

Figure 7.1 X-linked recessive inheritance.
Examples: Colour blindness, Duchenne muscular dystrophy, Fragile X syndrome, Haemophilia A and B, Ectodermal dysplasia.

The abnormal gene is carried on the X chromosome with the result that:

- The trait is normally passed from a carrier female to her male offspring
- Half the female carrier's sons will inherit the gene and therefore develop the disease
- Half the female carrier's daughters will be carriers like mother
- An affected male cannot pass the disease to his sons, but all his daughters will be carriers
- Daughters of affected males can pass the disease to their sons
- In the female carrier, the normal X chromosome protects her so that she doesn't manifest the condition or has mild symptoms

The first stage in the assessment and diagnostic process is a detailed medical, developmental and family history. The important areas are:

- **Sex:** learning difficulties are more common in boys and X-linked conditions causing learning difficulties need to be considered – the most common being fragile X and Duchenne muscular dystrophy (Figure 7.1 and Table 7.1)
- **Pregnancy:** any untoward event can have an effect on the developing fetus. Note gestation, occurrence of threatened miscarriage, infections, medication, alcohol
- **Delivery and neonatal period:** mode of delivery, fetal distress and treatment required, Apgar

Table 7.1 Duchenne muscular dystrophy

Incidence: 1/3500 male births

Cause: X-linked recessive condition; 30 per cent caused by new mutations. A deletion of chromosome material on the short arm of the X chromosome that codes for a protein called dystrophin, which maintains the integrity of the muscle cell wall

Presentation: abnormal gait, frequent falls, difficulties with steps. First symptoms noted between 1 and 3 years, but the diagnosis is often late

Findings on examination: waddling gait, Gower's sign present, firm enlargement of the calf muscles (pseudohypertrophy) as a result of replacement of muscle fibres by fat and fibrous tissue, proximal muscle weakness and absent reflexes, although ankle reflexes may be preserved

Associated problems: mild learning difficulties, scoliosis

Diagnosis: creatine kinase 50–100 times that of normal value, molecular genetics studies (gene for dystrophin in the Xp21 region), muscle biopsy

Management: genetic advice, physiotherapy, use of orthoses, appropriate aids and adaptations, and monitoring from a specialist clinic

Prognosis: most boys die of respiratory failure, cardiomyopathy or infection in late teens or early 20s

Family support: Family Care Officers, employed by the Muscular Dystrophy Campaign, provide practical support and information and can help families liaise with their local services

scores. Problems in the neonatal period such as hypotonia and slow feeding may indicate Prader–Willi syndrome, whereas irritability with slow feeding may suggest withdrawal from intrauterine exposure to drugs or alcohol

- **Medical history:** previous illness, accidents, detailed systemic review, fits
- **Family history:** anyone with any form of developmental or behavioural problems, miscarriages, stillbirths

- **Developmental history and current abilities:** access parent-held and health visitor records for information if required

History

Paul is the only child of James (aged 32 years) and Liz (aged 30 years). Both are healthy. Liz has idiopathic epilepsy that is well controlled. She has been taking sodium valproate for a number of years, which is monitored by her GP. Paul was a planned pregnancy. Liz was well during the pregnancy, she didn't smoke or drink alcohol and continued with her usual dose of anticonvulsant – she didn't have any fits. Paul was born at 39 weeks' gestation by normal delivery and weighed 3.4 kg. He cried immediately, was well after birth, and Liz and Paul were discharged home 24 hours later.

Previous illnesses

Paul is healthy, he isn't taking any medication and hasn't had any hospital attendances or admissions. He has occasional coughs and colds but hasn't had any serious illnesses or accidents.

Development

Paul sat independently at 9 months and walked at about 18 months of age. He walks upstairs and comes down on his bottom. He cannot pedal a tricycle.

Paul said his first word at 14 months of age. He now uses approximately 20 words to ask for things and to label toys and objects of interest. He has not started to link words together. His parents thought that he had a good understanding of what was said to him, but, on more specific questioning, Paul was only reliably understanding at a one-word level and needs visual cues to aid understanding of unfamiliar things (see Chapter 12).

Paul is very lively and 'into everything'. He loves climbing into cupboards and playing with things he shouldn't. He has no awareness of danger and requires constant supervision. Paul will 'talk' into a toy phone and 'helps' his mum around the house. He likes scribbling and looking at books. He pushes toy cars along the floor making brum-brum noises and is 'into' *Thomas the Tank Engine*. Paul's parents do not have any worries about his vision or hearing.

Paul is still in nappies and doesn't yet indicate whether he has wet or soiled. His parents tried toilet training a few months ago, but without any success. Paul can take his clothes off but needs help to dress. He can feed himself with a spoon and drink from a cup.

Social

Liz is a legal secretary and gave up work after she had Paul. James is an accountant. Paul doesn't have much opportunity to mix with other children except at the weekly toddler group, where he runs around after the other children but doesn't really play with them.

Family history

There is no family history of developmental delay.

Self-test 1: What factors in the history could be relevant in the aetiology of Paul's developmental delay?

Answer: Sodium valproate taken in pregnancy can result in congenital malformations and also learning difficulties.

Self-test 2: What is Paul's developmental age?

Answer: His developmental age is approximately 21 months, although his language is a bit more immature.

Interpretation of the history

The paediatrician interprets the developmental history using a developmental scale, together with his or her detailed knowledge of child development. A developmental scale is a means of arranging information about the mean ages at which children achieve various milestones. Information can be conveniently categorized as follows:

- Posture and large movements
- Vision and fine movements
- Hearing and language
- Social behaviour and play

Meaning of the history in Paul

Posture and large movements

Paul has been somewhat 'late' in achieving motor developmental milestones. There is a wide range of normality for learning to walk (11–18 months). Paul walked at 18 months, which wouldn't be a cause for concern in itself unless there was associated weakness or an abnormality to the gait. Paul is still crawling up and down stairs and cannot yet push himself along on a tricycle, which suggests an immaturity, rather than an abnormality, in gross motor skills.

Vision and fine movements

Paul's fine motor skills appear to be delayed. However, this has to be interpreted with caution. This apparent delay may also be the result of cognitive delay, poor vision, ataxia or lack of previous experience. Poor vision seems unlikely because Paul's parents have described normal visual behaviour (see Chapter 8). Children are usually managing a spoon and are able to mark paper with a pencil at 18 months of age.

Hearing and language

Paul's parents haven't any concerns about his hearing (see Chapter 12). Paul's language is delayed. A child of 2½ years should have over 100 words and be joining three and possibly more words together. Paul's receptive and expressive language is at an 18-month level.

Social behaviour and play

Helping around the house is usually demonstrated by children from 18 months of age. Being 'into everything' or exploratory play is usually seen as children start to move independently. Children often talk into a real phone from 12 months of age. Being able to play with a toy phone suggests slightly more advanced developmental skills and the emergence of early symbolic or pretend play. Boys are often later to achieve continence than girls, but by 2 years should be aware that they have wet or soiled. Paul's social interaction is delayed. He should be starting to play interactively with other children.

Cause of the developmental delay

The family history is negative. However, parents often aren't aware of a family history until their child is identified as having difficulties, when they ask specific questions of their relatives. Paul hasn't had any illnesses such as meningitis or a head injury that could account for a postnatal cause of developmental problems. There aren't any risk factors from the birth. It is important to remember that prescribed medication can have an adverse effect on the developing fetus, not just alcohol and drugs of abuse. Anticonvulsants are known to cause congenital abnormalities in the developing fetus and, more recently, it has been recognized that there is an increased risk of developmental delay with subsequent learning difficulties. However, it would be important to clarify the aetiology of the mother's epilepsy – she may have a genetic condition that is causing her epilepsy and her child's delay.

Self-test 3: Name a dominantly inherited condition that could account for a mother's epilepsy and her son's learning disability.

Answer: Tuberous sclerosis.

Examination

The examination consists of a full physical examination, including a search for dysmorphic features and examination of the skin for signs of neurocutaneous syndromes. Assessment of development by involvement of Paul in simple play and observation of his spontaneous play and interaction with his parents.

Physical examination

- Height and weight – 50th centiles
- Head circumference – 10th centile
- Examination of cardiovascular system (CVS), gastrointestinal tract (GIT) and respiratory system is normal
- Examination of neurological system essentially normal, although minimal hypotonia; immature gait and coordination
- No skin stigmata to indicate tuberous sclerosis or neurofibromatosis
- Dysmorphic features – minor dysmorphic facial features

Development

Paul took an interest in the toy box, very quickly tipping all the toys on to the floor. He pushed a toy car along the floor saying 'car', kicked a ball and said 'ball'. He pretended to drink from a toy cup when shown, but didn't give it to mummy when asked. Paul fetched a few familiar toys when asked, but did not point to body parts on request, apart from his hair. When offered a pencil and paper, Paul held the pencil with a palmar grip and marked the paper with the pencil, then quickly pushed it to one side. Paul spent a lot of time running around and climbing on and off the chairs and couch. He banged his head at one point and went to his mother to be comforted.

Self-test 4: Which other professionals could assist in a more detailed assessment of Paul's development?

Answer: Speech and language therapist, occupational therapist, physiotherapist, psychologist.

How to assess development

- Take a detailed developmental history from the parents including information on the child's current abilities. Obtain additional information from the nursery, childminder or grandparents if appropriate
- Observe the child playing: which toys does he play with and how does he play with them and for how long? Does he chatter as he plays and how does he respond when spoken to? How does he interact with his parents? Can he see and can he hear? If necessary, visit his nursery – this is particularly helpful to assess social interaction with the child's peers
- Engage the child in semi-structured play. Use a restricted range of toys for which you are familiar with the range of normal responses to them. Bricks, jigsaws, paper and crayons, and dolls' house toys and teasets can be used in a variety of ways (Figure 7.2)
- Interpret the information using a developmental scale with which you are familiar – the Denver Developmental Screening Test provides a

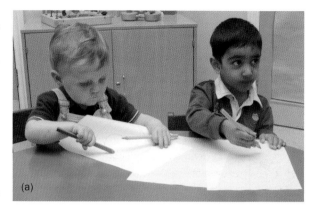
(a)

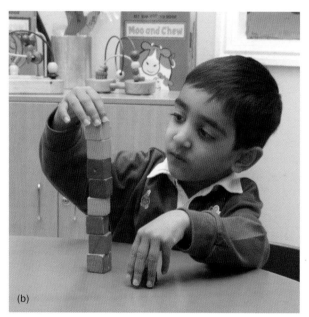
(b)

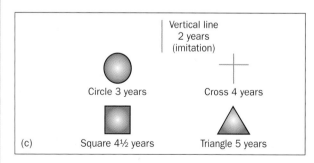

(c)
Vertical line 2 years (imitation)

Circle 3 years   Cross 4 years

Square 4½ years   Triangle 5 years

Figure 7.2 Assessment of fine motor skills and manipulation (a) pencil grip in an 18 month old and 3 year old child; (b) building a tower of bricks: tower of 3 at 18 months, 6 at 2 years, 8 at 2½ years, 9–10 at 3 years; (c) ages at which children can copy different shapes.

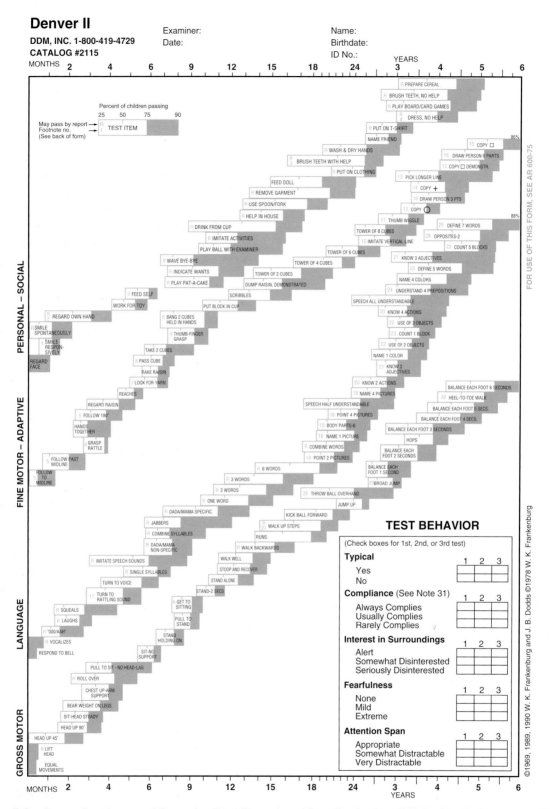

Figure 7.3 Denver Developmental Screening Test. (Reproduced from Frankenburg WK, Dodds JB. *Pediatrics* 1992; 89(1) with permission.)

convenient reference summary of important developmental milestones (Figure 7.3). It is, however, important to have a good understanding of normal child development

- Refer for hearing and vision assessment if indicated
- Use of standardized psychometric tests and scales: used by doctors, psychologists, and speech and language therapists when it is necessary to quantify the observations accurately. Most of these tests give an overall IQ or developmental quotient. However, it is much more useful to look at results in different areas because the child may have an uneven profile of development

The paediatrician discusses Paul with the other members of the child development team. Members of the team will vary, but usually include those listed in Table 7.2. The speech and language and occupational therapists arrange to see Paul for a detailed assessment of his language, play, self-help and fine motor skills. The physiotherapist didn't consider that she needed to assess Paul's motor skills. The findings of the paediatrician suggested a delay in motor skills in keeping with Paul's overall delay, rather than an abnormality. However, the physiotherapist joins the other therapists for part of the assessment, to ensure that nothing is missed.

Interpretation of the examination

Developmental assessment carried out in a clinic should be interpreted with caution. Much will depend on the child's cooperation generally and how he or she feels on the day – it is just a snapshot.

In clinic Paul performed much as his parents have described at home. Paul has a short attention span. Paul's social interaction with his parents was appropriate. The therapists confirmed the findings of the paediatrician.

The history and assessment have found that Paul's development is approximately 9 months delayed. Paul therefore fits within the MLD category – a developmental level less than half his chronological age would place him in the SLD group. In addition, Paul has a number of minor dysmorphic features and short attention span. These

Table 7.2 Child development team

Developmental paediatrician: special medical expertise in neurodevelopmental problems and management of complex disability

Physiotherapist: assesses patterns of movement. Advises on activities to promote normal patterns of movement and mobility and to limit skeletal deformity

Occupational therapist: assesses fine motor skills and functional tasks such as dressing, toileting and feeding. Provides aids to improve hand and manipulation skills, advises on seating, wheelchairs and housing adaptations. Works with the speech and language therapist to assess and advise on play

Speech and language therapist: assesses feeding and swallowing, communication and language. Advises on promoting communication using language and if necessary alternative methods using symbols or signs

Psychologist (clinical/educational): assesses abilities using standardized tests (e.g. Bayley Scales of Infant Development, Wechsler Intelligence Scale for Children), advises on difficult behaviour. The educational psychologist advises on educational provision

Social worker: acts as advocate for children and their families, provides advice on allowances and arranges practical support

Specialist health visitor/children's nurse: coordinates care by liaising with all professionals. Often visits the family before assessment at the Child Development Centre (CDC) to tell them about the process. Provides emotional support and may take on the role of key worker (see Chapter 27)

findings plus the history of exposure to sodium valproate *in utero* raises the possibility of fetal valproate syndrome as a cause for Paul's problems.

Investigations

There are no routine investigations for developmental delay and the yield is low in children with mild delay. Investigations should be determined by the findings in the history and examination. For some children it is better to plan investigations when more information is available, such as results of assessments by the therapists or response to specific intervention programmes.

Many paediatricians usually carry out a metabolic screen to exclude some conditions that could easily be missed (Table 7.3).

The paediatrician discussions his conclusions so far with Liz and James. He doesn't consider that investigations are indicated at this stage. Instead he obtains their consent to take photographs of Paul and discuss him with the clinical geneticist.

Investigations in Paul

- Assessment by clinical geneticist
- Hearing and vision assessments – normal

Diagnosis

Fetal valproate syndrome. The geneticist explains what is known about fetal valproate syndrome to Liz and James. The couple are planning a further pregnancy and so Liz is referred to a neurologist with an interest in epilepsy to review her medication.

Treatment and follow-up plan

Paul returns to the CDC where a programme of intervention is planned with his parents:

- The therapists plan a block of intervention to promote Paul's communication and play.
- Paul's social skills need to be addressed. In the short term, he needs to have increased opportunities to mix with other children and help him prepare for nursery. In the longer term, an appropriate nursery placement will help to prepare for school. The planning needs to start now, so the preschool advisory teacher from the education team is involved. Arrangements are made for the family to visit a nursery group. The therapy programmes can be carried at nursery and the advisory teacher is able to assess Paul. All are in agreement that Paul should move on to a mainstream educational nursery when he is 3, but that he will require some extra support.

Other members of the child development team have an equally important role. Behavioural problems are common in children with learning difficulties and sleep problems in particular can be exhausting for parents. Financial advice and support for the family in promoting the welfare of their child are key areas of responsibility for the social worker, who has statutory duties to 'children in need' (The Children Act 1989).

The paediatrician plans regular follow-up with the therapists to review Paul's progress and coordinate services. Liz and James are encouraged to contact the CDC should problems or worries arise between planned appointments. Once Paul starts in full-time school, it is likely that further review will be carried out by the school health team, with advice from the child development team should problems arise.

Children who have more significant developmental delay and complex needs will continue to be reviewed by the developmental paediatrician. Most developmental paediatricians hold clinics in the special schools, which improves communication and provides better holistic care.

Prognosis

Individuals with an IQ in the MLD range (50–70) will be able to undertake unskilled or semiskilled labour. The majority should be able to live independently unless they have additional problems.

Those with an IQ between 35 and 50 are unlikely to acquire much more than very basic literacy and numeracy skills. They will need supervision at work and are most unlikely to be able to live independently.

Adults with an IQ under 35 will be dependent on others for all their needs and will require close supervision.

Clinicians should be cautious in giving a prognosis in a very young child unless they are severely disabled. Prediction of long-term intellectual functioning in young children is inaccurate. Tests in the under-2s usually measure motor achievement and performance rather than cognitive functioning. Results are affected by many factors within the child and assessor.

Table 7.3   Investigations in developmental delay

Tests frequently carried out in children with severe developmental delay (no recognizable physical or behavioural phenotype)

Blood calcium: pseudohypoparathyroidism may present with developmental and speech delay

Creatine phosphokinase (CPK): Duchenne muscular dystrophy may present with developmental and speech delay before the motor regression

Urinary mucopolysaccharides: Sanfilippo's syndrome may present with developmental delay before coarsening of the features

Thyroid function tests: hypothyroidism, although there are usually other signs

Blood and urine amino acids

Chromosomes and DNA analysis for fragile X

Routine tests in children with mild developmental delay

CPK

Chromosomes and DNA analysis for fragile X

Tests in child with dysmorphic features/family history of learning difficulty

Specific test if recognizable phenotype

Karyotype if non-recognizable phenotype

Test for telomeric deletions if karyotype normal (discuss with geneticist)

Additional investigations that may be indicated

Magnetic resonance imaging (MRI) of brain – may be useful if the delay is profound, the size or shape of the head is abnormal, and the child also has cerebral palsy or epilepsy

EEG: essential if status epilepticus suspected, a syndrome that has specific EEG findings (e.g. Angelman's syndrome) or possible regression

Assessment by a clinical geneticist: particularly useful if the child has dysmorphic features or a particular pattern of behavioural difficulties (the behavioural phenotype). Also of use in any child with profound delay, to exclude any recognizable syndrome

Blood ammonia, uric acid, cholesterol, white cell enzymes

Maternal phenylalanine: in unexplained microcephaly

'TORCH' screen (toxoplasmosis, rubella, cytomegalovirus, herpes) if history of possible congenital infections, but difficult to interpret. Computed tomography (CT) of brain may show calcification

Further assessments indicated for all children

Hearing assessment

Vision assessment

Background information

Epidemiology

The prevalence of severe learning disability is 3.7 per 1000 children. Accurate figures for the prevalence of mild learning disability are not available. Three per cent of the population have an IQ in this range, but whether this poses a problem requiring services will depend on family support, educational achievement and management, and social abilities.

Causes of learning disability

- **Mild learning disability:** a biological cause is rarely found and it is commonly the result of a combination of genetic and environmental factors. However, many syndromes and disorders can cause this level of learning disability. Other factors may compound a child's difficulties, such as fluctuating hearing loss and social disadvantage.
- **Severe learning disability:** it isn't always possible to identify an exact cause, although often there are pointers to a prenatal origin. Identified causes are:
  - chromosome disorders – 20–25 per cent
  - identifiable disorders or syndromes – 20–25 per cent
  - SLD with cerebral palsy, microcephaly or infantile spasms – 10–20 per cent
  - postnatal insults (meningitis, trauma) – 10 per cent

Anticonvulsant drugs and teratogenicity

One in 200 babies with a learning disability is born to a mother who has epilepsy. The incidence of structural birth defects in their offspring is about two to three times that of the general population – neural tube defects, congenital heart defects, orofacial clefting and genitourinary malformations. Minor anomalies include hypoplastic digits and nails and dysmorphic facial features.

Infants exposed to anticonvulsants *in utero* often have withdrawal symptoms in the neonatal period, and may have feeding problems and hypoglycaemia. Hypotonia and joint laxity are frequent and may lead to mild delay in motor milestones. More recently, it has been suggested that these children are more likely to have learning disabilities.

Fetal valproate syndrome is recognized as a clinical entity characterized by abnormalities of the face (thin upper lip and everted lower lip, grooves under the eyes, fine arched eyebrows and prominence of the midline metopic suture of the forehead), developmental disabilities and occasional major organ abnormalities. Associated cognitive and behavioural problems have included poor concentration, delayed motor milestones and poor coordination, speech and language delay, and difficulties with social interaction.

Further sources of information

Book

Illingworth RS. *Basic Developmental Screening: 0–4 years*, 3rd edn. London: Blackwell Scientific Publications, 1982

Articles

Whiting K. Investigating the child with learning difficulty. *Current Paediatrics* 2001; **11**: 240–7

Turk J. Fragile X syndrome. *Archives of Disease in Childhood* 1995; **72**: 3–5

Self-test 5: Two and a half-year-old George is assessed by his health visitor. George started walking at 14 months of age but still falls frequently and struggles a bit to get up stairs. He has lots of single words, but doesn't link words together. He understands simple commands. George likes helping his mum around the house and is starting to interact in play with other children.

A What level of learning difficulty does George have?

B On examination Gower's sign was present. What is it and what does it indicate?

C Figure 7.4 is a photograph of George's legs – what does it show?

D What is the diagnosis?

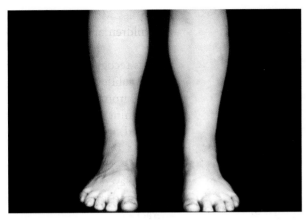

Figure 7.4   Self-test 5, question C.

Answers:

A Mild learning disability

B Gower's sign indicates proximal muscle weakness, not a specific diagnosis. To get off the floor from lying on his back, the child rolls on to his front, gets into four-point kneeling and 'walks' his hands up his thighs to get into the upright position

C Enlargement of the calf muscles – pseudohypertrophy

D Duchenne muscular dystrophy

A child with a squint

Presentation

The following is a referral letter from the health visitor to the ophthalmology clinic.

> Please would you see 8-month-old Peter who has a right convergent squint. His mother had noted an intermittent squint for some time, particularly when Peter was tired. She had been reassured by granny that it was probably because he has quite wideset eyes!
>
> Peter's development is satisfactory. He has normal visual responses – when I offered him a small sugar sweet, he promptly picked it up. I couldn't detect a squint myself.

Initial considerations and action

Squint (strabismus) is a common condition, in which the visual axis of one eye (the squinting eye) is not directed to the object being looked at by the other eye. (The visual axis is the line from the fovea to the point of fixation.) This interferes with the development of binocular single vision – when we look at an object, the view seen by the right eye is slightly different from the view seen by the left eye. These two dissimilar retinal images are fused in the visual centres of the brain to give a three-dimensional picture – an appreciation of depth (stereoscopic vision) as well as height and width. Binocular single vision will not develop unless there are reasonably clear and similar images in the two eyes, the brain is able to fuse the images and there is precise coordination of eye movements. Figure 8.1 shows how rays of light are focused on the retina of the eye.

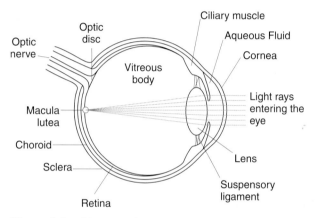

Figure 8.1 Diagram of the eye showing rays of light being brought to a focus on the retina.

Squints may affect one or both eyes. The eye may turn in, out, up or down. The squint may be constant or intermittent, with the latter possibly seen under stressful conditions such as when ill or tired.

Newborn babies often give the appearance of having a squint because of over-convergence. A wide nasal bridge or broad epicanthic folds may give the illusion of a convergent squint by hiding part of the sclera (pseudosquint – Figure 8.2).

Any infant with a fixed squint or any squint persisting beyond 2 months of age should be referred for a specialist ophthalmological opinion.

Self-test 1: Why should a child with a squint be referred as soon as it presents?

Answer: To detect treatable defects such as cataract and retinoblastoma and to prevent amblyopia.

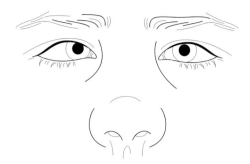

Figure 8.2   Diagram showing a right pseudosquint.

Squints are usually divided into paralytic and concomitant.

Paralytic squints are rare and are caused by paralysis of the motor nerves. The angle of the squint alters with different positions of gaze. A rapid onset may be sinister because of the possibility of a space-occupying lesion such as a brain tumour.

Concomitant squints are common. The angle of the eye is the same in all directions of gaze and whichever eye is fixing. This is usually the result of refractive error, but can occur in any form of severe eye disease. Squints are common in children with developmental delay.

Peter's mother has observed a squint, which should be taken seriously even though the health visitor didn't see it. The squint has been there for some time, so it is unlikely to have a sinister aetiology such as a tumour. Peter's vision for near objects such as a small sweet is reassuring. The ophthalmologist arranges to see Peter in the clinic within the next few weeks.

History

Peter is seen in the outpatient clinic with his mother. The history of the appearance of the squint is similar to that outlined by the health visitor in her letter. Mother has noticed that both eyes move, but that the right one turns in more than the left. Peter's mother describes normal developmental visual behaviour (Table 8.1). Useful questions to help determine whether young children have adequate vision are listed in Table 8.2. She has noticed that Peter will look at objects across their sitting room and will smile at his father when he comes into the room.

Table 8.1   Development of normal visual responses

Neonate	Pupils react to light
	Lids close against intense light
	Eyes and head turn to diffuse light
	From 3 to 4 weeks watches mother's face intently
4–6 weeks	Smiles at mother
1–3 months	Scans surroundings when held upright
	Follows slowly moving object 15–25 cm from face
	Converges eyes for finger play from 3 months
4–6 months	Visually alert for near and far
	Reaches for toys
	Adjusts position to see objects
7–12 months	Follows dangling ball in all directions
	Picks up tiny pellet

Table 8.2   Normal visual behaviour – questions to ask parents

1	Do you think your child can see?
2	Does your child recognize you before you speak to him or her?
3	Does he or she look at windows and bright lights?
4	Does he or she look at his or her hands and feet?
5	Does he or she take an interest in the surroundings?
6	Does he or she hold objects close to the eyes?
7	Does he or she reach out for toys?
8	Does he or she feel for objects?
9	Does he or she pick up tiny things such as bits of fluff?
10	Does he or she bump into things?
11	Does he or she sit very close to the television?
12	Has his or her vision got worse?
13	Have you noticed a squint, unusual eye movements or your child holding his or her head in an unusual position to look at things?

Answer: The visual behaviour is appropriate and suggests acceptable functional vision. However, it does not exclude a visual defect in one eye.

Peter is a healthy boy who was born at term by normal delivery, weighing 3.2 kg. He is the youngest of three children, there is no history of squint and he is reaching his developmental milestones.

Interpretation of the history

The key areas to consider are:

- Neurological disorder
- Eye disease
- Refractive error
- Defective cerebral fusion
- Family history

Meaning of the history in Peter

Neurological disorder

The squint is caused by impaired function or paralysis of one or more of the extraocular muscles as a result of a congenital or acquired cranial nerve palsy. This is commonly found in children with cerebral palsy and severe neurodisability.

This seems unlikely in Peter's case. Normal gross and fine motor development makes cerebral palsy unlikely. The history of the eye movements is suggestive of a concomitant squint rather than a paralytic squint.

Eye disease

Binocular single vision is needed to maintain alignment of the eyes. The brain is unable to control the alignment of an eye that does not receive a clear image. Squint is therefore commonly seen in young children with:

- Cataracts
- Corneal scars
- Optic atrophy

- Retinal disease, including retinoblastoma
- Blockage of the eye, e.g. trauma, ptosis

Note the association of Down's syndrome and cataracts and the importance of family history in retinal disease – neither is present in Peter. Many of these problems are bilateral, often resulting in bilateral vision impairment.

Peter picks up small objects without hesitation and recognizes people across a room, indicating that his near and distant vision is adequate.

Refractive errors

Refractive errors that produce blurred or unequal images may also cause a squint as a result of failure to develop binocular single vision. Hypermetropia (long-sightedness) is commonly associated with squint because the child has to accommodate excessively to obtain a clear image of near objects. The excessive accommodation is reflexly associated with excessive convergence activity, which may lead to a convergent squint. Less commonly, myopia (short-sightedness) may be associated with a divergent squint, particularly when looking at distant objects. However, the presence of a convergent squint does not mean that there is definitely hypermetropia and myopia may not be present with a divergent squint.

Peter's normal visual behaviour is a good indicator that he has adequate vision, but doesn't tell us whether he has a defect in one eye, which is compensated for by the other.

Defective cerebral fusion

This has little direct evidence, but may be the explanation for the high prevalence of squint in children with learning difficulties or cerebral palsy, even though they do not have cranial nerve involvement. Abnormal visual behaviour can be a manifestation of learning disability or autism rather than an ophthalmic disease.

Peter's development is age appropriate.

Family history

There may be a hereditary element in the aetiology of squint.

Examination

- **Facial appearance**

  Normal, no broad epicanthic folds or facial asymmetry to cause a pseudosquint, no dysmorphic findings

- **Corneal reflections:** this test is carried out by holding a small source of light about 30 cm from the eyes to produce reflections on both corneas simultaneously

  Asymmetrical

- **Ocular movements:** ocular movements are tested in both horizontal and vertical axes using a small object for the child to fix on and follow

  Normal in Peter and excludes a paralytic squint

- **Cover test:** when a squint is present and the fixing eye is covered, the squinting eye moves to take up fixation (Figure 8.3). This test is difficult to perform and is reliable only when carried out by an ophthalmologist or orthoptist. Note that, if the vision in the squinting eye is very poor, the eye may not move

  Demonstrates a right convergent squint

- **Head tilt:** compensatory head tilt occurs in order to attempt to maintain binocular fixation. Head

tilts are also seen in the presence of field defect, ptosis and torticollis

Not apparent

- **Eye and optic fundi**

  Normal, no cataracts, retinoblastoma, optic atrophy

- **Refraction**

  Hypermetropic refractive error in both eyes, but more marked in the right

In young children who cannot cooperate by fixing on a distant object, the amount of accommodation is constantly changing and therefore the refractive power of the eye can be measured only when this reflex has been paralysed (cycloplegia). Atropine or cyclopentolate is used for this purpose; these agents also dilate the pupil (mydriasis), which makes examination of the fundi much easier. Refraction is measured objectively using a retinoscope. In older children and adults, the refractive power of the lens can be assessed by determining the power of the spectacle lens that gives the clearest vision of a distant or near target. This is called subjective refraction. It gives a measure of visual acuity, i.e. it defines how much the individual can see. Objective refraction, on the other hand, determines whether spectacles would produce a sharper retinal image, but doesn't tell us what the individual actually sees.

Interpretation of the examination

Peter doesn't have evidence of a paralytic squint or underlying neurological cause for the squint. Examination reveals a right convergent squint, and objective refraction reveals hypermetropia of the squinting eye and to a lesser degree in the other eye. Examination of the fundi did not reveal any other abnormalities.

Investigations

No further investigations are indicated for Peter. If there had been concerns about his visual acuity, then further assessment would have been required.

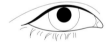
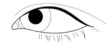
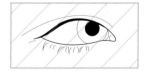
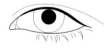
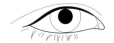
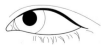

Figure 8.3   Cover test showing a left convergent squint.

Self-test 3: How is visual acuity assessed in a school-aged child?

Answer: Using a Snellen chart.

Visual acuity (VA) is a measure of the ability to separate visual stimuli, i.e. to distinguish the details and shapes of objects. This ability is dependent on the cerebral cortex as well as the eyes and VA can therefore be assessed accurately only if the child can tell us what he or she sees. Electrophysiological methods can provide an estimate of VA without the individual's direct cooperation.

How to assess visual acuity in a school-age child

- Use a Snellen letter chart (Figure 8.4). The Snellen letter chart is the criterion against which all other VA measures are standardized and gives a measure of distance vision. Similar charts are used to assess near vision
- First, check that the child knows his or her letters. If in doubt, get the child to match the letters on the Snellen chart with a card held in the hand
- The chart is placed 6 m from the child, in a well-lit room
- The VA for distance vision is expressed as a fraction, e.g. 6/60 means that the individual can see a letter at 6 m that a normal person could see at 60 m. Thus 6/6 is normal vision. If the test is done at 3 m, normal vision would be 3/3
- Test each eye separately. Use a patch to cover each eye rather than the child's hand, to avoid false results by peeping through fingers
- Be aware that some children may go to any lengths to pass or fail the test – rotate the charts in case the child has learned the sequence of letters on the bottom lines

Measurement of visual acuity is difficult in young children. Letter matching can aid a 4 or 5 year old to perform the Snellen test at the standard 6 m. A visual acuity test called Lea symbols is being increasingly used. It can give an accurate VA in children as young as 3 years.

Testing the VA of children under the age of 2½ years is very difficult. The simplest tests attempt to establish the smallest object visible to the child. They are not sensitive enough to detect minor visual defects and they cannot be converted to a Snellen equivalent. More precise estimates of VA can be obtained using forced-choice preferential looking, but this requires a greater degree of participation by the individual. Qualitative tests looking at visual function are best used in the significantly visually impaired or cognitively delayed child.

Electrophysiological tests are useful in the investigation of some visual disorders such as the inherited retinal degenerations.

Magnetic resonance imaging is useful when structural lesions of the ocular pathways or occipital cortex are suspected.

Diagnosis

Right convergent squint and hypermetropia.

Treatment and follow-up plan

Treatment depends on the cause of the squint, but usual treatment options are:

- Prescription of spectacles. Correction of the refractive error by spectacles may be all that is required in many cases of squint
- Occlusion, or patching, is the treatment for amblyopia
- Orthoptist intervention: the orthoptist is primarily involved with amblyopia therapy and assessment of binocular vision. Orthoptic exercises are of doubtful value in convergent squints. They also require cooperation, which means that they would be suitable only for the older preschool child

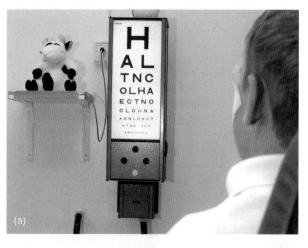

(a)

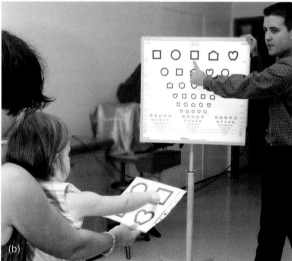

(b)

Figure 8.4 Vision testing using (a) Snellen chart and (b) Lea symbols.

● Surgery: surgical correction is often necessary, but in many cases the benefit is cosmetic

Peter is prescribed spectacles and the orthoptist provides advice and support in encouraging Peter to wear them. When he wears them, his squint is corrected and it is considered that he hasn't got amblyopia. It is important that Peter continues to wear his glasses all day long, because amblyopia could develop if the eye is allowed to continue to squint. Peter will therefore continue to be monitored in the ophthalmology and orthoptic clinics for a number of years.

Background information

Common vision problems

Prevalence

Minor anomalies of visual function are among the most common defects found in children: up to 10 per cent of children have some visual defect. Between 4 and 7 per cent of 5 year olds have a squint and between 3 and 5 per cent have amblyopia. Squint is more common in children born pre-term. The prevalence of refractive errors is not known. Myopia is rare in the first few years but becomes increasingly common in the school years. A significant number of disabled children have visual problems.

Pathophysiology

Abnormalities of refraction (Figure 8.5)
Hypermetropia (long-sighted) The eyeball is slightly shorter than normal so that parallel rays of light are

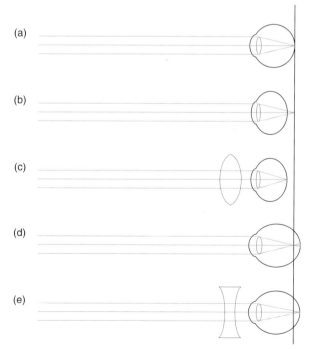

(a)

(b)

(c)

(d)

(e)

Figure 8.5 Common refractive errors of the eye and corrective lenses: (a) normal eye (b, c) hypermetropia; and (d, e) myopia.

brought to focus behind the retina. Hypermetropia is the normal state in the infant and diminishes with growth. Minor degrees of hypermetropia may be overcome by the normal powers of accommodation. If it is too great, difficulty will be experienced on normal vision screening when distant vision is tested. In severe hypermetropia near vision is usually quite good, although the child may need to bring his or her eye very close to the object at which he or she is looking. Hypermetropia may produce frontal headache or a convergent squint, and may be associated with astigmatism. It is treated with spectacles using convex lenses to aid convergence of the light source.

Myopia (short-sighted) The eye is marginally too long so that parallel rays of light are brought to focus in front of the retina. The myopic child has difficulty with distant vision. Myopia usually develops between the ages of 5 and 15 years as a result of excessive growth of the eye and there is often a family history. It is treated with spectacles using concave lenses. Rarely, congenital myopia occurs and may be associated with retinal detachment.

Astigmatism This arises when the curvature of the cornea and lens is different in the horizontal and vertical planes. Minor degrees of astigmatism have no significant effect but greater degrees of astigmatism produce difficulties in focusing horizontally and vertically simultaneously. This produces difficulties in reading and a dislike of prolonged close work. Some children screw up their eyes in an attempt to improve acuity.

Amblyopia (commonly known as lazy eye) This is a defect in acuity that is not corrected by spectacles. It can cause a permanent loss of vision with associated loss of stereoscopic vision. Amblyopia causes more visual impairment in the under-40 age group than all other eye problems (including trauma) combined. It arises from suppression of a poor image received by that eye. It develops in a child under the age of 7 years and is caused by defective development of vision during the critical period of rapid brain maturation. It is not yet clear what is the peak age for development of amblyopia or how early the predisposing factors need to be recognized to prevent its development.

- **Detection:** it usually occurs in one eye only and children therefore may be unaware of its presence. Many districts have screening programmes to detect it early, but there has been a poor clinical evidence base underpinning the programmes. There is now emerging evidence that early treatment is more effective than later treatment
- **Aetiology:** anything that interferes with clear vision in either eye during the critical period can result in amblyopia – refractive errors, cataract, ptosis, etc. Squint is the most common cause, where the retinal image is displaced away from the fovea (the most sensitive part of the retina). In an attempt to avoid double vision, the brain disregards or suppresses the image of one eye
- **Management:** occlusion of the non-amblyopic eye by patching to encourage the amblyopic eye to fix and so develop better vision

Further sources of information

Book

Rowe F. *Clinical Orthoptics*. London: Blackwell Science, 1997

Article

Williams C, Northstone K, Harrad RA et al. Amblyopia treatment outcomes after screening before or at 3 years: follow up from randomised trial. *British Medical Journal* 2002; **324**: 1549–51

Self-test 4: Nicola is a 6-month-old child with Down's syndrome who is being reviewed by the health visitor. Her mother has noticed that her right eye turns inwards. Nicola's mother hasn't any particular concerns about her visual development. However, on direct questioning, she has observed that Nicola doesn't recognize her mother across a room until she calls her name, or moves up close to her. Nicola is starting to reach out for toys and will readily try to get large colourful objects. She doesn't seem to take much interest in small, less colourful toys.

A Is Nicola's vision development age appropriate?

B What is the likely cause of the squint?

C What should the health visitor do now?

D Why should squints be treated early?

Answers:

A No, she should be able to recognize her mother across a room and see small objects. Children with Down's syndrome may have significant developmental delay with associated delay in visual behaviour. Nicola's ability to reach for toys suggests age-appropriate development.

B Cataract: as her vision appears to be impaired, the cataract is most likely to be bilateral.

C Refer urgently for an ophthalmological opinion.

D To reduce the likelihood of amblyopia developing.

CHAPTER 9

Acute presentation

Cold, cough and wheeze in a young child

Age: 15 weeks

LEENA PATEL

Presentation

Billy-Jo, 15 weeks old, is taken to the accident and emergency department (A&E) by her mother one winter evening because she has been struggling with her breathing that day. She has been coughing and wheezing for 2 days. In A&E, she is seen promptly by the triage nurse who made the following observations: temperature: 37.8°C; pulse: 180/min; respiratory rate: 60/min; arterial oxygen saturation (Sao_2): 97 per cent.

Self test 1: What are the two main acute respiratory illnesses in children?

Answers:

1 Respiratory tract infections – more troublesome in infants and toddlers and bronchiolitis caused by respiratory syncytial virus (RSV) is most common
2 Asthma – more troublesome after the first few years

Initial considerations and action

Wheezing is a symptom of:

- Lower respiratory tract obstruction
- Pulmonary venous congestion

The site of obstruction may be anywhere from the intrathoracic trachea to the small bronchi or large bronchioles (see Figure 9.1). Infants and toddlers are prone to wheezing (Table 9.1 and Figure 9.2, p. 78) and are especially severely affected by diseases involving the smaller airways.

Initial assessment

As Billy-Jo has presented with an acute history of difficulty breathing associated with cough and wheeze, the severity of her respiratory disease is first assessed (Table 9.2, p. 79). This reveals:

- Respiratory distress but no hypoxia
- Stable circulation
- No signs of impending respiratory failure (Table 9.3, p. 80)

She does not require any immediate resuscitation or treatment and is allowed to sit in her mother's lap while a history is obtained.

Self test 2: Explain the following clinical features:

A **Tachycardia**
B **Nasal flaring**
C **Inspiratory recessions**

Answers:

A Tachycardia is caused by increased sympathetic drive. Factors that contribute to this include hypoxia, hypercapnia, anxiety, increased metabolic work of breathing, fever and dehydration

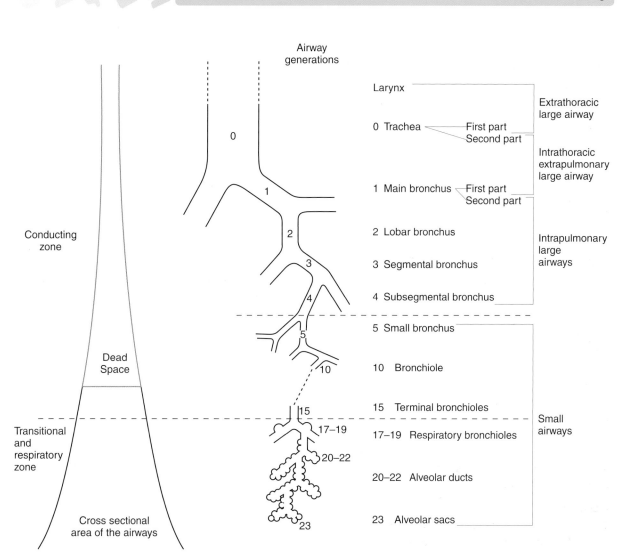

Figure 9.1 The structure of the airways. Redrawn with modifications from Sly PD and Hayden MJ, Applied clinical respiratory physiology, in Taussig LM and Landau LI (eds) *Paediatric Respiratory Medicine*, 1st edn, pp. 94–110, Copyright 1999, with permission from Elsevier.

B Nasal flaring occurs in an attempt to reduce upper airway resistance

C Inspiratory recessions occur when high negative intrathoracic pressure is generated during inspiration as a result of airway obstruction (e.g. bronchiolitis, asthma) or poor compliance (e.g. pneumonia or pulmonary oedema). Breaths are generally rapid and shallow when compliance is poor, and slower and deeper with airway obstruction. Intercostal and subcostal recessions are prominent in infants and young children because their chest wall is much more compliant than that of older children and adults

History

The history and examination help towards:

- Making a diagnosis
- Determining how unwell Billy-Jo is
- Determining what supportive treatment she requires

Table 9.1 Causes of acute and recurrent wheeze in infants and older children

	Acute wheeze	Recurrent wheeze
Infants	Bronchiolitis	Chronic lung disease of prematurity
	Bacterial and non-viral lower respiratory tract infections	Recurrent/chronic respiratory infection
	Inhaled foreign body	Cystic fibrosis
		Ciliary dyskinesia
		Primary immunodeficieny
		Aspiration secondary to gastro-oesophageal reflux
		Congenital narrowing of a bronchus
		Pulmonary congestion from left-to-right shunt
Older children	Respiratory infection	Asthma
	Inhaled foreign body	Recurrent/chronic respiratory infection
	Acute allergic reaction	Cystic fibrosis
	Enlarged hilar and mediastinal lymph nodes, e.g. lymphoma	Bronchiectasis

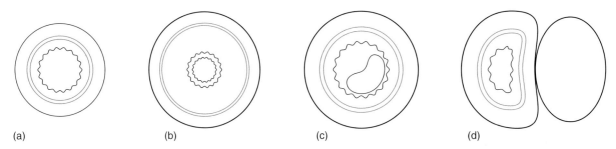

(a)   (b)   (c)   (d)

Figure 9.2 Pathological processes that result in airway obstruction and wheezing: (a) muscle spasm, e.g. asthma, infection; (b) swelling of wall from oedema and inflammation, e.g. infection, asthma; (c) in the lumen, e.g. excessive mucus (cystic fibrosis), inhaled foreign body, gastric contents or fluid (e.g. heart failure); and (d) extrinsic compression, e.g. enlarged lymph node, vascular ring.

Billy-Jo caught a cold from her mother a few days earlier. A 'chesty' cough and wheeze followed. The cough has been quite distressing. Today she has struggled more and more with her breathing, has not finished her feeds, has vomited after bouts of coughing, and has slept more than usual. She has felt hot at times. Her mother tried but was not able to get an appointment at the general practice. She has not had any treatment other than paracetamol syrup.

In the past, Billy-Jo has had a few colds but no cough, wheeze or 'chestiness'. She has not had a skin rash or persistent diarrhoea. The pregnancy and delivery were normal, she was not born prematurely and she did not have any breathing problems after birth. Her birth weight was 3.1 kg and mother has been pleased with her growth and development. She has had two lots of her baby jabs. Mother is single and lives with her parents. They do not smoke and do not have any pets. There is no family history of asthma or other chest problems.

Interpretation of the history

It is important to ascertain whether the major symptoms (cough and wheeze) are acute or chronic/recurrent

Table 9.2   Initial assessment of Billy-Jo

Airway and breathing	Sign indicates
• Sao_2 97 per cent in air	No hypoxia
• Alert infant (as opposed to irritable or drowsy)	
• Tachypnoea (respiratory rate 60/min vs normal 30–40)	Respiratory distress
• Nasal flaring	
• Use of accessory muscles	Increased work of breathing
• Head bobbing (caused by use of sternomastoid muscle)	
• Inspiratory intercostal recessions	Airway obstruction and poor compliance
• Expiratory wheeze	Lower airway narrowing
• Tachycardia (heart rate 180/min vs normal 110–160)	Physiological response to respiratory distress and fever
Circulation	
• Warm hands and feet	
• Capillary refill <2 seconds	Stable circulation
• Radial and femoral pulses easily felt	

(see Table 9.1). Billy-Jo's presentation is acute and the illness followed a cold. Viral infections and bronchiolitis are common during the winter months. The history does not indicate:

- Factors that might predispose to serious lower respiratory tract problems such as:
  - prematurity, mechanical ventilation and chronic lung disease
  - previous respiratory problems
  - cystic fibrosis
  - immunodeficiency
- Conditions that might deteriorate with a respiratory infection such as:
  - congenital heart defect
  - chronic lung disease

Examination

A general examination is undertaken while Billy-Jo is in her mother's lap. The following are noted:

- Snuffly
- Moist 'mucousy' cough

- Not agitated, drowsy or floppy
- Cries when examined
- No deterioration from the initial assessment
- No limb oedema
- No dehydration
- Weight 5.3 kg

The respiratory and cardiovascular systems are examined thoroughly:

- Bilateral end-expiratory crackles and wheeze which is louder in expiration than inspiration
- Precordium not hyperactive, no prominent precordial bulge and no thrill
- Heart sounds normal and no murmurs
- Liver palpable 4 cm below the costal margin and soft

Interpretation of the examination

Making a diagnosis

The cough in bronchiolitis is characteristically moist or wet in nature and difficult to differentiate from the

Table 9.3 Clinical features of respiratory muscle fatigue and impending respiratory failure

1	Loss of respiratory reserve required to perform non-ventilatory functions:
	Not able to pause breathing voluntarily to cry, talk, feed or eat
	Not able to cough (it requires a deep breath, an inspiratory hold and a forceful expiration)
2	Use of accessory muscles – sternocleidomastoid, pectoralis major
3	Respiratory rate, regularity and pattern of breathing:
	Rapid respiratory rate – cannot be sustained for long and leads to exhaustion
	Very shallow breathing
	Deep breaths with a brief pause to rest exhausted inspiratory muscles
	Grunting: produced by expiring against a partially closed glottis, results in increased end-expiratory pressure which improves oxygenation in small airway diseases (bronchiolitis) and in alveolar diseases (bronchopneumonia, pulmonary oedema)
	Paradoxical thoracic–abdominal breathing: deep thoracic breathing (abdomen paradoxically draws in as the diaphragm rests) alternates with deep abdominal breathing (chest paradoxically draws in as the accessory muscles rest)
4	Impending respiratory failure:
	Cyanosis: pre-terminal sign of hypoxia
	Irregular breathing
	Silent chest: sign of ineffective breathing
	Apnoea
	Drooling in absence of airway obstruction: cannot pause to swallow saliva
	Confusion, drowsiness or impaired consciousness: signs of cerebral hypoxia
	Bradycardia: a sign of severe or prolonged hypoxia
	Absent peripheral pulses and weak central pulses: signs of hypotension and advanced shock

cough associated with a:

- Bacterial lower respiratory tract infection
- Heart failure associated with a left-to-right shunt such as a large ventricular septal defect (VSD) or atrial septal defect (ASD)

Further difficulty arises as a viral infection (cold) may:

- Precede a bacterial infection and
- Precipitate heart failure in an infant with a heart defect

In addition, the findings on auscultation of the chest (bilateral wheeze and crackles) may be similar. However, an infant with a bacterial lower respiratory tract infection (LRTI) would be expected to have a high fever (temperature >38°C) and signs of sepsis. Infants with a heart defect and failure (e.g. moderate-to-large VSD) typically present at 6–8 weeks of age. This is because pulmonary vascular resistance is relatively high in the first few weeks of life, and it restricts the amount of shunting through the defect. Heart failure occurs when pulmonary resistance drops sufficiently to allow significant shunting from left to right. Although the presentation may be acute, the history may reveal symptoms, preceding by days to weeks, of tiring with feeds, difficult to settle, sweating, poor weight gain and fast breathing. Wheezing may be associated with heart failure and careful auscultation of the heart is required to appreciate the heart murmur.

Although Billy-Jo has a palpable liver, it is most likely to result from lung overexpansion. Percussion of the upper edge of the liver in an older child helps differentiate whether a palpable liver is pushed down or enlarged but is difficult in an infant.

Determining how unwell Billy-Jo is and what supportive treatment she requires

At this stage there are no signs of impending respiratory failure or dehydration. Billy-Jo does not require oxygen, respiratory support or intravenous fluids. However, she requires close observation because of:

- Worsening respiratory symptoms over 2 days
- Inability to complete feeds
- Vomiting

Infants with bronchiolitis generally deteriorate over 48–72 hours before showing signs of improvement. Billy-Jo is therefore admitted to hospital for close monitoring of her respiratory status, oral intake and general condition.

Indications for admitting a child with bronchiolitis to hospital

- Moderate-to-severe respiratory distress
- Apnoeas
- Arterial oxygen saturation (Sao_2) $\leq$92 per cent in air
- Difficulty feeding

Investigations and results

Billy-Jo has a nasopharyngeal aspirate (NPA), of secretions containing epithelial cells, for RSV (by immunofluorescence or enzyme-linked immunofluorescence assay or ELISA). The result is usually available within 24 hours.

At this stage, a chest radiograph is not indicated (Table 9.4 and Figure 9.3).

Table 9.4   Indications for a chest radiograph in suspected bronchiolitis

- Sudden deterioration
- Localized chest signs
- Failure to improve within 2–3 days
- Severe illness
- Atypical features
- Bacterial pneumonia suspected
- Abnormal heart sounds or murmur

Diagnosis

Billy-Jo is a 15-week-old girl with an acute history of moist cough, wheezing and difficulty breathing following a cold. She has worsening symptoms, bilateral crackles and wheeze, and signs of respiratory distress but not of impending respiratory failure. She has bronchiolitis causing moderate-to-severe respiratory distress. She has been previously healthy and there is nothing to suggest that she has a coexisting condition.

Management and follow-up

The most important aspects of management of bronchiolitis are:

- Careful monitoring
- Good supportive care until there are signs of improvement and the illness resolves

Billy-Jo is admitted to a cubicle on a general paediatric ward to prevent spread within the ward because RSV is contagious.

Monitoring

Monitoring is aimed at detecting apnoea, hypoxia and exhaustion, and includes:

- Continuous oxygen saturation and apnoea monitoring

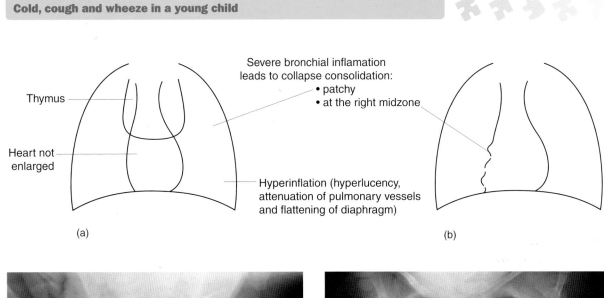

Thymus

Heart not enlarged

Severe bronchial inflamation leads to collapse consolidation:
• patchy
• at the right midzone

Hyperinflation (hyperlucency, attenuation of pulmonary vessels and flattening of diaphragm)

(a)

(b)

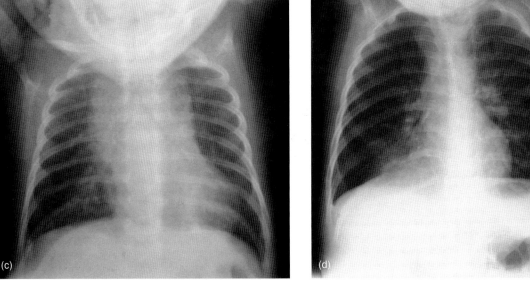

(c)

(d)

Figure 9.3   Chest radiograph in bronchiolitis. (a) and (b) are line drawings illustrating the findings in (c) and (d).

- Respiratory rate, pattern of breathing and heart rate every hour
- Feeding and hydration at regular intervals

Blood gas monitoring (for CO_2 retention and respiratory acidosis) will be necessary if there is significant worsening or any signs of severe respiratory failure.

Supportive treatment

Hypoxia caused by ventilation–perfusion mismatch is common. Billy-Jo will need oxygen if her Sa_{O_2} falls to <92 per cent. Supplemental humidified oxygen with nasal prongs or headbox (30–40 per cent) is usually sufficient to maintain Sa_{O_2} >94 per cent.

- Minimal handling helps reduce the likelihood of exhaustion
- Mechanical ventilation is required in a small number of infants admitted to hospital
- Dehydration is probably the result of increased loss from tachypnoea, fever and/or vomiting, and poor intake owing to respiratory distress. Adequate fluid intake needs to be ensured

Billy-Jo is initially offered small frequent feeds orally. However, she coughs, splutters, and gets more breathless and tachypnoeic when she feeds. To relieve her of the effort to feed she is given nasogastric feeds. (Orogastric feeding is preferred in infants <12 weeks of age because nasogastric tubes may increase airway resistance.) If a full stomach compromises her breathing or she deteriorates, she will require intravenous fluids (two-thirds of maintenance requirements with 0.45 per cent sodium chloride and 5 per cent dextrose). Antibiotics are not generally indicated in infants with mild or moderate-to-severe respiratory distress because secondary bacterial infection is rare (see below).

No proven benefit in bronchiolitis

Chest physiotherapy to assist clearing of secretions, adrenaline (epinephrine) and bronchodilators (ipratropium bromide and β_2 agonists) have not been found to be of significant benefit. There is a risk of hypoxia and deterioration with the last. Treatment with inhaled glucocorticoids is controversial.

Indications for intravenous antibiotics

- Seriously ill infants
- Atypical features
- At risk of severe illness
- Secondary bacterial infection suspected:
  - signs of sepsis
  - temperature persistently >39°C

Infants at risk of severe bronchiolitis (apnoea, severe respiratory failure)

- Neonates: the younger the infant, the more serious the symptoms
- Pre-term babies
- Cardiopulmonary disease:
  - congenital heart defect (especially left-to-right shunts)
  - chronic lung disease
  - cystic fibrosis
- Immunodeficiency
- Neurological abnormality

Specific treatment

Ribavirin, an antiviral drug, has not been found to be of clear benefit. It should be considered in seriously ill infants and those at risk of serious illness because it may bring about rapid improvement (see above).

Information to parents

In addition to the diagnosis, natural history of bronchiolitis and management, the parents are told that Billy-Jo will need to stay in hospital until:

- She shows improvement and maintains her oxygen saturation >93 per cent in air for at least 24 hours
- She feeds well orally

Billy-Jo's progress

On the ward-round the following day, Billy-Jo has less respiratory distress. The mother feels that she is brighter and coughing less. She takes some feeds with a bottle but has the remainder through the nasogastric tube. Two days later, she has minimal intercostal recessions and is fully bottle-fed. She still has a cough and wheeze but they do not seem to distress her. Parents are reassured that these are not serious but may continue for a few weeks. Billy-Jo is discharged and as no major complications are likely, follow-up in hospital is not arranged. Parents are told that some infants with bronchiolitis go on to have recurrent wheeze for a few years but it is not possible to predict this in an individual infant. They should consult their general practitioner if symptoms are worrying or troublesome (Figure 9.4).

Background information

The anatomical segments of the lungs:

- Anteriorly most of the area is occupied by the middle and upper lobes on the right and the upper lobe on the left (Figure 9.5)

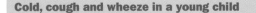

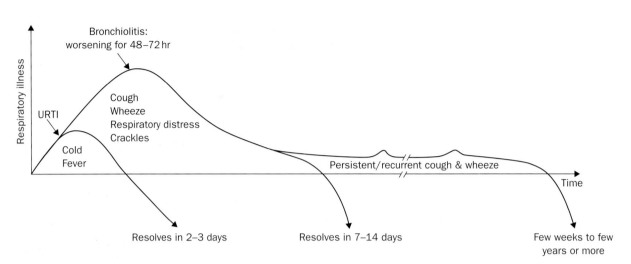

Figure 9.4 Natural history of bronchiolitis. URTI, upper respiratory tract infection.

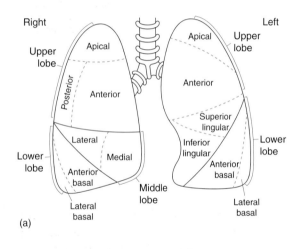

(a)

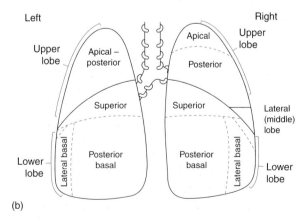

(b)

Figure 9.5 The anatomical segments of the lungs:
(a) anterior; (b) posterior.

- The middle lobe on the right and the lingular lobes on the left are adjacent to the heart
- Posteriorly, most of the area is occupied by the lower lobes
- The right main bronchus is more vertical than the left. Therefore, inhaled foreign bodies are more likely to lodge in the right bronchus
- The trachea is reinforced with C-shaped cartilages on the front and sides. This maintains an open passageway for air

Cough

Cough is a protective reflex that helps clear excess secretions and foreign material from the airways. Like any other reflex response, it is effected by means of a reflex arc (Figure 9.6) composed of:

- Cough receptors and vagus nerve sensory fibres in the afferent limb
- Integrating centre in the brain
- Vagus, phrenic and spinal motor nerves (C3–S2) to the larynx, inspiratory and expiratory muscles in the efferent limb

The different stimuli that elicit coughing are shown in Table 9.5. Table 9.6 (p. 86) shows common and less common causes of coughing.

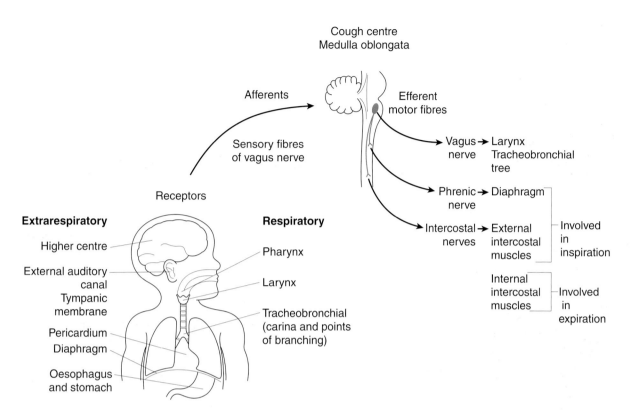

Figure 9.6   The cough reflex arc.

Table 9.5   Stimuli that cause coughing

Central

Psychogenic: anxiety, habit

Large airways

Irritation: cigarette smoke, dust, foreign body,
            postnasal drip

Inflammation: infection, asthma, aspiration

Abnormal mucus: cystic fibrosis

Extrinsic compression: lymphadenopathy,
                       vascular ring

Non-pulmonary

Stimulation of the auricular branch of the
vagus nerve

Irritation of pleura, diaphragm or pericardium

Differentiation of infants/young children from older children

The following show how infants and young children differ from older ones and why they are particularly affected by diseases involving the small airways:

- Lungs lack elastic recoil and the airways are less well supported
- Chest wall is more compliant (threefold greater than lung compliance) and stiffens as the child gets older (when chest wall compliance is comparable to lung compliance)
- End-expiratory volume or functional residual capacity is actively maintained – expiration is interrupted by active glottic narrowing or onset of inspiration, otherwise the compliant chest wall would allow complete collapse of the lungs.

In older children, end-expiratory volume is set passively by the balance between the recoils of the lungs and the chest wall

Table 9.6 Common and less common causes of coughing

	Very brief	Acute (<3 weeks)	Episodic	Chronic
Common causes	Clearing something in the throat	URTI, e.g. common cold, middle-ear infection, sinusitis, laryngotracheobronchitis	Asthma	Smoking
	Environmental irritant, e.g. smoke, fumes	LRTI, e.g. bronchiolitis, pneumonia		
Less common causes		Pertussis	Gastro-oesophageal reflux	Cystic fibrosis
		Inhaled foreign body		Pulmonary tuberculosis
		Acute allergic reaction		Congenital heart defect with congestive failure
				Psychogenic

LRTI, lower respiratory tract infection; URTI, upper respiratory tract infection.

- Chest wall 'caves in' during obstructed inspiration and paradoxical respiration develops, contributing to increased work of breathing (Figure 9.7)
- Airway walls are thicker and the diameter of the lumen of the conducting airways relative to the thickness of the walls is small (Figure 9.8).
  Bronchospasm, mucosal oedema and excess mucus cause greater airway narrowing in infants
- Small peripheral airways may contribute as much as 50 per cent of the total airway resistance (<20 per cent in adults). Infants and young children are severely affected by diseases involving the smaller airways as resistance is increased further
- Small airways are compressed during forced expiration (dynamic airway narrowing) and this results in airflow limitation (flow does not increase with increased expiratory effort) (Figure 9.9, p. 89)

Acute respiratory illnesses

Respiratory disease is an important cause of morbidity and mortality in childhood. Acute respiratory illness accounts for:

- Up to 80 per cent of presentations to the general practitioner within the first year of life; the most

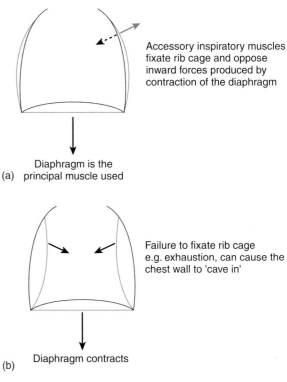

Accessory inspiratory muscles fixate rib cage and oppose inward forces produced by contraction of the diaphragm

(a) Diaphragm is the principal muscle used

Failure to fixate rib cage e.g. exhaustion, can cause the chest wall to 'cave in'

(b) Diaphragm contracts

Figure 9.7 Paradoxical respirations: inspiration (a) under normal resting conditions and (b) in the presence of airway obstruction.

What to look at when interpreting a chest radiograph

- Patient's name and date of examination
- Marker for right and left sides
- Position of clavicles to identify any rotation
- **Phase of respiration**

	Full inspiration	**Expiratory phase**
Mediastinum	Relatively narrow	Wide
Heart size		Exaggerated
Diaphragm	Over fifth to seventh anterior rib ends	High
Lung fields	Occupy large portion of the chest	Disproportionately small and prominent vascular markings

- Artefacts, tubes and drains – external, endotracheal, nasogastric, pleural, central venous, ventriculoperitoneal
- Thoracic cage – rib fracture or other lesions
- **Part of the chest**

	Appearance	**Points to consider**
Mediastinum	Widening	Differentiate normal thymus in infants from abnormal masses (see Chapter 13)
Hilar regions	Enlargement	Lymphadenopathy
Heart	Size and shape	Normal heart is approximately 60% of the transverse diameter of the thorax
Diaphragm	Flattened	Overinflation
	Elevation	Collapse of lung
		Paralysis
Costophrenic angle	Obliterated	Pleural effusion (see Chapter 24)
Trachea	Shift from midline	Collapse, pleural effusion or pneumothorax
Bronchial wall	Thickening, streaky shadows	Chronic inflammation, e.g. cystic fibrosis (see Chapter 36)
Lungs	Increased translucency	With flattened diaphragm suggests air trapping and is localized or bilateral depending on site of airway obstruction (see Chapters 13 and 35)
		Compensatory overinflation if other segments or lobes are collapsed
		If unilateral, differentiate from pneumothorax
	Opacification	Alveolar infiltrates or consolidation, e.g. bacterial infection, bronchiolitis
		Interstitial infiltrates, e.g. fibrosis, pulmonary oedema, *Mycoplasma pneumoniae*
		Collapse (shift of mediastinum towards it)
		Pleural fluid (shift of mediastinum away from it)
		Tumour
Pulmonary vascularity	Distribution	Branches of the pulmonary arteries are not normally seen in the peripheral third of the lungs

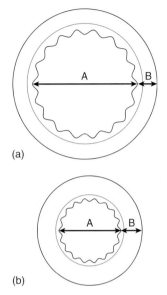

(a)

(b)

Figure 9.8 Airway wall thickness and diameter in adults (a) compared with infants (b). The diameter of the lumen of the conducting airways A relative to the thickness of the walls B is small in infants compared with adults.

common reason for hospital admission is bronchiolitis

- One-fifth of all admissions to hospital in the first 5 years of life

Death results mainly from:

- Acute LRTI in infancy
- Cystic fibrosis and asthma in later childhood

Bronchiolitis – a snapshot

This is a common and serious viral respiratory infection in early childhood.

Epidemiology

- Age: 90 per cent patients are aged 1–9 months; rare after 1 year
- Winter outbreaks occur each year

Cause

A virally induced acute inflammation of the bronchioles:

- Most common: RSV (over 70 per cent cases)

- Other viruses include parainfluenza, influenza, adenovirus, rhinovirus

The incubation period is 2–8 days.

Clinical features

- Varies from mild self-limiting disease to serious life-threatening illness (apnoea in neonates)
- Initial symptoms resemble those of the common cold: runny nose, nasal congestion, irritation in the back of the throat ('tickly throat'), mild cough and fever
- Predominant symptoms are:
  – a sharp moist irritating cough
  – wheezing and signs of airway obstruction
- Reinfection is common but the illness is less severe owing to some immunity acquired from the previous infection

Pathogenesis

Respiratory syncytial virus replicates in the nasopharynx. Fusion of the virus with host cells and formation of syncytium allows the virus to propagate and spread from infected to uninfected cells. The major sites of replication are bronchial epithelial cells and alveolar macrophages. The pathological findings include necrosis of bronchiolar epithelium and ciliated cells, submucosal oedema, excess mucus secretion and obstruction of small bronchioles (Figure 9.10, p. 90). This leads to hyperinflation or collapse of distal lung tissue.

Bacterial and non-viral LRTIs (pneumonias) – a snapshot

A pathogen is found only in 20–60 per cent of suspected bacterial lower respiratory tract infections (Table 9.7, p. 90).

Radiology

A chest radiograph is indicated:

- At presentation if bacterial pneumonia is suspected clinically

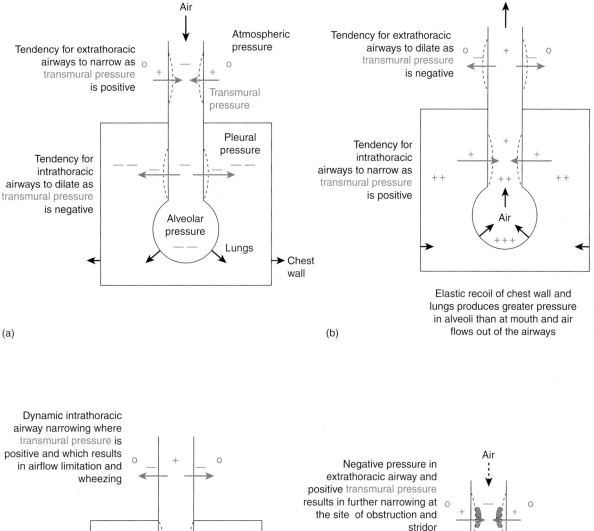

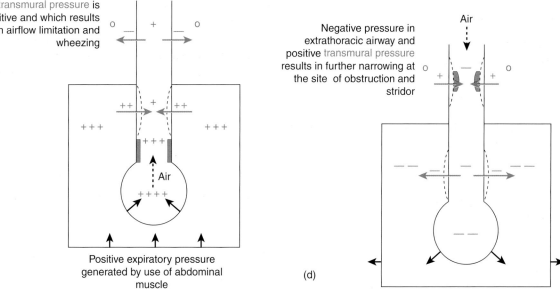

Figure 9.9 Dynamic changes in airway calibre during (a) inspiration and (b) expiration; (c) shows forced expiration or the presence of intrathoracic airway obstruction and (d) inspiration in the presence of upper airway obstruction.

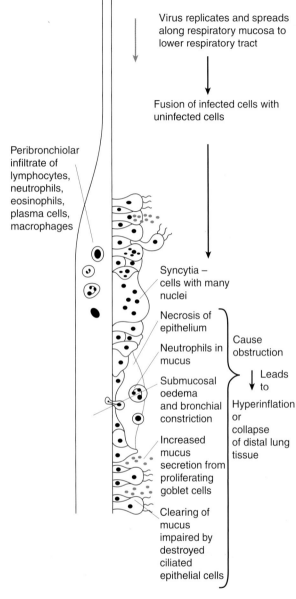

Virus replicates and spreads along respiratory mucosa to lower respiratory tract

Fusion of infected cells with uninfected cells

Peribronchiolar infiltrate of lymphocytes, neutrophils, eosinophils, plasma cells, macrophages

Syncytia – cells with many nuclei

Necrosis of epithelium

Neutrophils in mucus

Submucosal oedema and bronchial constriction

Cause obstruction

Leads to

Hyperinflation or collapse of distal lung tissue

Increased mucus secretion from proliferating goblet cells

Clearing of mucus impaired by destroyed ciliated epithelial cells

Figure 9.10 Pathogenesis of bronchiolitis.

- During the acute phase of a respiratory illness if there is deterioration
- After 6 weeks in children with an abnormality on an initial chest radiograph (e.g. consolidation, collapse, pleural effusion) or persistent respiratory symptoms

Table 9.7 Features of bacterial and non-viral lower respiratory tract infections (LRTIs)

Features common to bacterial LRTIs and bronchiolitis	Features suggestive of bacterial pneumonia
Tachypnoea	Fever >38°C but usually >39°C
Respiratory distress	Slow capillary refill
Irritability or lethargy	Bronchial breathing
Crackles	Unilateral wheeze
Reduced breath sounds	Consolidation on chest radiograph

Microbiological investigations

- Cough swab in infants and young children and sputum sample in children old enough to expectorate should be taken for bacterial culture (Table 9.8). A negative result does not exclude bacterial pneumonia. A positive result does not necessarily indicate that the organisms are from the lower respiratory tract
- Blood cultures should be taken in infants <3 months age and those with signs of septicaemia

Bacterial and non-viral LRTIs secondary to other pathology

The following features of bacterial/non-viral LRTIs indicate that other pathology such as cystic fibrosis (incidence 1 in 2500 live births) or primary immuno-deficiency (incidence 5 in 100 000 population, e.g. agammaglobulinaemia, severe combined immuno-deficiency) should be considered:

- Persistent infection with persistent chest radiographic changes
- Recurrent infection especially with organisms that usually cause isolated infection (e.g. *Streptococcus pneumoniae, Haemophilus influenzae*)
- Severe infection
- Unusual infection (e.g. *Pseudomonas aeruginosa, Burkholderia cepacia, Pneumocystis carinii*)

Table 9.8 The likely organisms causing lower respiratory tract infection (LRTI) in different age groups

Organism	Antibiotic of choice pending bacterial sensitivity result
Neonates	
Staphylococcus aureus	Flucloxacillin
Group B β-haemolytic streptococci	Benzylpenicillin
Gram-negative	Gentamicin
Preschool-age	
Viruses are more common (RSV, influenza, parainfluenza, adenovirus, rhinovirus, coronavirus, cytomegalovirus, herpes simplex virus, enteroviruses)	None
Streptococcus pneumoniae	Benzylpenicillin
Haemophilus influenzae	Amoxicillin
School-age	
Mycoplasma pneumoniae	Erythromycin
Streptococcus pneumoniae	Benzylpenicillin
Uncommon	
Bordetella pertussis	Erythromycin
Legionella pneumophilae	Erythromycin ± rifampicin
Chlamydia pneumoniae	
Varicella-zoster	Aciclovir

- Associated with poor weight gain, diarrhoea, skin rash or unusual lesions

Further sources of information

Book

Patel RM, Simoes EAF. Respiratory syncytial virus infection: pathogenesis and its implications for prevention. In: David TJ (ed.) *Recent Advances in Paediatrics* 19. Edinburgh: Churchill Livingstone, 2001: 197–210.

Articles

Balfour-Lynn IM. Why do viruses make infants wheeze? *Archives of Disease in Childhood* 1996; **74**: 251–9

Irwin RS, Madison JM. The diagnosis and treatment of cough. *New England Journal of Medicine* 2000; **343**: 1715–21

Self test 3: Why might a child cough when you examine the ears with an auroscope ?

Answer: The auricular branch of the vagus nerve is stimulated.

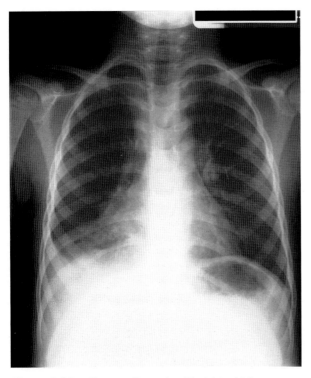

Figure 9.11 Chest radiograph with right middle zone shadowing and small left pleural effusion.

Self test 4: Interpret this chest radiograph of a 4-year-old girl (Figure 9.11). The mother is worried because the phlegmy cough, which started after a runny nose a week ago, is not getting better and her daughter has had a fever for 2 days.

Answer: The right heart border is not clear and the adjacent opacification is in the right middle lobe. The right costophrenic angle is obliterated suggesting a small pleural effusion.

Self test 5: A 3-month-old boy presented to hospital with acute symptoms: runny nose, moist cough, wheeze, poor feeding and respiratory distress. Chest radiograph showed consolidation of the right upper and middle lobes. As he was quite unwell and required intensive care, he was investigated for a primary underlying condition. Interpret the results of two of the tests:

Sweat test: Weight of sweat 126 mg, chloride 20 mmol/L, sodium 22 mmol/L

Immunoglobulins: IgG 1.1 g/L (normal range 2.31–5.89)
IgA 0.03 g/L (normal range 0.1–0.46)
IgM 0.13 g/L (normal range 0.25–0.57)

Answer:

The sweat test is normal. A minimum of 100 mg sweat is required for reliability.

Sweat chloride and sodium levels:

- <35 mmol/L is normal
- Between 35 and 60 mmol/L are equivocal and the test should be repeated
- >60 mmol/L and chloride > sodium are diagnostic for cystic fibrosis

The immunoglobulin levels are low, suggesting agammaglobulinaemia.

Lymphocyte subsets showed normal number of T cells but no B cells. Molecular genetic studies confirmed X-linked agammaglobulinaemia.

Chronic disorder

He never stops! An overactive child

Age: 6½ years

JACKIE GREGG

CHAPTER

10

Presentation

Referral letter from GP:
Please see this 6½-year-old boy who is always on the go and is constantly naughty. His mum hoped that things would settle down once he started school. He has just moved to year 2 and the teacher is complaining that he is disrupting the class and not making much academic progress. James's parents are becoming exhausted and frustrated that they haven't been able to improve his behaviour.

Initial considerations and action

All children go through phases when they are naughty or don't pay attention. At times, children can exhaust their parents and teachers by being constantly 'on the go'. All of this is normal and is part of healthy child development. The situation with James seems different. The problem appears to have been there for some time and is more than just a phase. The teacher has highlighted concerns, which may indicate that he is behaving differently from his peers.

An appointment is therefore made for James to see the community paediatrician.

History

James attends the clinic with his mother and father who are concerned that he has attention deficit hyperactivity disorder (ADHD).

Self-test 1: What are the core symptoms of ADHD?

Answer: Inattention, hyperactivity, impulsiveness.

James was born at term after an uneventful pregnancy. He weighed 3.4 kg and didn't develop any neonatal problems. He was a somewhat unsettled baby, but the problems really seemed to start when James began walking at 14 months of age. He never seemed to stop and was constantly running around and climbing without any awareness of danger. His parents had to watch him all the time, but even so he managed to fall and break his right radius and ulna at 3 years of age and needed stitches in his forehead 6 months later. James doesn't settle down to sleep until 11pm, but once he has settled he sleeps all night. He has a good appetite and has achieved all his developmental milestones.

James has never played appropriately with toys because he constantly flits from one activity to the next. This has improved a bit, but he quickly becomes frustrated with toys and often ends up breaking them. James can spend up to 20 minutes watching his favourite cartoons, but even then he is fidgeting. He is always doing silly things without thinking, which irritates the whole family and he gets very upset when told off. His parents are very frustrated, because he doesn't seem to learn from his mistakes.

James attends the local primary school with his siblings. James makes friends easily, but more recently he has annoyed some of the other children by spoiling their work accidentally as he is rushing at things. School has found a similar behaviour pattern to home. James's teacher is very experienced and it was she who indicated to his parents that there may be an underlying problem requiring investigation.

James had started to attend Beavers, but his parents withdrew him. He tended to 'run wild' and become over-excited which had proved challenging for the leaders.

James has two older siblings. His 10-year-old sister hasn't caused any concern and his 8-year-old brother has mild dyslexia with minor attentional difficulties.

Interpretation of the history

Three types of behaviour characterize children with ADHD. These are:

1 Inattention
2 Hyperactivity
3 Impulsiveness

A child with ADHD may not demonstrate all three types of behaviour. Some children have little trouble sitting still, but may be predominantly inattentive and as a result have great difficulty becoming, or staying, focused on a task. Other children may be able to pay attention to a task but lose focus because they have trouble controlling their physical activity and impulse behaviour. In most cases, all these features are combined.

The following conditions may also present with hyperactive, impulsive and inattentive behaviours:

- Developmental delay/specific learning difficulties/advanced development without adequate stimulation
- Language disorder
- Autistic spectrum disorder
- Obsessive–compulsive disorder
- Anxiety disorders
- Major affective disorders
- Sleep disorders
- Absence seizure disorder
- Management problems
- Family dysfunction/child abuse
- Unrealistic parental expectation

It is very important to identify environmental factors that may be contributing to the ADHD-type behaviours. Physical, emotional or sexual abuse and severe family discord may also produce symptoms of inattention, impulsivity and hyperactivity. A high index of suspicion for alternative diagnoses must be present when older, previously normally functioning children develop ADHD symptoms. An ADHD diagnosis should not be given in such instances.

Meaning of the history in James

A history of normal developmental milestones makes a developmental problem an unlikely cause for James's difficulties. This doesn't exclude more specific learning difficulties, which will need to be explored with school. Normal sleep pattern, good appetite and absence of other symptoms make a mental health disorder unlikely to be the underlying diagnosis. James's parents appear to have realistic expectations of their children's behaviour and there are no indications of family dysfunction, but this would need further exploration. James's siblings do not have behavioural problems, which suggests that his parents know how to manage a child's behaviour successfully. James therefore seems more than just a naughty boy whose parents don't know how to handle him. ADHD appears to be a possible diagnosis.

Self-test 2: How do children with ADHD present?

Answer: Many children present with hyperactivity. Many others are regarded as naughty, because they are unable to control their behaviour. They are very easily bored and distracted and can be disruptive in the classroom and at home. They do not respond to the normal methods of discipline and as a result many are excluded from school.

The symptoms associated with ADHD are:

- **Inattention:**
  - careless mistakes
  - difficulty sustaining attention
  - seems not to listen
  - fails to finish school work or other tasks
  - difficulty in organizing tasks and activities
  - avoids, dislikes, or is reluctant to engage in tasks that require sustained mental effort
  - loses things
  - easily distracted
  - forgetful
- **Hyperactivity:**
  - fidgets
  - unable to remain seated
  - moves excessively, restless

- difficulty playing or engaging in leisure activities quietly
- 'on the go', acts as if 'driven by a motor'
- talks excessively

● **Impulsivity:**
  - blurts out answers before questions have been completed
  - difficulty in awaiting his or her turn
  - interrupts or intrudes on others (e.g. butts into conversations or games)

James's inability to play with any toy for long suggests inattention. Doing silly things without thinking suggests impulsiveness and the almost constant movements and accidents because of carelessness are likely to be a result of hyperactivity.

To meet the diagnostic criteria, it is essential that symptoms:

- have their onset before the age of 6 years
- have persisted for at least 6 months
- must be pervasive (present in more than one setting)
- have caused significant functional impairment
- are not better accounted for by other mental disorders

The first three are evident from the history, but further assessment of the fourth and fifth criteria will be required.

James has some of the additional emotional, social and family-related features associated with ADHD:

● **Emotional:**
  - easily frustrated, no patience
  - temper outbursts, anger
  - sadness or mood swings
  - anxiety or nervousness
  - poor self-esteem
● **Social and family related:**
  - unpopular, with few friends
  - bossy, overbearing
  - difficulty in following rules
  - disorganized
  - underachieves at school

These additional problems are usually a consequence of the behavioural problems and result from the frustrations and failures that the child experiences at home and at school.

Self-test 3: How is a diagnosis of ADHD made?

Answer: The diagnosis is a clinical one based on a detailed history from parents and school and observation of the child in the clinic setting and at school.

Examination

- Physical examination normal
- Growth normal
- Development is within normal limits
- Social interaction with parents and doctor appropriate, but somewhat immature
- Behaviour was acceptable and James was polite. However, he was very fidgety and didn't settle to any activity for longer than 5 minutes. He kept interrupting while his mother was talking

Interpretation of the examination

Developmental delay has been excluded. James's social interaction is appropriate, which excludes an autistic spectrum disorder. It is difficult to assess the severity of behaviours in a clinic setting, but James's inability to stay focused on a task for longer than 5 minutes is indicative of significant attentional difficulties in a child of this age.

Assessment

A flow chart outlining the assessment and management of children with possible ADHD is shown in Figure 10.1.

ADHD is diagnosed primarily by evaluation of the child's history and from observations made by parents, teachers and others who know the child – contributions from grandparents and Cub or Scout leaders can be extremely helpful. Family assessment requires detailed information about the core symptoms of ADHD in various settings, the age of onset, duration of symptoms and the degree of functional impairment. Questionnaires to rate children's behaviour, concentration, social

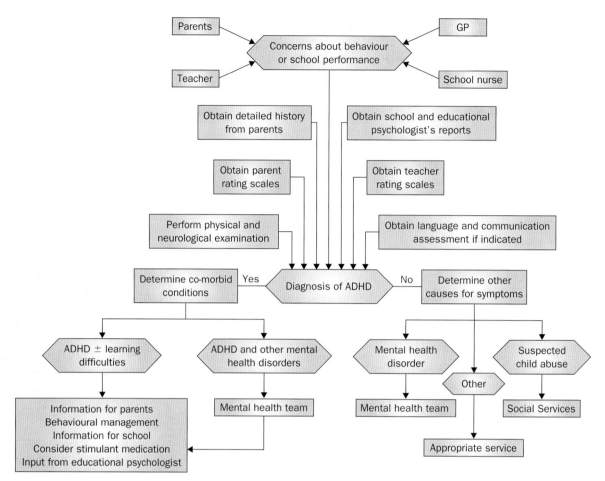

Figure 10.1 Flow chart outlining the assessment and management of young people with suspected attention deficit hyperactivity disorder (ADHD).

skills and mood swings are widely used as part of the assessment.

In view of the complexity of the condition and associated co-morbidity (Table 10.1), James is further assessed in the ADHD clinic run by the community paediatrician and clinical psychologist, with input from the school nurse.

The psychological assessment does not reveal any coexisting conditions or cognitive deficits. The family give permission for the Beaver leader to be contacted, who confirms James's overactivity at Beavers.

School assessment is crucial. Details of the child's behaviour, learning patterns and degree of functional impairment must be obtained. Teacher versions of the

Table 10.1 Conditions co-morbid with attention deficit hyperactivity disorder

- Oppositional defiant disorder
- Conduct disorder
- Anxiety
- Depression
- Specific learning difficulties, e.g. dyslexia
- Language-based difficulties
- Developmental coordination disorder (dyspraxia)
- Gilles de la Tourette's syndrome
- Obsessive–compulsive disorder
- Autistic spectrum disorders

questionnaires can be helpful. Ideally assessment by an educational psychologist should be carried out to detect any subtle learning difficulties. Information on interventions carried out in the classroom and their success is important.

The school nurse liaises with James's class teacher, who has assessed him as being an intelligent boy who is underachieving. He is very easily distracted and only completes work if he has one-to-one support. It is not unusual for James to get up and wander around the classroom, which distracts the other children. James has been sitting at the front of the class with three other children, but, more recently, he has been moved to sit at a desk on his own, which has helped somewhat.

James is described as a pleasant and likeable boy. He easily gets upset when reprimanded and his teacher is concerned that his self-esteem is poor. James becomes frustrated when he can't complete his work, he is aware of his difficulties and he has had the occasional angry outburst in class. The school is at a loss about what to do next.

Diagnosis

Attention deficit hyperactivity disorder.

Treatment and follow-up plan

There is no cure or 'quick fix' for ADHD. The aim when considering treatment is to create a situation in which the child can flourish and be educated, and in which his or her self-esteem is improved. Managing ADHD involves:

- Support of families in their management at home
- Help for the school and the class teacher
- Boosting self-esteem and developing outside interests
- Consideration of other therapies
- Medication

Self-test 4: What is the role of stimulant medication in the management of ADHD?

Answer: Stimulant medication can have a significant effect on the three main behaviours. This can provide a window of opportunity to implement other behavioural therapies, to improve self-esteem and to develop friendships.

Self-test 5: Which of the following are thought to be implicated in the aetiology of ADHD?
A Food additives
B Genetic factors
C Imbalance of neurotransmitters
D Poor parenting
E Sleep deprivation

Answer: B/C.

Behavioural management

Parents have first to accept that their child with ADHD is different. They need a careful explanation of the condition and advice on where to obtain further information. Family support groups can be a useful resource.

Normal behaviour techniques work poorly in children with ADHD – their impulsiveness means that they act before they have thought of the consequences. As a result of this, many parents feel that they have failed. They have to learn to be patient and keep calm – heated arguments will quickly get out of control. Children require routine and behaviours can be changed using small, well-planned steps. Rewards should be frequent and will need to be constantly repeated.

Many families need advice and support in modifying their child's behaviour and benefit greatly from behavioural or psychological therapy. Family-based psychosocial interventions of a behavioural type are recommended for the treatment of co-morbid behavioural problems.

School

Many schools are experienced in dealing with children with ADHD, whereas others may have very little knowledge about the condition. Written information is helpful. A crucial first step is for the school to accept that the child's behaviour is not naughtiness – the child can't help it.

The child needs consistency – a firm but encouraging teacher who will be there every school day, all year.

The child should sit near the front of the class, away from distracting influences, and be given clear stepwise instructions and constant feedback. Special supervision at times of change, such as coming in from break when the child may be 'high' or on a school trip, is needed.

The child's progress must be carefully monitored. Extra help may be required in the classroom, assessment and advice from the school's educational psychologist may be required and the curriculum may need to be modified. Some children who have associated learning difficulties may need to attend a special unit or special school.

Self-esteem

Parents and schools should aim to help the child have successful experiences, so that he or she gains confidence and improves his or her self-esteem. By understanding the child's strengths, parents can encourage success, such as finding a sport or activity that the child is good at. Local clubs, Scouts or Brownies can suit many children, but leaders need to be fully informed. Friendships may need to be encouraged, by involving them in the child's favourite activity.

Other therapies

Dietary factors do not cause ADHD. Less than 10 per cent of children with ADHD are affected by additives or colourings, and parents can often identify a few foods that have to be avoided. Many fizzy drinks contain caffeine, a known stimulant. Multi-vitamins and natural products are unproven in treatment.

Medication

The main medications used in ADHD are the stimulants methylphenidate and dexamphetamine. These have been shown to be effective in over 80 per cent of children in the short to medium term by:

- Increasing the attention span
- Reducing impulsiveness
- Decreasing hyperactivity
- Reducing negative social interactions

Medication is a valuable addition to other management strategies. There has been much adverse publicity about medication, particularly methylphenidate, yet it has been used since 1958 and its safety profile has been well documented.

How to use and monitor methylphenidate

When to use

- Diagnosis of ADHD
- When educational and psychological therapies have not produced, or are unlikely to produce, sufficient benefits – medication can provide 'a window of opportunity'
- With parental and child agreement

Monitor

- Dose – titrate to achieve optimal therapeutic response with minimal side effects
- Growth – some reports of decreasing height velocity, although rare in practice
- Blood pressure – may cause hypertension
- Side effects – the most common are insomnia, loss of appetite and emotional lability, which can usually be controlled by adjusting the dose or by changing the time that it is given
- Effectiveness – is the dose appropriate? Is it no longer needed?

Management of James

James's parents feel that they will be able to modify their behavioural approach to suit James's needs now that they have a diagnosis and have some pointers of what is likely to work. They don't feel that they need any input from the psychologist at present. James's parents are keen to discuss the role of medication. The nurse attached to the ADHD clinic had visited the school to explain the condition to them. Although school didn't feel that they knew much about ADHD, they had introduced many appropriate measures, which, however, hadn't helped James's academic progress. It was therefore considered that a trial of methylphenidate was indicated. Baseline measurements of height, weight and blood pressure were taken and James was started on a 5 mg dose in the morning.

The paediatrician contacts the family by phone a week later. James is tolerating the medication and there has been some improvement in his concentration. The dose is doubled and, when the paediatrician speaks to the family a week later, they report that school have seen a very marked improvement in James's attention and for the first time he has completed a piece of work. The effects, however, have worn off by midday, so a lunchtime dose is introduced. (The therapeutic effects of methylphenidate usually last 3–4 hours. Slow-release preparations are being evaluated.)

James is reviewed a month later and already his parents have noticed an improvement in his reading and hand-writing. They would like James to return to Beavers and take a small dose of methylphenidate to see if his behaviour will be more manageable. If that works, they would like him to have medication on a Saturday, so that he can also go to Beaver football.

Three months later, James is continuing to catch up with his school work. His parents have noticed that he is getting invited to more parties and to friends' houses. Beavers, too, is proving a success.

Young people on methylphenidate are usually reviewed 4- to 6-monthly in the clinic. School will be asked to provide regular reports. It will be important to consider whether medication is still indicated at regular intervals, by deliberately stopping it for a week and getting reports from school. Often this is unnecessary because even one accidentally missed dose results in a noticeable deterioration in the child's concentration. It is likely that James will need to be on treatment for several years.

Background information

Attention deficit hyperactivity disorder

Epidemiology

Attention deficit hyperactivity disorder is a relatively common behavioural disorder in childhood, diagnosed more frequently in boys than girls by a ratio of 4:1. In the USA, where slightly different guidelines for the diagnosis of ADHD apply, some 10–20 per cent of schoolchildren appear to be affected. In Britain, the condition is reported less frequently, with the prevalence in the range of 2–5 per cent.

Aetiology

Until relatively recent times, professionals blamed parents' attachment or relationships for causing ADHD. Others blamed food additives. It is now recognized that neither of these is the cause, although poor parenting and some food substances may influence already existing ADHD. ADHD is a biological condition, which is strongly hereditary – most children have a parent or close relative who has experienced many of the same difficulties. There are a number of conditions that frequently have features of ADHD and may have a common aetiology:

- Traumatic brain injury
- Fetal alcohol syndrome
- Fragile X syndrome
- Chronic lead poisoning
- Untreated phenylketonuria
- Post-infectious encephalopathy
- Cerebral palsy
- Neurocutaneous syndromes

Pathophysiology

Imaging studies, including functional magnetic resonance imaging (fMRI), as well as quantitative electroencephalography (EEG) and positron emission tomography (PET), provide evidence of brain dysfunction in the behaviour inhibition areas of the brain (the frontal lobes and their connections). The mechanism seems to be an imbalance of the neurotransmitters dopamine and noradrenaline (norepinephrine). It is thought that the stimulant medications used in treatment increase dopamine and noradrenaline levels in the brain.

Prognosis

It had been thought that most children with ADHD grow out of it. However, it is now recognized that 50 per cent of children with ADHD will have some symptoms in adult life. It is usually less noticeable in adults because they have learned how to camouflage the symptoms by organizing their lives around them. It is not unusual for a parent to understand their own social, learning and behavioural weaknesses when their child is diagnosed as having ADHD.

Further sources of information

Books

Green C, Chee K. *Understanding Attention Deficit Disorder*. London: Vermilion, 1995

Website

www.nice.org.uk

National Institute for Clinical Excellence's 'Guidance on Methylphenidate for ADHD'.

Guidelines

Scottish Intercollegiate Guidelines Network. *Attention Deficit and Hyperkinetic Disorder in Children and Young People. A national clinical guideline*. Edinburgh: SIGN, 2001

Self-test 6: Joseph aged 11 years attends clinic. He has been taking methylphenidate in a dose of 10 mg twice daily for 2 years with good effect. He has just moved to secondary school and is refusing to take his medication because he says that he doesn't need it any more – his parents feel that he does.

A Why do you think that Joseph is refusing to take his medication?

B What information will you request to help you decide if treatment is still indicated?

C How could you make taking the treatment more acceptable to Joseph?

Answers:

A He may not want to appear different; bullying or teasing because of the treatment may be occurring

B Assessments and reports from school about his attention and concentration and progress with his work

C Suggest that Joseph administers it himself at lunchtime, consider the sustained-release preparation, and reassure Joseph that you will regularly plan a drug-free period to see whether he still needs to take it

A boy with persistent diarrhoea

Age: 14 months

LEENA PATEL

Presentation

The following is a GP's referral letter to a general paediatrician:

> Asim is a 14-month-old boy who has had diarrhoea for the past 2 months. His appetite has not changed but his mother is concerned about his weight. His parents are first cousins. Physical examination revealed nothing abnormal. Haemoglobin is 8.1 g/dL. Stool culture showed no growth.
> Kindly see this patient.

Self-test 1: What might be the cause of this little boy's diarrhoea? Do clinical features, such as the age of the patient, name and consanguinity, and the duration of diarrhoea and associated low haemoglobin, give clues to the underlying diagnosis? While reading Asim's history and examination, pick out other cues and try to connect them.

Answer: How the important features from Asim's history and examination might be linked is shown in Figure 11.1, p. 102. Positive and negative findings help to consider and eliminate various diagnoses.

Initial considerations and action

Diarrhoea as a symptom

Diarrhoea is a common paediatric problem. It may be defined as an increase in the frequency or decrease in the consistency of stool:

- Acute diarrhoea is more common than chronic diarrhoea
- Chronic diarrhoea is defined by the World Health Organization as diarrhoea that continues for more than 2 weeks

There are considerable normal variations in bowel habits and stool number, volume and consistency throughout childhood. It is important to differentiate:

- Normal stool frequency and consistency from abnormal, e.g. breast-fed infants may have frequent watery stools of varying colour
- Genuine diarrhoea from constipation and overflow or soiling (encopresis)

Self-test 2: What factors determine stool volume and consistency?

Answer: Stool volume and consistency are determined by:
- Diet and fibre intake
- Normal function of the gastrointestinal (GI) tract, which includes (Figure 11.2, p. 103):
  - motility (regulated by enteric and autonomic nervous systems, GI hormones and neuropeptides)
  - secretion (of enzymes, fluid and electrolytes, immunoglobulins)
  - digestion
  - absorption

Disruption of one or more of these functions occurs in diseases of the GI tract and leads to diarrhoea with or without malabsorption (Figure 11.3, p. 104). An understanding of the normal functions of the GI tract and the consequences of disruption of these

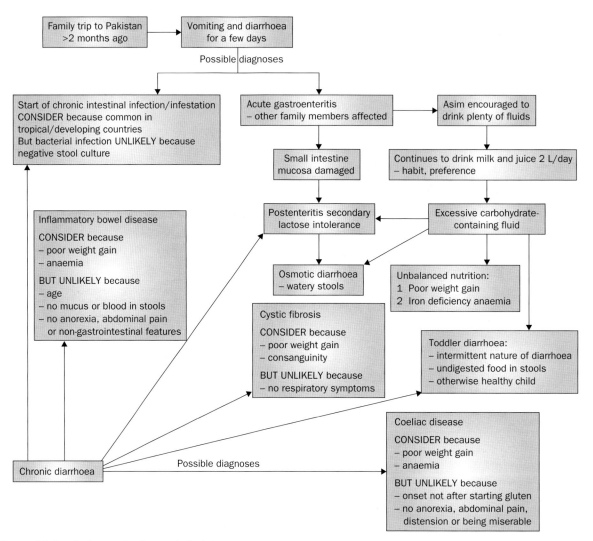

Figure 11.1 Pathways to diagnosis in Asim.

functions helps to approach the clinical assessment of this child with chronic diarrhoea (see Background information).

Initial thoughts about the differential diagnosis

The most frequent cause of chronic diarrhoea in pre-school children in developed countries is toddler diarrhoea (chronic non-specific diarrhoea) (Table 11.1), but it is important not to overlook:

- Pathology, such as coeliac disease and cystic fibrosis
- Complications such as malnutrition

Asim is offered an appointment within 1 week.

History and examination will provide information about:

- The GI tract disorder
- Secondary effects of deranged GI function, such as failure to thrive, anaemia or rickets, water and electrolyte imbalance
- Associated non-GI features, such as lung disease

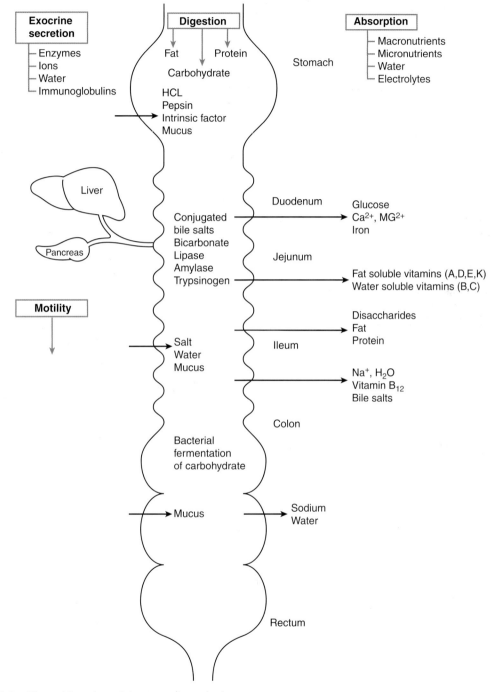

Figure 11.2 Normal function of the gastrointestinal tract.

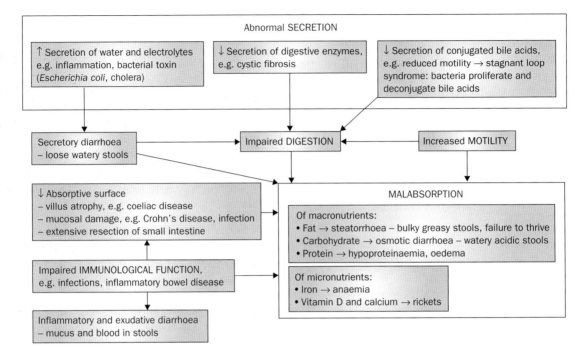

Figure 11.3   Abnormal functions of the gastrointestinal tract.

Table 11.1   The differential diagnosis of chronic diarrhoea in different age groups

	Infancy	Toddler, preschool	School
Common	Toddler diarrhoea	Toddler diarrhoea	Inflammatory bowel disease
	Postenteritis: small intestinal mucosal injury after rotavirus or *Escherichia coli* acute gastroenteritis	Postenteritis	
		Coeliac disease	
	Cows' milk intolerance	Ulcerative colitis	
	Cystic fibrosis	Repeated courses of broad-spectrum antibiotics such as amoxicillin	
	Coeliac disease		
Rare	Intractable diarrhoea of infancy	Bacterial: *Salmonella*, *Shigella* and *Yersinia* species, tuberculosis	
	Congenital microvillus atrophy	Parasitic: *Giardia* species, *Entamoeba histolytica*, *Cryptosporidium* species	
	Hirschsprung's disease		
	Munchausen's syndrome by proxy (e.g. laxatives)	Opportunistic infections in immunocompromised individuals	
	Congenital chloridorrhoea	Hyperthyroidism	

History

Asim had been a healthy child until the family trip to Pakistan over 2 months ago. He has had intermittent diarrhoea, with up to three mushy stools on some days and three to six watery stools on other days, but none at night, since the holiday. There has not been any blood in the stools. He and the rest of the family had a 'tummy bug' while they were in Pakistan: they had vomiting for a day and then several very loose motions for 2–3 days. At that time, a doctor in Pakistan advised the family to drink plenty of fluids. Mother therefore encouraged Asim to have even more drinks than before. Since then, he has preferred drinks to food. He has six bottles (8 oz each) of milk or juice during the day and two bottles at night, and has a tantrum if he is given water instead. The little that he does eat seems to go straight through and it is possible to identify the food in his stools. His mother feels that Asim has not gained weight since the holiday. He is 'full of energy', very inquisitive and 'into everything'.

Self-test 3: The most likely causes of the initial symptoms in Pakistan are:

A A food allergy

B Food poisoning

C Cholera

D Typhoid

E Acute gastroenteritis

Answer: B and E are true. A and D are excluded because other family members were affected at the same time and had similar symptoms. Cholera is characterized by profuse diarrhoea and severe dehydration necessitating intravenous fluids.

Self-test 4: Acute gastroenteritis with blood in the stools is well recognized with the following:

A Rotavirus

B *Campylobacter* species

C *Shigella* species

D *Salmonella* species

E *Escherichia coli*

Answer: B, C, D and E are true.

Interpretation of the history

Comparing the present weight with previous weight measurements (using the parent-held record known as the 'Red book') will reveal whether mother's concerns about Asim's weight are real. If weight gain is indeed poor, then (1) malabsorption of major nutrients as in cystic fibrosis and coeliac disease and (2) inadequate intake in an otherwise healthy but 'fussy' eater (excess consumption of juice and drinks) will have to be considered (see Figure 11.4, p. 106). Asim's history favours the latter.

- Children with cystic fibrosis may have a good appetite and adequate intake but weight gain is poor as a result of malabsorption
- Anorexia is common in coeliac disease (see Chapter 6)
- Autosomal recessive conditions are more likely to manifest when there is consanguinity, e.g. cystic fibrosis

History in a child presenting with chronic diarrhoea

- Clarify parent's perception of diarrhoea
- Duration of diarrhoea – is it chronic?
- Onset:
  - after acute gastroenteritis or insidious onset
  - after change in diet, e.g. starting excessive carbohydrate-containing fluids (osmotic diarrhoea), cows' milk (intolerance) or cereals (coeliac disease)
- Nature of the stools:
  - loose and contain recognizable undigested food (toddler diarrhoea)
  - profuse and very watery stools (secretory diarrhoea)
  - frothy and watery (osmotic diarrhoea, carbohydrate malabsorption)
  - blood and mucus in stools (infective colitis or inflammatory bowel disease)
  - pale, large and offensive (cystic fibrosis, coeliac disease)
- Time pattern:
  - nocturnal (inflammatory bowel disease)

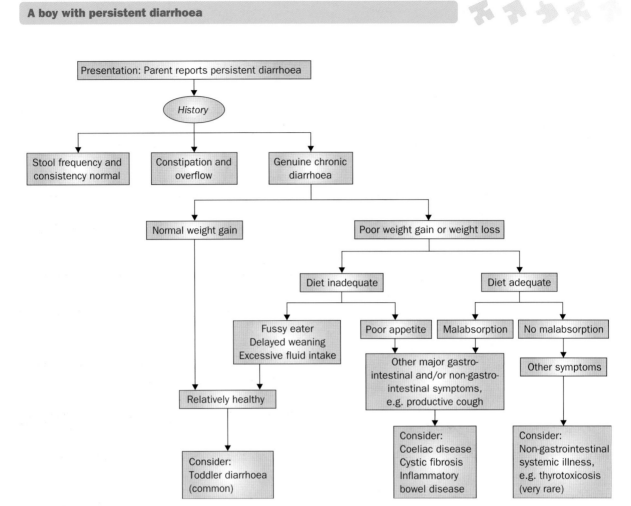

Figure 11.4 Clinically differentiating conditions that present as persistent diarrhoea.

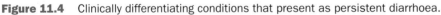

- – continues with starving (secretory diarrhoea)
- – stops when starved (osmotic diarrhoea)
- History of weaning and diet:
  - – prolonged breast-feeding beyond 6–9 months of age
  - – high intake of carbohydrate-rich drinks (toddler diarrhoea)
  - – adequate in calories, macronutrients, vitamins and minerals
- Growth:
  - – normal weight gain (toddler diarrhoea)
  - – failure to gain weight (inadequate diet; malabsorption of macronutrients as in coeliac disease, cystic fibrosis or inflammatory bowel disease)
  - – short stature (coeliac disease, Crohn's disease)

- Associated gastrointestinal symptoms:
  - – abdominal distension (malabsorption as in coeliac disease, cystic fibrosis; reduced motility)
  - – vomiting, abdominal pain (infection, inflammatory bowel disease; uncommon in toddler diarrhoea)
- Associated non-gastrointestinal symptoms:
  - – puffiness of hands and feet (hypoalbuminaemia as in coeliac disease, cystic fibrosis)
  - – fever, rash, mouth sores or joint pain (systemic manifestations of inflammatory bowel disease)
  - – anorexia (coeliac disease, inflammatory bowel disease)
  - – recurrent productive cough (cystic fibrosis)
  - – goitre, tremor, palpitations, eye signs (hyperthyroidism)

- Development:
  - delayed motor milestones from muscle wasting, reduced power and hypotonia (coeliac disease)
- Foreign travel (tropical infection from bacteria such as *Salmonella* or *Shigella* species)
- Contact with animals: farm animals (infection with *Campylobacter* species, brucellosis)
- Medication: antibiotics
- Family history: coeliac disease, cystic fibrosis, inflammatory bowel disease

Examination

Asim plays happily with toys in the consulting room. He does not appear scrawny. However, his weight is on the 10th centile and has indeed been static for the past 2 months. His height is on the 25th centile. His conjunctiva and mucous membrane are pale, but there is no jaundice, oedema, lymphadenopathy or hepatosplenomegaly. There is no clubbing and nothing else abnormal on general, abdominal and systemic examination.

The important components of the examination in a child presenting with chronic diarrhoea

- General appearance:
  - happy, playful (toddler diarrhoea)
  - unhappy, irritable, clingy (coeliac disease)
  - subdued (inflammatory bowel disease)
- Growth: weight and height measured and plotted on a growth chart, serial recordings are more useful than single measurements
- State of hydration: sunken eyes, sunken anterior fontanelle, dry tongue, reduced skin turgor, rapid pulse, reduced urine output (dehydration)
- Clubbing (cystic fibrosis, inflammatory bowel disease, chronic liver disease)
- Pallor (anaemia)
- Jaundice (liver or biliary disorder)
- Uveitis, mouth ulcers, rash, arthritis (inflammatory bowel disease)
- Lymphadenopathy (intestinal tuberculosis, lymphoma, AIDS)
- Generalized oedema (coeliac disease, cystic fibrosis)
- Muscle wasting (coeliac disease, inflammatory bowel disease)

- Abdominal:
  - inspection: distension (coeliac disease, cystic fibrosis)
  - palpation: right iliac fossa mass, tenderness, perianal lesions (inflammatory bowel disease)
  - auscultation: borborygmi (carbohydrate malabsorption)
  - perianal region:
    perianal excoriation (carbohydrate/lactose malabsorption)
    mucosal tag, fissure or fistula (Crohn's disease)

Interpretation of the examination

The nature of the stools, diet history and good general health differentiate toddler diarrhoea from GI pathology.

Pallor suggests anaemia. This and the static weight are most probably the result of a nutritional intake poor in calories and micronutrients.

Investigations and results

Investigations in a patient presenting with chronic diarrhoea

Although toddler diarrhoea is diagnosed clinically, the diagnosis of other causes of chronic diarrhoea is based on a composite of findings including clinical, laboratory and radiological (see below). Investigations may be necessary to do the following.

Establish a diagnosis

Diagnostic and supporting tests for specific conditions should be undertaken according to the probability from history and examination.

Gastrointestinal tract infection or infestation
- Bacterial screen: aerobic and anaerobic cultures and tests for particular bacterial toxins can be done
- Virology: by immunofluorescence or electron microscopy
- Parasites: fresh stool samples or duodenal/jejunal aspirate is needed to look for ova and cysts of *Giardia* species

Post-enteritis lactose malabsorption
- Stool pH and reducing substances: acidic stool that is positive for reducing substances is the result of undigested sugars in the stool as in lactase (a disaccharidase in the brush border) deficiency, most often seen in postviral enteritis (or any disease affecting small intestinal mucosa)

Cystic fibrosis
- Sweat sodium and chloride: raised >60 mmol/L and chloride >sodium
- DNA for cystic fibrosis gene mutations
- Plasma immunoreactive trypsin in infants <6 weeks old: raised in pancreatic insufficiency
- Stool chymotrypsin: low in pancreatic insufficiency

Coeliac disease
- Anti-endomysial antibodies
- Jejunal biopsies: villous atrophy in coeliac disease; partial villous atrophy in giardiasis

Inflammatory bowel disease
- Barium meal and follow-through; contrast enema: diagnostic significance and to determine extent of involvement
- Upper and lower gastrointestinal (GI) endoscopy

Assess the secondary effects of deranged GI function

- **Plasma protein and albumin:** low in protein malabsorption (cystic fibrosis) and protein-losing enteropathy (coeliac disease, Crohn's disease)
- **Full blood count:**
  - haemoglobin may be low as a result of iron deficiency (coeliac disease, Crohn's disease), chronic blood loss (ulcerative colitis), malabsorption of folic acid (coeliac disease, Crohn's disease), chronic disease (inflammatory bowel disease)
  - peripheral blood smear shows microcytic/hypochromic anaemia with iron deficiency or a macrocytic anaemia with folic acid deficiency
  - white cell count can be high as a result of infection, inflammation or a malignancy; a low

white count may be found in the immunocompromised host
- **Zinc protoporphyrin:** high in iron deficiency anaemia
- **Serum vitamin B_{12}:** low in vitamin B_{12} deficiency
- **Serum folate:** low in folic acid deficiency
- **Serum calcium, phosphate, alkaline phosphatase and parathyroid hormone (PTH):** calcium and vitamin D deficiency with secondary hyperparathyroidism (coeliac disease)
- **Prothrombin time:** prolonged in vitamin K deficiency (a fat-soluble vitamin)
- **Vitamin A and E levels:** other fat-soluble vitamins that may be malabsorbed

The final assessment is of water, electrolytes and acid–base imbalance.

The diagnosis of toddler diarrhoea is clinical. As Asim is anaemic, he has a full blood count (FBC), blood film and zinc protoporphyrin (ZPP) taken (see below). Negative stool culture excludes bacterial infection. Asim's investigation results are shown in Table 11.2. The conclusion is that Asim has iron deficiency anaemia. Iron deficiency anaemia is common in otherwise healthy toddlers who drink a lot of milk but may occur with malabsorption, e.g. coeliac disease or GI blood loss, e.g. colitis (see Chapters 6 and 18).

Self-test 5: What is ZPP?

Answer: ZPP (zinc protoporphyrin) is a metabolic intermediate of the haemoglobin synthetic pathway. Its level is raised when there is iron deficiency. The ZPP level is inversely related to plasma ferritin and stainable iron in the marrow.

Diagnosis

Asim has the following:

- Toddler diarrhoea: this followed acute gastroenteritis when his parents encouraged fluids to prevent dehydration, and thereafter Asim continued to have carbohydrate-containing fluids

Table 11.2 Asim's investigation results and what they mean

Result	Interpretation	Causes
Full blood count (FBC)		
Hb 7.5 g/dL (normal range 11.5–15.5)	Anaemia	Defect in RBC production
		Increased RBC breakdown
RBC 4.3 × 10^{12}/L		Chronic blood loss
MCV 72 fl (normal range 77–95)	Microcytosis	Iron deficiency, thalassaemia trait, chronic
		Inflammation (macrocytosis with folate or vitamin B_{12} deficiency, aplastic anaemia)
MCH 21 pg/RBC (normal range 23–31)	Hypochromia	Iron deficiency
MCHC 32 g Hb/dL RBC (normal range 30–36)	Normal	
WBC 8.5 × 10^9/L	Normal	
Platelets 230 × 10^9/L	Normal	
Blood film		
Anisocytosis, poikilocytosis	RBCs vary in size and shape	
Zinc protoporphyrin (ZPP)		
200 μmol/mol of haem (normal range 30–80)	High	Iron deficiency

Hb, haemoglobin; MCH, mean corpuscular haemoglobin; MCV, mean corpuscular volume; RBC, red blood cell count; WBC, white blood cell count.

- Poor weight gain associated with inadequate calorie intake as a result of excessive consumption of milk and juice
- Iron deficiency anaemia associated with inadequate dietary intake of iron

Toddler diarrhoea (chronic non-specific diarrhoea) – a snapshot

- The most frequent cause of chronic diarrhoea in preschool children in developed countries
- Usual age 6 months to 2 years
- More common in boys than in girls
- Associated with a diet low in fat and a high fluid intake (fruit juices) rich in carbohydrate (i.e. high osmolality)
- Rapid transit, especially through colon
- Absorption of nutrients intact leading to normal growth, provided that dietary intake is adequate

- Intermittent diarrhoea:
  - varies from a few mushy to 6–10 watery stools a day
  - unusual at night
  - forcefully expelled, foul (but not like steatorrhoea)
  - contains undigested vegetable matter (thus 'the peas and carrots syndrome')
- Family history of irritable bowel syndrome

Management and follow-up

The management of toddler diarrhoea requires:

- Reassurance to parents
- Normalization of the diet according to the 'four Fs': limited fluid and fruit juice (to reduce dietary osmolality), more fibre and fat (fat retards GI motility)

Reassurance to Asim's parents

Asim's parents are informed about these and are reassured that:

- Toddler diarrhoea is not a serious GI tract disease
- Improvement is likely with appropriate changes in the diet

Advice from a paediatric dietician

Asim is referred and assessed by a paediatric dietician. Parents are advised to:

- Reduce his intake of fluids to a pint of milk a day, to meet his calcium requirements
- Reduce his intake of fruit, fizzy and sugary drinks to one beaker after each meal
- Encourage him to have set meals and snacks to meet his calorie and fibre requirements
- Include red meat, cereals (e.g. ReadyBrek) and pulses in his diet to meet his iron requirements

Oral iron

Asim is given an oral iron syrup until his Hb, ZPP and red cell indices return to normal.

Asim's progress

When Asim is reviewed in clinic after 6 weeks, his parents appear pleased with him. He is reported to have reduced stool frequency (three to four per day) but they are still loose at times. He has been eating better, has gained weight (now between the 10th and 25th centiles) and his height is following the 25th centile.

Background information (Figure 11.5)

Pathophysiology of diarrhoea (see Figure 11.3)

One or more of the following pathophysiological processes contribute to diarrhoea depending on the disease process and site involved, e.g. the diarrhoea in inflammatory bowel disease affecting the small intestine has osmotic, secretory and exudative components.

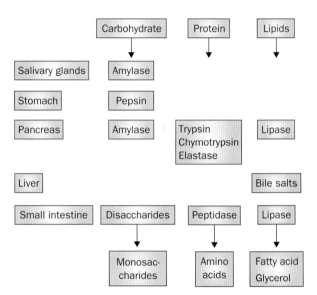

Figure 11.5 The enzymes involved in digesting macronutrients.

Osmotic diarrhoea (Figure 11.6)

Undigested carbohydrate creates an osmotic load. Water is passively drawn into the gut and fluid losses in the stool are increased. The diarrhoea characteristically stops when the patient is starved. Stools are also acidic (pH < 5.5) as lactic acid is released from bacterial fermentation of malabsorbed carbohydrate, for example, where there is:

- High carbohydrate feeding as in toddler diarrhoea
- Disease affecting the intestinal mucosa ('brush border') where disaccharidases (e.g. lactase) are located, as in coeliac disease, viral gastroenteritis, giardiasis, inflammatory bowel disease

The most common carbohydrate malabsorbed is lactose (lactose intolerance).

Common causes of secondary lactose intolerance

- Viral gastroenteritis
- Coeliac disease
- Giardiasis
- Cows' milk protein intolerance

Secretory diarrhoea (Figure 11.7)

Secretory diarrhoea results when fluid and electrolytes are secreted abnormally into the small intestine and

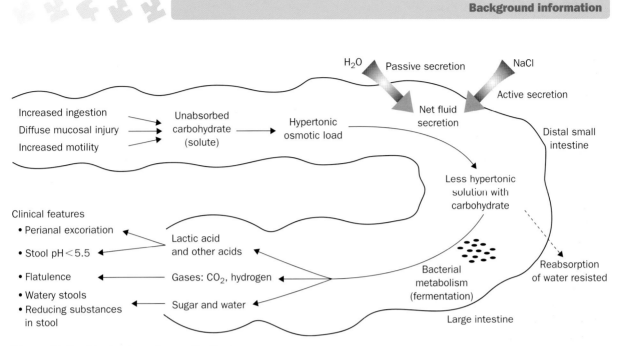

Figure 11.6 Mechanism of osmotic diarrhoea.

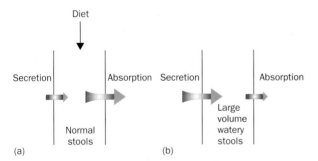

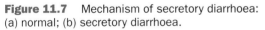

Figure 11.7 Mechanism of secretory diarrhoea: (a) normal; (b) secretory diarrhoea.

secretion exceeds absorption. It is characterized by profuse (large volume of) watery stools, which persist even when the patient is starved, for example, caused by:

- Bacterial toxin: cholera, some strains of *Escherichia coli*
- Villus destruction from inflammation
- Congenital chloridorrhoea, neuroblastoma

Inflammatory or exudative diarrhoea

Exudation of mucus, protein and blood occurs in inflammatory conditions. Stools typically contain mucus and blood, and may be watery as a result of secretory and osmotic components, e.g. inflammatory bowel disease

Motility disturbances

Rapid transit through the intestine, as in toddler diarrhoea, results in watery diarrhoea. Slow transit leads to stasis and bacterial overgrowth (e.g. stagnant loop or contaminated small bowel syndrome). As intestinal bacteria deconjugate bile salts and use vitamin B_{12} and folic acid, steatorrhoea and megaloblastic anaemia occur.

The classification of chronic diarrhoea according to site is as follows:

- **Proximal small intestine:**
  - giardiasis
  - postviral enteritis
- **Small intestine:**
  - coeliac disease
  - intestinal lymphangiectasia
  - short bowel syndrome
  - blind loop syndrome
- **Large intestine:**
  - inflammatory bowel disease
  - Hirschsprung's colitis

- **Pancreas:**
  - cystic fibrosis

Giardiasis – a snapshot

Oral–faecal transfer. *Giardia lamblia* is a protozoon that is endemic in Asia and parts of eastern Europe.

Presentation
Asymptomatic or present with:

- Watery diarrhoea (osmotic diarrhoea from lactose malabsorption)
- Steatorrhoea and weight loss caused by mucosal injury of the proximal small intestine

Investigations
See 'Investigations in a patient presenting with chronic diarrhoea'.

Treatment
Metronidazole is the treatment of choice.

Cows' milk protein intolerance – a snapshot

Onset is within the first 6 months of life. Hypersensitivity to cows' milk protein manifests as acute (within 45 minutes) or delayed reactions (more than 20 hours after ingestion).

Clinical features
- **Symptoms that:**
  - occur or are made worse after ingestion of cows' milk
  - improve within 1–14 days of withdrawing cows' milk from the diet
- **Gastrointestinal:** chronic diarrhoea, vomiting, poor weight gain
- **Skin:** urticarial rash, angio-oedema
- **Respiratory:** stridor (laryngeal spasm), cough, wheeze and difficulty breathing (bronchospasm)
- **History of atopy:** eczema, asthma or rhinitis

Investigations
Diagnosis is based on a thorough history and confirmation may require cows' milk exclusion for 2 weeks, followed by milk challenge.

Management
- A strict cows' milk-free diet supervised by a dietician
- Adequate intake of a cows' milk substitute to ensure that calcium requirements are met

Most patients have transient intolerance and are able to tolerate cows' milk by 3 years of age. Rechallenge with cows' milk should be undertaken in hospital after 12 months of age.

Cystic fibrosis – a snapshot (see Chapter 36)

Cystic fibrosis (CF) is the most common autosomal recessive disorder in the developed countries. The gene encodes a protein (called cystic fibrosis transmembrane conductance regulator or CFTR). Mutations (over 1000 mutations reported) in the gene affect chloride transport and are also likely to affect Na^+, HCO_3^- and other ions. The defect in ion transport affects all epithelial tissues, but mucus secretion is enhanced in some tissues and not in others.

Presentation
Neonatal screening for CF is currently undertaken only in a few regions in the UK. Children may present with symptoms at different ages.

Soon after birth Acute intestinal obstruction from meconium ileus (acutely ill, abdominal distension, bilious vomiting, failure to pass meconium).

In infancy and childhood
- Poor weight gain/failure to thrive associated with frequent offensive stools (90 per cent of affected children have pancreatic insufficiency)
- Recurrent productive cough ('chestiness' which may be misdiagnosed as virus infections or asthma)
- Purulent nasal discharge or obstruction associated with sinusitis or polyps (nasal polyps are rare in children except those with CF)
- Family history

Investigations
See 'Investigations in a patient presenting with chronic diarrhoea'.

Management
The aims of management are:

1 To provide support for patients and families (essential for any complex chronic disease)
2 Maintain nutrition with pancreatic enzyme supplements, high-calorie diet (fat is a high source of calories compared with carbohydrate and protein) and fat-soluble vitamin supplements
3 To prevent respiratory infections and lung damage with:
   – chest physiotherapy
   – oral antibiotics for prophylaxis against *Staphylococcus aureus*
   – antibiotics (oral, inhaled or intravenous) for treatment of bacterial respiratory tract infections

Inflammatory bowel disease – a snapshot

Incidence
Five per 100 000 children under 16 years of age in the UK.

Aetiology
Although not precisely known, an inappropriate immune response or breakdown of normal immuno-regulatory mechanisms is likely to contribute to the pathogenesis. The most important risk factor is a family history. The prevalence of Crohn's disease among first-degree relatives is 5–30 times higher than in the general population.

Clinical features
As any part of the gastrointestinal tract may be affected, clinical features vary with the extent of involvement. The colon, as well as the small intestine, is more likely to be involved in children than in adults.

Presentation
Presentation may be abrupt, insidious or ill defined and varies according to site and extent of GI involvement. Typical presentation is in late childhood or adolescence (10–14 years) with the triad of:

- Chronic diarrhoea (mucus and/or blood in the stools)
- Abdominal pain (periumbilical and colicky, worse after eating)
- Poor linear growth and weight loss

Growth failure may be the sole initial feature at presentation. The factors contributing to poor growth include:

- Reduced nutrient intake
- Avoiding meals to minimize symptoms (abdominal pain, bloating, diarrhoea)
- Anorexia from zinc deficiency
- Malabsorption
- Increased metabolic demands
- Corticosteroid treatment

Delayed puberty may be a feature in adolescence. Anorexia, vomiting, anaemia and unexplained fever are common.

Extraintestinal manifestations
- **Related to colonic disease activity:**
  - joints: clubbing, arthritis, ankylosing spondylitis, sacroiliitis
  - skin: erythema nodosum, pyoderma gangrenosum, psoriasis
  - eyes: uveitis, conjunctivitis, episcleritis
- **Related to small intestinal disease activity:**
  - malabsorption
  - liver: cholangitis, hepatitis
  - kidneys: stones, hydronephrosis, fistula
- **Non-specific:**
  - vascular disease processes

Investigations
Investigations are carried out to:

- Exclude other disorders
- Determine severity and clinical course
- Determine response to treatment

Screening laboratory tests
- Full blood count: iron deficiency or normocytic/normochromic anaemia, neutrophil leucocytosis, high platelet count
- Inflammatory markers raised: erythrocyte sedimentation rate (ESR), C-reactive protein (CRP), serum α_1-antitrypsin
- Low plasma albumin

Endoscopy and biopsy Helps to determine extent of involvement and to differentiate Crohn's disease from ulcerative colitis (Table 11.3).

Table 11.3 Differentiating Crohn's disease and ulcerative colitis

Measure	Crohn's disease	Ulcerative colitis
Incidence	Twice that of ulcerative colitis	
Rectal bleeding	Less common	Common and associated with tenesmus
Involvement	Segmental	Not segmental
	Rectum often spared	Diffuse confluent inflammatory process begins at anorectal margin and extends proximally
Radiology		
● Granular mucosa	Absent	Present
● Continuity	Discontinuous	Continuous
● Symmetrical involvement	Absent	Present
● Terminal ileum	Usually involved	Usually normal
● Rectum	Occasional ulcers	Most often involved
● Mucosal ulceration	On normal mucosa	On granular mucosa
Histology	Non-caseating granuloma is pathognomonic	Inflammation confined to mucosa and submucosa with loss of normal crypt architecture and presence of crypt abscesses
	Transmural disease	Friable granular mucosa
		Normal vascular pattern of the mucosa is lost

Radiological, to assess extent of involvement

● **Barium meal and follow-through:** signs in the small intestine include thickened mucosa (oedema), granular mucosal pattern, dilated and narrow segments, narrowing of terminal ileum, increased peristalsis

● **Barium enema:** findings typical of ulcerative colitis include loss of haustral markings, irregular mucosal pattern and marginal ulceration. Thumbprinting of the mucosa and toxic dilatation may be present in severe colitis. The findings in Crohn's disease include diffusely narrowed colon and asymmetrical loss of haustral pattern

Management

The aim of treatment is to induce remission and relieve symptoms. Treatment involves:

● Support for patients and families
● Acetylsalicylate, corticosteroids (oral or rectal) and other immunosuppressant drugs
● Nutritional support with enteral feeding or total parenteral nutrition
● Surgical resection for localized lesions

Further sources of information

Articles

Branski D, Lerner A, Lebenthal E. Chronic diarrhoea and malabsorption. *Pediatric Clinics of North America* 1996; **43**: 307–31.

Hoekstra JH. Toddler diarrhoea: more a nutritional disorder than a disease. *Archives of Disease in Childhood* 1998; **79**: 2–5.

Hyams JS. Crohn's disease in children. *Pediatric Clinics of North America* 1996; **43**: 255–77.

Kirschner BS. Ulcerative colitis in children. *Pediatric Clinics of North America* 1996; **43**: 235–54.

Mäki M, Collin P. Coeliac disease. *The Lancet* 1997; **349**: 1755–9.

Self-test 6: Can you think of another explanation for Asim's anaemia in the context of his ethnic origin and consanguinity?

Answer: Thalassaemia trait.

Self-test 7: Eddie is a 2-year-old with a history of:
- Five to eight smelly greasy stools per day, which are difficult to flush, since his first birthday
- Tummy getting bloated 'like a football'
- Eats 'everything' and usually has a good appetite
- A cough with yellow–green phlegm for the past year

His mother had initially been told that Eddie had 'toddler diarrhoea' and 'asthma'. The notable findings on examination are pallor, mild generalized oedema, clubbing, weight on the 10th centile and height on the 75th centile. He is diagnosed to have cystic fibrosis from the sweat test. Which of the following are the most likely explanations for his clinical features?

A Abdominal distension is caused by ascites
B Generous appetite is the result of malabsorption
C Productive cough is the result of coexisting asthma
D Pallor is caused by iron deficiency anaemia
E Mild generalized oedema results from hypoalbuminaemia

Answer: True: B and E.
A Abdominal distension is caused by bloating of intestine with fluid and gas
C Eddie has clubbing and the productive cough is most likely to be the result of cystic fibrosis lung disease
D Anaemia in cystic fibrosis tends to be macrocytic with acanthocytes and associated with vitamin E deficiency (not absorbed because it is fat soluble)

CHAPTER

12

Community

A boy with poor language
and hearing problems

Age: 2½ years

JACKIE GREGG

In this chapter, the histories obtained led the paediatrician down two separate paths – case 1 and case 2.

Presentation

Referral letter from GP:

Please could you see this 2½-year-old boy whose parents are concerned about his speech. David is a healthy boy and otherwise appears to be developing normally. His parents are becoming increasingly concerned that his language is not progressing. At times they think he is in a world of his own and wonder if he has a hearing problem. He has had two ear infections and had two courses of antibiotics. I've therefore referred him to the ENT clinic.

David had bacterial meningitis at 18 months of age. He was admitted to hospital for a week and treated with antibiotics.

Self-test 1: Is there any significance in the history of meningitis?

Answer: Yes. Meningitis can cause sensorineural hearing loss. All children should have a hearing assessment after they have recovered from the infection.

Initial considerations and action

Parental concern about delay in speech is common. The principal conditions, which need to be considered in a child presenting with language delay, are:

- Global developmental delay, i.e. delay in all aspects of development. Parents of young children usually focus on development of motor skills and may not recognize that cognitive skills are delayed. Referral is usually prompted when the child isn't saying as much as his or her peers
- Hearing impairment: it is essential that this be considered in all children who have language delay
- Environmental and emotional deprivation: language development is fairly robust, but children from families where there is less spoken language may be slower to acquire speech. Children who have experienced severe deprivation are at risk of language delay as well as delay in other skills, but usually catch up as soon as they are placed in a more stimulating environment
- Elective mutism or selective mutism: in this condition the child does not talk in certain selected situations, most commonly at school or nursery
- Autistic spectrum disorder (ASD): children may present in many ways, but often with delay/loss of speech, concerns about possible deafness or behaviour problems
- Specific language disorder/impairment: a significant discrepancy between language development and non-verbal skills. This may affect expressive language or both expressive and receptive language. Language impairments are more common in boys. There is a strong genetic component. Some dysmorphic syndromes are linked with language impairments

- Normal variation: there is a wide degree of variation in the rate of language acquisition

The letter from the GP refers to normal early development but doesn't give details of David's play and social skills, which would help to clarify whether this is a general delay, a specific language disorder or an ASD. The referrer indicates concerns about possible hearing impairment – meningitis is a risk factor. It will be important to clarify whether there has been a loss of other skills, which would suggest a degenerative condition such as a metabolic disorder, or a neoplasm.

Self-test 2: What are the three key areas of difficulty in autistic spectrum disorder?

Answer: Social interaction, social communication and imagination.

A clinic appointment with the community paediatrician is arranged for 4 weeks' time.

History: case 1

In the clinic the paediatrician obtains further details from David's parents.

David was born at term following a planned and normal pregnancy. David's mother had been in good health, hadn't required any medication and had taken only occasional alcohol. His birth weight was 3.7 kg, he had no neonatal problems and was breast-fed for 9 months. He is fully immunized.

Previous illnesses

David has had two ear infections, tends to be catarrhal and sometimes snores. He had bacterial meningitis at 18 months of age. His mum thought that it had been 'caught early' because he seemed to improve quickly once antibiotics were started. His parents were not clear whether or not a referral to audiology had been mentioned. They hadn't received an appointment, but they had moved house shortly after David's discharge.

Development

There were no parental concerns about early developmental milestones. David had always been a vocal child, babbling tunefully from about 8 months of age. He passed the routine hearing assessment at 8 months.

Self-test 3: What is the routine hearing assessment at 8 months?

Answer: The health visitor distraction test is used as a screening tool at 8–9 months in some areas. In other areas, surveillance methods such as a hearing questionnaire have replaced the health visitor distraction test.

By 13 months David was walking and enjoyed peek-a-boo games and was described as very sociable. Just before he developed meningitis he was saying about 15 words and carrying out simple verbal commands. Since the meningitis he has gradually stopped using words. He is not responding to speech or his name and his parents do not think that he can hear anything but very loud noises. He enjoys playing with his siblings and likes to pretend to feed and care for his teddies; however, he is becoming increasingly frustrated and irritable because of his communication difficulties.

Family history

Nil of note. Both parents are teachers and mum works part-time. David is cared for by his grandmother. David is the youngest of three children – his two older siblings are at infant school and making good progress.

Interpretation of the history

David's parents have given a history of concerns about delay in language and hearing impairment. There are a number of important areas that need to be addressed:

- Developmental milestones, including auditory and language development
- Factors predisposing to hearing loss
- Social skills and behaviour
- Family history

Meaning of the history in David

Developmental milestones

David had normal early developmental milestones. Table 12.1 outlines the early development of hearing, listening and language:

- Hearing is the reception of sound by the ear and its transmission to the central nervous system
- Listening is paying attention to what is heard with the object of interpreting its meaning

Global developmental delay could explain a lack of or delayed response to sound; however, the history of normal play suggests that David's non-verbal ability is age appropriate.

Table 12.1 Early development of hearing, listening and language

Birth	Startles and blinks at sudden noise
4–6 weeks	Turns head to nearby speaker, coos
8–10 weeks	Attends to meaningful sounds (e.g. spoon in a cup)
4–7 months	Consistently turns to voice and sounds, frequent vocalizations
8–12 months	Tuneful babble, imitates adult playful sounds
	Listens attentively, responds to own name
12 months	May respond to familiar words such as 'bye bye' and 'no', may use one or two words with meaning
18 months	Responds to one key word, e.g. 'where's your *nose*?'
	Uses 8–10 words
2 years	Joining two to three words together
	Responds to two key words
2½ years	Knows full name, sex
3 years	Constantly asking questions, using short sentences

Factors predisposing to hearing loss

Early normal speech development and apparently normal hearing at 8 months indicate that a congenital hearing loss is unlikely, although some forms of genetic hearing loss may not develop until later. Routine surveillance of hearing is carried out as part of the programme of child health promotion within primary care. Parents are asked about their child's responses to sound and are referred for audiological assessment if concerns are identified. The health visitor distraction test is used as a screening tool at 8–9 months in some areas. In other areas, surveillance methods such as a hearing questionnaire have replaced the health visitor distraction test. Neonatal screening is becoming increasingly available, but this will miss deafness in children who have acquired or late-onset deafness. Mum had a normal pregnancy with no suggestion of infection, such as rubella or cytomegalovirus (CMV), which are recognized causes of hearing loss. David did not have a hearing assessment after the meningitis illness and he may therefore have an acquired sensorineural hearing loss secondary to meningitis. There may also be a fluctuating conductive loss in view of the history of catarrh, but this on its own would be unlikely to account for the loss of speech.

Social skills and behaviour

Children with an ASD may at first appear to be deaf. David's frustration suggests that he wants to communicate and this, linked with his sociability, makes an ASD unlikely.

Family history

Fifty per cent of congenital hearing loss is genetic and a careful family history of hearing impairment and conditions associated with hearing impairment is essential.

Examination: case 1

- Normal growth
- Normal physical examination
- Eardrums slightly pink and retracted
- No response when spoken to unless given visual cues; no response to other sounds

Self-test 4: Which type of hearing test will the audiologist perform on a child of this age?

Answer: This is a difficult age. The child may be able to manage a performance test where he or she has to make a specific response every time he or she hears a sound. The McCormack Toy Speech Discrimination test may be easier to perform. The child is required to point to a named toy to indicate that he or she has heard.

David had been rather anxious about coming into the examination room and looked to his parents for reassurance. They responded by smiling at him and showing him familiar toys. He soon started to play with the toy teaset and pretended to feed a teddy. During the examination, David said a few words, didn't respond to any verbal instructions, but did respond to gesture.

Interpretation of the examination

- The paediatrician has confirmed the parents' reports of age-appropriate play and normal social interaction
- David didn't respond to any sound at all during the examination, which raises concerns that he has significant hearing loss
- The pink and retracted eardrums suggest that David has a degree of glue ear
- David relates well to his parents and they appear to be intuitive to his needs. Environmental or emotional deprivation seems highly unlikely

Differential diagnosis

The most likely diagnosis is acquired sensorineural hearing loss secondary to meningitis. A receptive language disorder is much less likely.

Investigations: case 1

David requires urgent diagnostic hearing assessment and is referred to the specialist paediatric audiology service. Assessing hearing reliably in young children is difficult unless carried out by experienced professionals. Optimal conditions are also necessary – there is

Table 12.2 Tests of hearing and auditory function

Age	Test
Birth–6 months	Behavioural observation
6–18 months	Distraction test
18 months–2½ years	Cooperative tests
	Visual reinforcement audiometry
2½–4 years	Performance testing
	Speech discrimination (toy) test
4 years +	Audiometry
All ages	Otoacoustic emissions[a]
	Brain-stem-evoked potentials[b]

[a]Measure of cochlear function.
[b]Measure of pathways up to brain-stem level.

little point trying to test hearing in a busy clinic on a main bus route.

Table 12.2 shows the assessment methods, which can be used at different ages. Which one can be successfully used will depend on the developmental stage of the child. The audiologist carried out a performance test (Figure 12.1). David demonstrated responses to very loud levels of sound only, following which brain stem-evoked potentials were carried out. The brain stem-evoked potentials show a profound hearing loss.

How to interpret an audiogram

- Audiometry is the standard method of accurately recording hearing. An audiometer generates pure tones, each having a single fixed frequency and known intensity. The sounds are fed to each ear via headphones and the individual is asked to indicate when the sound is heard. The results are plotted graphically as an audiogram. At each frequency, the quietest sounds heard by the individual are recorded (Figure 12.2)
- Frequency of a soundwave is measured in hertz (Hz). The human ear is able to perceive frequencies of between 16 Hz and 20 000 Hz; however, the range important for speech is

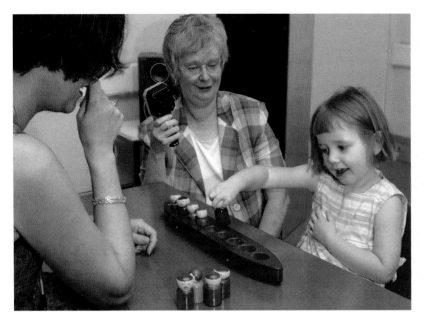

Figure 12.1 Hearing assessment using a performance test – when the child hears the sounds produced by the hand-held device, she puts the figure in the boat, indicating that she has heard.

250–4000 Hz. The frequency is plotted along the horizontal axis of the audiogram
- Intensity of a soundwave refers to the transmission of sound energy. Intensity is measured on a logarithmic scale in decibels (dB), and is plotted along the vertical axis on the audiogram. The audibility threshold (0 dB) is the intensity of the softest sound audible to the average person. Intensity of everyday experiences:
  - a whisper: 20–30 dB
  - background noise in an average home: 40–50 dB
  - conversational voice: 60 dB
  - a shout: 105–110 dB
  - low-flying aircraft: 110–120 dB
  - heavy machinery: 120–140 dB
  - the pain threshold: 140 dB.

The audiogram of a child with normal hearing and with a profound bilateral sensorineural hearing loss is shown in Figure 12.3.

Diagnosis: case 1

Sensorineural hearing loss secondary to meningitis.

Treatment and follow-up plan: case 1

The significance of the hearing loss and its management needs to be explained to the parents. Sensorineural hearing loss is permanent. Hearing aids do not restore normal hearing. The main reason for provision of a hearing aid is to allow the child access to the speech spectrum. For some children with severe or profound losses, this may not be possible even with the most powerful hearing aid. For these children the use of cochlear implants will be considered.

Hearing aid use requires careful supervision and parents need education in their use. Some children accept hearing aid use straight away; for others, it may take some time to achieve regular use.

Significant hearing loss can affect all aspects of a child's functioning, including development and behaviour, and lead to specific educational requirements. From the time of diagnosis an advisory teacher for hearing-impaired children will visit David and his family. A multidisciplinary approach is essential, with input from the advisory teacher for hearing impairment, the educational psychologist, speech and language therapist, paediatric audiologist and clinical psychologist.

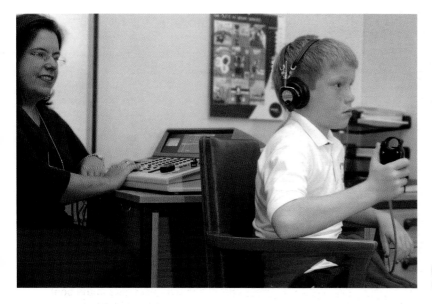

Figure 12.2 Hearing assessment using pure-tone audiometry.

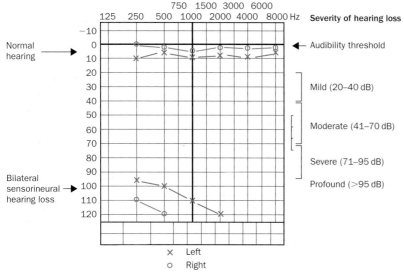

Figure 12.3 Audiogram showing normal hearing and profound bilateral sensorineural hearing loss.

Prognosis

David's hearing loss is acquired. He was known to be developing normally, has experienced everyday sounds and had started to acquire speech. Provided that David can have adequate amplification, he is likely to acquire speech. Increasingly most hearing-impaired children are educated in mainstream school with support. For many children, sign language is useful in the early stages to allow them to communicate with their families. This does not adversely affect their ability to develop spoken language.

Background information: case 1

Anatomy

The ear may be divided into:

- **The external ear** – auricle and external auditory meatus
- **The middle ear or tympanic cavity** – an air-filled cavity in the petrous part of the temporal bone, containing the auditory ossicles (malleus, incus and stapes)
- **The internal ear or labyrinth** – medial to the middle ear, consisting of the bony labyrinth (which includes the cochlea) in which the membranous labyrinth is lodged. The spiral organ of Corti, which contains the sensory receptors for hearing, is situated within the cochlea

Pathophysiology

The ear converts sound waves in the external environment into action potentials in the auditory nerves. The waves are transformed by the eardrum and auditory ossicles into movements of the footplate of the stapes. These movements set up waves in the fluid of the inner ear. The action of the waves on the organ of Corti generates action potentials in the nerve fibres. Clinical hearing impairment may result from impaired sound transmission in the external or middle ear (conductive deafness) or from damage to the cochlea or the neural pathways (nerve or sensorineural deafness).

Epidemiology

Sensorineural hearing loss is uncommon – 1–2 per 1000 live births and 1 in 100 in extremely low-birthweight infants. Enquiring about family history is very important, because 50 per cent of congenital hearing loss is genetic. Hearing loss is often present at birth. However, 16 per cent of permanent childhood hearing impairment is not present at birth. This group includes acquired hearing loss and genetic loss that is progressive or of later onset. Evidence of normal hearing and/or language development in the early months or years does not exclude genetic deafness.

The loss of hearing is the result of abnormalities of or damage to the cochlea, auditory nerve and/or higher pathways. The hearing loss can be of any severity, including profound. Children with severe-to-profound hearing loss may require special education. Children with sensorineural hearing loss may also have an added conductive element to their deafness.

Conductive hearing loss from middle-ear disease can be up to 60 dB. It is very common and may occur in 5–10 per cent of the total population. Many children have episodes of hearing loss, which are self-limiting in association with upper respiratory tract infections. Some children can suffer from prolonged loss. Conductive loss is often acquired in the first few years of life and may be recurrent. Passive smoking is a recognized risk factor and children with Down's syndrome, cleft palate and atopy are particularly prone to middle-ear disease.

Any concern about hearing loss should be taken seriously. A child with delayed language or speech, learning difficulties or behavioural problems should have his or her hearing tested, because a mild hearing loss can be the underlying cause or exacerbating factor.

Aetiology

The causes of hearing loss are listed in Table 12.3.

Table 12.3   Causes of hearing loss

Sensorineural	Conductive
Genetic	Wax (rarely)
Perinatal	Otitis media with effusion (glue ear)
Congenital infection	Foreign body
Pre-term birth	
Birth asphyxia	
Hyperbilirubinaemia	
Postnatal	
Meningitis/encephalitis	
Head injury	
Drugs, e.g. aminoglycosides	

In the clinic the paediatrician obtains further details from David's parents.

David was born at term following a planned and normal pregnancy. David's mother had been in good health, hadn't required any medication and had taken only occasional alcohol. His birth weight was 3.7 kg, he had no neonatal problems and was breast fed for 9 months. He is fully immunized including MMR (measles/mumps/rubella).

Previous illnesses

David has had two ear infections, tends to be catarrhal and sometimes snores. He had bacterial meningitis at 18 months of age. He had his hearing assessed in the audiology department following discharge and it was found to be normal. No history suggestive of epileptic seizures.

Development

No parental concerns about early developmental milestones. David was described as a very good and undemanding baby and toddler. He passed the routine hearing assessment at 8 months of age. By 13 months David was walking and had started to say one or two words. However, he didn't seem to take much notice of other children, apart from playing chase with his siblings. By 2 years David used words extremely rarely. If he did use a word, it might not be repeated for weeks, but at times he could be heard singing a nursery rhyme or repeating chunks from his favourite video. He didn't respond to his name but occasionally would surprise his parents by responding to a verbal instruction – they thought he probably understood more than he let on. At one stage, David's parents thought that he might be deaf, but as he responded to some words and seemed to be hypersensitive to sounds such as the vacuum cleaner and washing machine, they no longer thought that this was a possibility. David likes to spend his time either watching his favourite video or doing jigsaws. He doesn't show any interest in playing with small figures, train sets or cars, apart from spinning the wheels.

Self-test 5: Is David's language typical of a 2½ year old?

Answer: No. A child of this age should have a vocabulary of over 100 words and be linking three and four words together to make short sentences. Children should be responding to commands with two to three key words.

Family history

A maternal male cousin was initially somewhat slow with language development. He attended mainstream school, but tends to be a bit of a loner.

Interpretation of the history

There are a number of important areas, which need to be explored in a child with a communication difficulty and atypical behaviours:

- Possible regression
- Social skills
- Receptive and expressive language and social use of language
- Non-verbal skills
- Behaviour
- Family history

Meaning of the history in David

Possible regression

Apart from not saying as much as he used to, David has shown no loss or regression of other skills, thus reducing the likelihood of a degenerative neurological condition.

Social skills

The early description of David being an undemanding baby suggests that, even at that early stage, he may have had little interest in social interaction. This continued with little interest in other children. Parents may interpret limited eye contact and solitary play as being shy and 'wanting to do their own thing'.

Receptive and expressive language and social use of language

David's language is very delayed. By 2½ years, children should be using lots of single words, joining three words together and relating two ideas such as 'Put the … in the …'. Repeating chunks from a video can falsely reassure families that language is progressing normally; however, when its use is analysed it is apparent that it is meaningless.

Non-verbal skills

David's imaginative or symbolic play is delayed, which is an indicator of developmental delay. However, the play is very limited and repetitive (watching videos and doing jigsaws) which is atypical of globally delayed children who would demonstrate a range of play appropriate to their developmental level. First-time parents often do not know what to expect and may interpret repetitive and basic play that may be seen in the ASD as normal.

Behaviour

David's apparent hypersensitivity to certain everyday sounds is somewhat unusual and is a feature not uncommonly seen in children with ASD.

Family history

The family history of a relative who showed language delay and is now a loner is of interest because genetic factors in ASD and language disorder are becoming increasingly recognized.

Examination: case 2

A key part of the examination apart from looking at David's general well-being is to search for a possible cause of his difficulties. Conditions such as fragile X syndrome, tuberous sclerosis, neurofibromatosis, phenylketonuria, Angelman's and Down's syndromes are linked with ASD.

David is appropriately grown with a normal head circumference, normal neurological system and his gross motor development is age appropriate. There are no skin findings to indicate tuberous sclerosis or neurofibromatosis. There are no dysmorphic signs that may be linked with developmental delay or an indication of a chromosomal defect or other syndrome.

David had been reluctant to come into the examination room and was carried in screaming. However, he quickly settled down and sat on the floor, taking an interest in the toy teaset, and repeatedly lining all the objects up. He amused himself for about 30 minutes and didn't make any demands on his parents. He ignored the examining doctor when he tried to engage him in play and turned away from him. He did not appear to respond to any spoken language until his mother said it was time to go home when he approached the paediatrician, kissed him and ran to the door. His mum commented that he always kissed adults when going home.

Interpretation of the examination: case 2

Many 2-year-olds are initially reluctant to enter the consulting room and may be somewhat shy at first. However, they soon relax and start to explore the toys while looking to their parents for reassurance. They can be wary at first of the doctor, looking at him from the comfort of a parent's knee, but may eventually approach him or her to show him or her things of interest. Children of this age have a short attention span and usually need some input from an adult to direct them to another activity. It is therefore unusual that David played for such a long time without any reference to his parents. Similarly, toddlers love to share things of interest with their parents.

David demonstrated unusual behaviours of ignoring the paediatrician, paying little attention to his parents and lining objects up rather than playing with them appropriately. Kissing the paediatrician on departure may seem quite sweet; however, it is socially inappropriate and reflects a repetitive behaviour carried out without regard to the social setting.

Differential diagnosis

Global developmental delay and a specific language disorder are possibilities; however, the associated behaviours such as the poor social interaction, limited play and unusual use of language make it much more likely that David has an ASD.

Investigations: case 2

The paediatrician explains that David has difficulties with social use of language and social interaction, which requires further detailed assessment. He discusses the differential diagnoses of autism and specific language disorder and provides the family with written information. By this stage many parents will have already asked 'is he autistic?'. The paediatrician refers David for the following investigations and assessments:

1 Hearing assessment
2 Detailed developmental history and medical assessment by a developmental paediatrician and/or paediatric neurologist with an interest in autism
3 Speech, language and communication assessment by a speech and language therapist
4 Cognitive assessment by educational psychologist and preschool teacher
5 Medical investigations will depend on the results of the assessment and medical findings. The yield of investigations in children with autism who have good cognitive ability is extremely low, but the developmental paediatrician would generally arrange chromosomal analysis, including fragile X syndrome, and an examination of the skin under Wood's light. (This transmits ultraviolet light under which depigmented patches, as seen in tuberous sclerosis, fluoresce.) The greater the degree of cognitive impairment, the greater the likelihood of finding an associated medical condition. Further investigations may include magnetic resonance imaging (MRI) of the brain, measurement of organic and amino acids, thyroid function tests (TFTs), creatine phosphokinase (CPK) and liver function tests (LFTs) (see Chapter 7). An EEG should be considered if there were suspicions of fits

Ideally (2), (3) and (4) should be carried out by a multiagency team experienced in assessing children presenting with social and communication difficulties and suspected ASD.

Results

- **Hearing:** normal
- **Language:** single word understanding, uses single words to ask for things he wants but impossible to assess further

- **Social use of language:** 'chunking' of excerpts from books and videos and used at inappropriate times; only uses words appropriately to get things he wants
- **Cognitive ability:** probably within average range
- **Play:** repetitive with delay in imagination
- **Medical assessment:** normal examination
- **Medical investigations:** normal chromosomes and CPK, normal examination of the skin

Diagnosis: case 2

Autistic spectrum disorder.

Treatment and follow-up plan: case 2

The developmental paediatrician meets with the family to feed back the conclusions from the assessments and discuss the diagnosis of autism. As David's family had been very much part of the assessments, the diagnosis didn't come as a surprise, although this didn't lessen the shock or distress. It is important that as much information as possible can be given to families and David's parents are given the contact number for the National Autistic Society (NAS) and a local parent support group. They are given information about a local programme for parents that teaches them about ASD, and gives them strategies to improve their child's communication and to manage behaviour.

Communication therapy

David needs ongoing intervention from a speech and language therapist experienced in autism to promote his communication and understanding of the world around him. Generally, visual skills are much better than verbal skills and pictures can be used to aid communication – the Picture Exchange Communication System (PECS) is widely used (Figure 12.4).

Behavioural management

There are many behavioural approaches that are claimed to have a considerable impact on autistic features; however, for most there is no evidence base to support such claims. Standard behavioural interventions, if

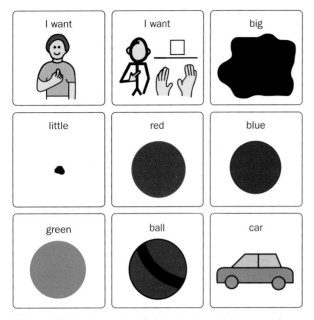

Figure 12.4 Example of pictures to assist expressive communication. The individual symbols can be arranged to make a sentence, e.g. 'I want the big blue car'.

intensive enough, can reduce difficult and repetitive behaviours, which may result in the child being more able to cope in a mainstream school. It is not clear at the moment how many hours of intervention are required to be 'intensive enough'. Families need access to experienced psychologists to help manage challenging behaviours, should they arise.

Medical review

Individuals with autism may have a very restricted diet, which is part of their rigidity. In such cases it is important to monitor growth with advice from a dietician if required. There is an increased incidence of epilepsy, with onset usually in the teenage years.

Education

The autistic spectrum covers a wide range of cognitive ability and of social and communication difficulties, so a spectrum of educational provision is necessary. The needs of some children can be met in mainstream with specialist advice and support. Others may need to be in a small group for teaching but within a mainstream setting, whereas others may need to attend a school for children with learning difficulties or even a specialist school for children with autism.

Alternative therapies

At present there is no cure for autism. Conventional therapy is limited and families therefore search for other interventions, which may help. Various drug therapies have been tried and at present gluten-free and milk-free diets are fashionable. There is no evidence for their effectiveness and randomized controlled trials are at present being carried out in the UK and the USA.

MMR

There is considerable concern among many parents about links between the MMR vaccine and autism, even though there is no scientific evidence to support it. This isn't an issue with David's parents.

Prognosis

This will depend on the individual's underlying cognitive ability and the 'severity' of the autism. Children with autism and severe learning difficulties will be unlikely to live independently, whereas individuals with Asperger's syndrome are much more likely to become independent with the possibility of employment.

How to advise parents about the MMR vaccine

- Acknowledge recent adverse publicity. Explore what the parents understand by vaccine causing autism, ask about personal experience of autism, mention that autism is commonly diagnosed after 18 months of age
- Discuss the lack of evidence linking MMR vaccine and autism – provide supporting evidence, e.g. health promotion literature, review and original articles from peer-reviewed journals (if appropriate)

- Explain why the MMR vaccine is given to children twice, i.e. at 13 months and at preschool entry – to ensure that those who did not seroconvert after the first immunization (5–10 per cent) have another chance to be protected and to boost the antibodies of those who did
- Discuss the dangers of not immunizing – measles, mumps and rubella are contagious and can have serious complications:
  - measles – death, pneumonia, deafness, encephalitis
  - mumps – meningitis, pancreatitis, orchitis
  - rubella – congenital rubella with deafness, blindness, heart defects and brain damage
- Explain that there can be some minor side effects with the MMR vaccine – fever, rash, joint pain
- Check that there were no problems with the primary vaccines and no contraindication to MMR
- Single vaccines are not recommended. Explain why:
  - no evidence of benefit with single vaccines
  - requires three times more injections
  - child vulnerable to disease between immunizations
  - increased chance of incomplete immunization
- Do not be coercive

Background information: case 2

Autistic spectrum disorder

Autism was first described by Leo Kanner in 1943. A year later Hans Asperger described a closely similar condition; however, his paper wasn't translated into English until the 1980s. In 1979 Wing and Gould introduced the terminology 'triad of impairments' when, in a large-scale epidemiological study, they found that difficulties in forming social relationships were associated with profound difficulties in communication and imagination. This now forms the basis for diagnosis in systems such as the *International Classification of Diseases* (Table 12.4). The term 'autism' covers a spectrum of difficulties within the triad and a wide spectrum of intellectual ability – up to 75 per cent of individuals have additional learning disability. Asperger's syndrome

Table 12.4 The triad of impairments

Social interaction: difficulty with social relationships, e.g. appearing aloof and indifferent to other people

Social communication: difficulty with verbal and non-verbal communication, e.g. not really understanding the meaning of gestures, facial expressions or tone of voice

Imagination: difficulty in the development of play and imagination, e.g. having a limited range of imaginative activities, possibly copied and pursued rigidly and repetitively

In addition to the triad, repetitive behaviour patterns are a notable feature as is resistance to change in routine

is generally ascribed to individuals with autism who are of average or above-average intellectual ability with good surface language skills.

Epidemiology

The prevalence of ASD is 58 per 10 000 (Wing) and of Asperger's syndrome 30 per 10 000. There has been a considerable increase in prevalence over the past 30 years. This is partly explained by increased identification and awareness, and using the broader definition of ASD. Experts are divided about whether or not there is a true increase in prevalence.

Aetiology

Autism is a neurobiological disorder, but its exact cause is not known. Research shows that genetic factors are important. Autism tends to run in families: 3–5 per cent of siblings will also develop the condition, with 10–15 per cent developing other significant learning difficulties. Identical twins are more likely to develop autism than dizygotic twins, with a 60 per cent concordance. It has been suggested that there is a genetic predisposition to autism in over 90 per cent of cases, with between 3 and 10 genes involved. How this predisposition is translated into autism is not fully understood and there are probably multiple influences. Fragile X syndrome, tuberous sclerosis and phenylketonuria are genetically inherited conditions associated with autism. Other associations include epilepsy, rubella, herpes encephalitis, birth trauma and intrauterine exposure to sodium valproate.

What is actually going 'wrong' in the brain of individuals with ASD has not been proved. Various structural abnormalities have been described, including irregularities of the cerebellum and brain stem, but most brain scans are normal. Other important brain structures linked with autism are the limbic system and frontal lobes. There is evidence of irregularities in the functioning of neurotransmitters, in particular serotonin.

Autism is diagnosed according to its behavioural manifestations – the triad of impairments – and there are various psychological theories to explain the behaviours. No theory has fully addressed all the issues, but the theory of mind and central coherence theory have accounted for some of them.

Further sources of information

Books

Hall DMB, Hill PD. Hearing tests. *The Child with a Disability*. Oxford: Blackwell Science, 1996: 67–85

Hall DMB, Hill PD. Communication disorders. *The Child with a Disability*. Oxford: Blackwell Science, 1996: 173–209

World Health Organization. *International Classification of Mental and Behavioural Disorders: Clinical descriptions and diagnostic guidelines*, 10th edn (ICD-10). Geneva: WHO

Websites

www.oneworld.org/autism_uk/

National Autistic Society.

www.immunisation.org.uk

Health Promotion England and Department of Health website on immunization.

Self-test 6: Three-year-old Sophie is seen in clinic because she says only 10 words. She may point to a familiar object on request, but this is inconsistent. Sophie finds it difficult to mix at play group, but likes playing in the home corner with her sister at home.

A What are the important features in the history?

B What investigation would you arrange?

C What is the diagnosis?

D Which health professional would you involve?

Answer:

A Delay in expressive and receptive language, relates well to sister, age-appropriate play

B Hearing test

C Specific language disorder

D Speech and language therapist

A boy with a croupy cough and breathlessness

Age: 20 months

LEENA PATEL

Presentation

Sameer is 20 months old. After seeing him in the evening surgery, the GP advises the mother to take Sameer immediately to the hospital accident and emergency department (A&E.) Over the course of the evening Sameer's breathing has become very noisy and he appears to have increasing difficulty breathing. The staff in A&E can hear his stridor as soon as his mother walks in with him.

Self-test 1: Which four conditions will you immediately consider in a toddler presenting acutely with noisy breathing as a result of stridor?

Answers:

1 Epiglottitis – rare but a medical emergency
2 Bacterial laryngotracheobronchitis – uncommon but serious
3 Inhaled foreign body – uncommon but serious
4 Viral laryngotracheobronchitis – common and less serious

Other causes are shown in Figure 13.1.

Initial considerations and action

- Stridor is a sign of upper airway obstruction. It is usually a harsh, low- to medium-pitched whistling sound, but can vary in intensity and may be higher pitched and musical. It results from increased velocity and turbulence to airflow from obstruction in the larynx or trachea. The stridor is predominantly inspiratory when the obstruction is extrathoracic and in the larynx, because negative airway pressure during inspiration causes further narrowing at the site of obstruction (see Figure 9.1, p. 77). A stridor is not heard during expiration, when the high positive pressure below the obstruction distends the airway and widens the obstructed area. A prolonged expiratory stridor indicates intrathoracic airway obstruction (e.g. tracheomalacia, bronchomalacia, foreign body in trachea or bronchus, or tumour compressing trachea)

- Epiglottitis is a serious life-threatening condition. It is rare and there has been a significant reduction in the incidence since the introduction of routine immunization with the *Haemophilus influenzae* b vaccine. However, it must not be forgotten because cases still occur as a result of vaccine refusal or vaccine failure. It can rapidly progress to complete airway obstruction and respiratory arrest if not diagnosed and managed promptly. The most striking feature is a stridor without cough

- Viral laryngotracheobronchitis is common in children aged between 6 months and 3 years. It is a benign, self-limited disease but rarely upper airway obstruction may be severe. The presenting features are stridor, a barking cough, and hoarse voice or cry. Hoarseness indicates inflammation of the vocal cords. Croup is a term used to describe the combination of these symptoms and is not a diagnosis.

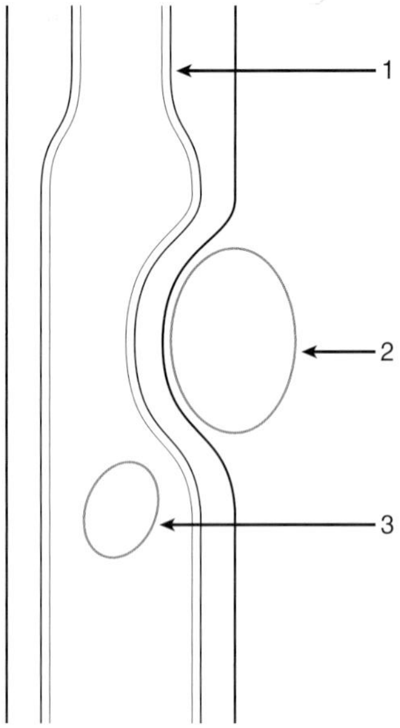

Site of pathology	Acute	Chronic/recurrent
1 In the mucosa and submucosa	Epiglottitis	Laryngomalacia
	Viral laryngotracheobronchitis	Atopic (spasmodic)
		Haemangioma
	Bacterial laryngotracheobronchitis	Congenital stenosis
		Acquired post-intubation stenosis
	Angio-oedema	
		Vocal cord palsy
2 Outside the wall	Enlarged lymph node	Vascular ring
	Retropharyngeal abscess	
3 In the lumen	Inhaled foreign body	Laryngeal web
	Diphtheria	Laryngeal papilloma
		Adenotonsillar hypertrophy

Figure 13.1 Causes of acute and chronic upper airway obstruction.

Immediate assessment of Sameer in A&E

As a result of the stridor and acute history of difficulty in breathing, Sameer is rapidly assessed for:

- Obvious signs of epiglottitis
- Severity of respiratory distress (see Chapter 9)

He is initially observed from a distance and approached cautiously to avoid upsetting him. Any action that upsets a child with epiglottitis or forcing the child to lie down can precipitate complete airway obstruction and respiratory arrest. Reassuringly, Sameer is alert, does not look seriously ill and is not drooling.

Children with epiglottitis prefer to sit upright with the chin up and mouth open and keep fairly still. This posture maximizes the size of the inlet to the upper airway. Sameer does not sit immobile in such a position but wriggles in his mother's lap and points to a toy in A&E that has grabbed his interest. The nurse gently proceeds with her observations and notes:

- Arterial oxygen saturation (Sao_2): 97 per cent
- Respiratory rate: 48/min
- Pulse: 170/min
- Ear temperature: 37.9°C, warm hands

Sameer is not thought to have epiglottitis and does not have severe respiratory distress. The senior house officer (SHO) now proceeds with the history and examination that will help with (1) further diagnosis and (2) assessing the severity of airway obstruction (Table 13.1).

Self-test 2: What sort of actions might upset a child with epiglottitis?

Answer: A stranger approaching suddenly, examining the child's throat, forcing the child to wear an oxygen mask, inserting an intravenous cannula or taking a lateral neck radiograph.

History

Important aspects of the history and examination in a child with acute stridor

- Onset acute over minutes, hours or days
- Precipitating event or condition and circumstances around it

Table 13.1 The clinical features of epiglottitis compared with viral laryngotracheobronchitis and bacterial laryngotracheitis

	Epiglottitis	Viral laryngotracheobronchitis	Bacterial tracheitis
Season	Throughout the year	Winter	Throughout the year
Most common age	2–6 years	6 months–3 years	6 months–12 years
Onset	Over hours	Over days	Over days
Preceding symptoms	None	Cold, runny nose, snuffles for a few days	
Stridor	Soft, muffled	Harsh, rasping	
Cough	Minimal or absent	Harsh, barking	Barking
Respiratory difficulty	Increases rapidly over a few hours	Gradual and worse at night	
Sore throat	Severe	No	Usually no
Drooling of saliva	Yes	No	No
Able to drink	No	Yes	Yes
Voice, cry	Muffled	Hoarse	Hoarse
Posture	Sits upright with chin raised and mouth open	Any posture	Any posture
Appearance	Seriously ill, toxic, poor peripheral perfusion	Unwell but not seriously ill	Seriously ill, toxic
Fever	High (>38.5°C)	Low (<38.5°C)	Usually high (>38.5°C)
Voice, cry	Muffled (throat sore)	Hoarse	

- Nature and course of stridor
- Associated symptoms:
  - choking
  - difficulty breathing
  - sore throat
  - refusal to swallow
  - unexplained drooling
  - hoarseness
  - cough
  - wheeze
  - high fever
- Past history of similar symptoms
- Allergies
- Immunizations

Mother's account

Sameer was snuffly and had a fever yesterday morning, which settled with paracetamol. He started with a barking cough and hoarseness in the morning. The cough was not too bad till this evening. His mother took Sameer to the GP in the evening because she was frightened by the awful noise that he made every time he took a breath. She thought he might suddenly stop breathing because he was struggling to breathe. His breathing got worse while she was waiting at the surgery. He has not had this sort of noisy breathing before.

His mother does not think that Sameer choked on anything. He has been eating and drinking but not as much as when he is well. He had one small vomit and one loose stool yesterday. He has not had any medicines other than paracetamol, has not had a rash and is not allergic to anything. He has had all his immunizations including the Hib and has been previously healthy. He has three siblings and there has been a cold going around in the family.

Interpretation of the history

- Sameer's history confirms that he does not have epiglottitis (Table 13.1)

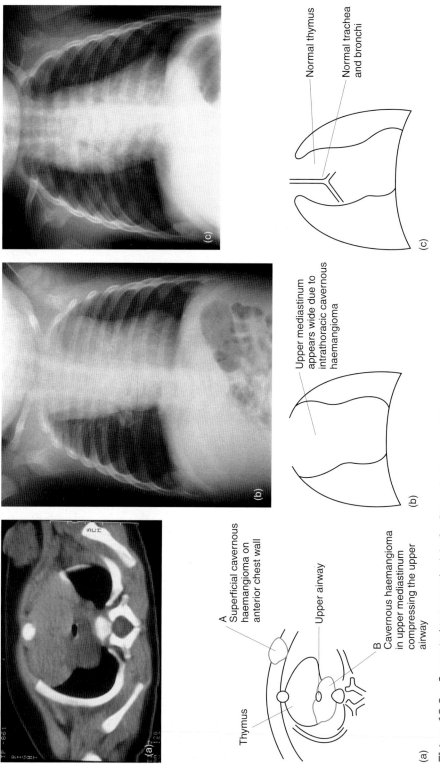

Figure 13.2 Computed tomography (a) of a 6-month-old baby with a cavernous haemangioma on the anterior chest (A) and also around the upper airway (B). The chest radiograph (b) showed mediastinal widening which differed in appearance from a normal thymus (c). (see Self-test 6). (Courtesy of Dr Julian Vyas.)

(a)

(b)

(c)

A
Superficial cavernous haemangioma on anterior chest wall

Upper airway

B
Cavernous haemangioma in upper mediastinum compressing the upper airway

Thymus

Upper mediastinum appears wide due to intrathoracic cavernous haemangioma

Normal thymus

Normal trachea and bronchi

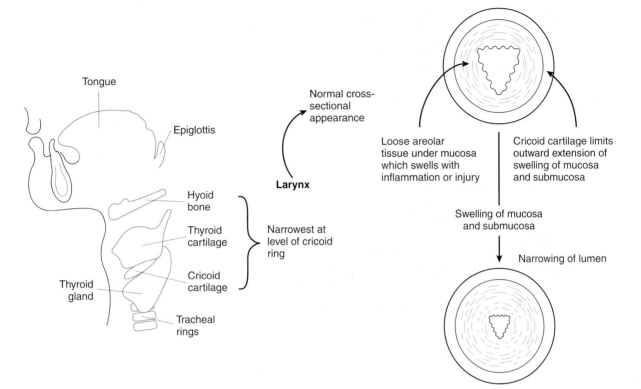

Figure 13.3 The larynx in infants and young children.

- The initial coryzal illness, vomiting, loose stool and family history of a cold suggest a viral infection
- The combination of barking cough, hoarseness and stridor, which gradually worsen in the evening, is typical of upper airway obstruction from acute viral laryngotracheobronchitis
- Bacterial laryngotracheitis is unusual in toddlers and a child with it would be expected to have a high fever
- Absence of drooling and the ability to drink exclude a severe sore throat, obstruction of the pharynx, difficulty in swallowing and dysphagia, as would be expected with epiglottitis or a retropharyngeal abscess
- Sameer has not had choking, rash or an allergy that might be expected with foreign body inhalation and laryngeal oedema associated with an acute allergic reaction
- A noisy stridor can be a frightening experience for parents, especially if it is perceived as a sign of respiratory failure

The absence of previous similar symptoms excludes the conditions associated with chronic upper airway obstruction (see Figure 13.1). Chronic upper airway obstruction is caused by:

- Congenital conditions (e.g. laryngomalacia, subglottic haemangioma, subglottic stenosis)
- Acquired conditions (e.g. prolonged intubation resulting from extreme prematurity, spasmodic croup with airway hyperreactivity)

With congenital conditions, the history reveals that the stridor started soon after birth (e.g. laryngomalacia) or within the first few weeks (e.g. subglottic haemangioma) (Figure 13.2). If the obstruction is mild, the child may first present acutely during a viral infection, when swelling of the upper airway lining causes significant narrowing (Figure 13.3). However, a careful history should reveal that parents have heard a mild stridor when the child is excited, crying or very active. It is important not to overlook this because a child with chronic airway obstruction, other than laryngomalacia, needs referral to an ear, nose and throat (ENT) surgeon for direct visualization of the airway.

Examination

Examination helps with:

- Immediate assessment of adequacy of airway, breathing and circulation
- Identifying the cause and site of airway obstruction:
  - general appearance: posture, mental state, colour
  - vital signs
  - mouth and pharynx provided that the child does not have epiglottitis
  - chest movements and auscultation

Further examination of Sameer, in addition to the initial observations, reveals the following:

- Good peripheral perfusion, capillary refill time less than 2 seconds
- Not drowsy, restless or agitated; fidgets a lot with his mother's bag and its contents
- No rash or swelling on the face, mouth or neck
- Wax in both ears
- Tonsils not enlarged, pharynx not congested, no bulge on the posterior pharyngeal wall
- No lymphadenopathy
- Stridor inspiratory and present even at rest
- Dry barking cough
- Intercostal recessions
- Chest auscultation: good air entry bilaterally, no crackles, no wheeze
- Heart sounds normal and no murmurs

Interpretation of the examination

The symptoms of bacterial laryngotracheitis resemble viral laryngotracheobronchitis but the major difference is that the child is usually older (school age), appears seriously unwell or toxic (no lethargy and poor peripheral perfusion) and has a high fever (>38.5°C) (see Table 13.1). Sameer's examination findings do not suggest bacterial tracheitis. Laryngeal oedema caused by an acute allergic reaction is also unlikely in the absence of a rash and angio-oedema of the face and mouth. There is no history of choking and no unilateral wheeze and/or reduced air entry to suggest an inhaled foreign body.

Only inspiratory stridor when a child is upset, crying or running around would suggest minor narrowing of the upper airway. Sameer has an inspiratory stridor even at rest and this indicates moderate obstruction. He is not likely to have severe obstruction of the larynx and obstruction of the trachea and bronchi because he does not have:

- An expiratory stridor or a wheeze
- Agitation
- Marked sternal and subcostal recessions
- Low Sao_2

Investigations

The diagnosis of viral laryngotracheobronchitis, epiglottitis and bacterial tracheitis is based on clinical features. Investigations are only necessary in the last two bacterial conditions to identify the pathogenic organism, i.e. culture of (1) airway secretions obtained at time of intubation and (2) blood.

Diagnosis

Sameer has viral laryngotracheobronchitis with moderately severe upper airway obstruction (Table 13.2). Mother is given an explanation about the diagnosis and reassured that Sameer is not likely to stop breathing suddenly.

Self-test 3: Match the clinical scenarios 1–7 with the most likely diagnosis.
A Bronchiolitis
B Asthma
C Virally induced wheezing
D Cystic fibrosis
E Immotile cilia syndrome
F Chronic lung disease of prematurity
G Viral laryngotracheobronchitis
H Epiglottitis
I Laryngomalacia

J   Inhaled foreign body

K   Tuberculosis

L   Agammaglobulinaemia

1   A previously well 18-month-old boy presents with a sudden onset of cough and wheeze. On examination wheeze is heard over the right lung

2   A 9-year-old boy has had a chronic cough for 6 weeks. His grandfather has had a chronic productive cough and haemoptysis. Sputum analysis shows organisms that stain positively with Ziehl–Neelsen staining

3   A 3-year-old girl presents with stridor at rest. She is drowsy and drooling

4   A 3-year-old girl has had recurrent purulent nasal discharge and ear infections. Her apex beat is on the right side of the chest

5   A 10-month-old boy has had a cold for 2 days and then develops a stridor and barking cough

6   A 3-month-old infant has had an intermittent stridor since the second day of life

7   A 3-month-old infant develops a cold and then has apnoea. Examination reveals hyperinflation and inspiratory crackles

Answers: 1J, 2K, 3H, 4E, 5G, 6I, 7A.

Management

Management is immediate treatment with cortico-steroids (Table 13.3). Budesonide and dexamethasone are equally effective in:

- Improving symptoms
- Shortening the time spent in hospital
- Reducing the need for additional intervention with nebulized adrenaline/epinephrine (5 ml 1:1000 adrenaline)

Dexamethasone can be given intramuscularly, but is likely to be unpleasant for the child. A single dose of budesonide or dexamethasone is usually sufficient to treat mild-to-moderate viral laryngotracheobronchitis. However, the dose can be repeated as necessary.

Management includes not upsetting the child because crying increases respiratory distress by increasing oxygen demand and may increase laryngeal oedema.

As a nebulizer as well as oral medication may upset a young child, Sameer's mother is asked which one of these she thinks he is most likely to tolerate. She thinks he will manage the oral medication and Sameer is given a dose of dexamethasone. Observations are continued in A&E.

Table 13.2   Severity of upper airway obstruction in viral laryngotracheobronchitis

Very mild	Inspiratory stridor on exertion (crying) but not at rest
Mild	Inspiratory stridor at rest but no intercostal recessions
Moderate	Inspiratory stridor at rest
	Intercostal recessions
Severe	Inspiratory and expiratory stridor
	Intercostal and suprasternal recessions
	Severe respiratory distress
	Hypoxia (restless, drowsy, irritable, impaired consciousness; cyanosis; bradycardia)

Table 13.3   Corticosteroid treatment for viral laryngotracheobronchitis

Preparation	Administration	Single dose	Comment
Budesonide	Nebulized	2 mg	Plasma half-life shorter than dexamethasone
Dexamethasone	Oral	0.15–0.6 mg/kg	Cheaper than budesonide
	Intravenous or intramuscular	0.6 mg/kg	

Observations and review in A&E

An hour later, mother thinks Sameer is better in that he is coughing less and struggling less with his breathing. He has continued to drink and observations confirm that there has been no deterioration. Sameer is admitted to the ward for observations because he still has an inspiratory stridor, tachypnoea, intercostal recessions and tachycardia. In addition, mother is anxious about taking him home (it is now 10 pm).

Progress overnight

The following morning, Sameer has improved markedly:

- No stridor and only the very occasional cough
- Afebrile
- Pulse and respiratory rate have come down (105/min and 26/min respectively), Sao_2 97 per cent in air
- No intercostal recession
- Chest clear on auscultation

His mother is pleased with him and no longer anxious.

Sameer is discharged and no follow-up is arranged. However, his mother is informed that:

- He may have a stridor as the day progresses, but it is not expected to be as severe as the previous evening
- He should be brought to A&E without delay if has difficulty breathing
- The cough may persist for as long as 2 weeks

Background information

The upper airway in infants and young children

The narrowest part of the upper airway is the subglottic region (see Figure 13.3, p. 133) and significant obstruction occurs even with mild inflammation.

Viral laryngotracheobronchitis – a snapshot

Incidence
- Three to five per cent in children aged 6 months to 6 years, with a peak in the second year of life

- More common in boys than in girls
- Occurs throughout the year, with a peak in autumn and winter

Cause
- Most common: parainfluenza virus types 1, 2 and 3
- Other: adenovirus, respiratory syncytial virus (RSV), rhinovirus, influenza A, enteroviruses
- The infection results in swelling of the glottic and subglottic region

Treatment
- As described above
- No proven benefit: mist therapy

Prognosis
- A self-limiting illness with symptoms most severe on the first and second nights
- Less than 2 per cent of children require admission to hospital

Complications
These are rare and include:

- Respiratory failure: of those admitted, only 0.5–1.5 per cent require intubation and ventilatory support; mortality is low
- Secondary bacterial infection leading to bacterial laryngotracheitis

Bacterial laryngotracheitis (pseudomembranous croup) – a snapshot

Uncommon but life threatening.

Cause
Infection with *Staphylococcus aureus*, streptococci and *Haemophilus influenzae* b results in inflammation, oedema and necrosis of the tracheal mucosa, and mucopurulent secretions.

Management
- Intubation, clearance of mucopurulent secretions (which may repeatedly block the airway) and mechanical ventilation: required in over 80 per cent of patients

- Intravenous antibiotics: flucloxacillin + cefotaxime in high doses until bacterial sensitivities are available

Epiglottitis – a snapshot

Uncommon but a true paediatric emergency.

Cause
Haemophilus influenzae type b results in a rapidly progressive cellulitis of the epiglottis and supraglottic region.

Management
- The priority is to secure the airway immediately. Intubation should be done by an experienced anaesthetist because the swollen epiglottis makes the procedure difficult. Most children can be extubated after 24–36 hours and full recovery is expected within 5 days
- Intravenous cefotaxime 30 mg/kg 8-hourly until bacterial sensitivities are available

Further sources of information

Book

Rothera MP, Woolford TJ. Identification and management of large airway disease in the first year of life. In: David TJ (ed). *Recent Advances in Paediatrics 15*. New York: Churchill Livingstone, 1997: 11–29

Articles

Ausejo M, Saenz A, Pham B, Kellner JD, Johnson DW, Moher D, Klassen TP. The effectiveness of glucocorticoids in treating croup: meta-analysis. *British Medical Journal* 1999; **319**: 595–600

Griffin S, Ellis S, Fitzgerald-Barron A, Rose J, Egger M. Nebulised steroid in the treatment of croup: a systematic review of randomised controlled trials. *British Journal of General Practice* 2000; **50**: 135–41

Self-test 4: How does the upper airway of infants and young children differ from that in adults?

Answer: In infants and young children:
- The tongue is relatively large in relation to the oropharynx and respiratory obstruction is more likely
- The epiglottis is softer, bulkier and floppier
- The larynx is situated higher in the neck (C3–4) and placed more anteriorly because the angle between the base of the tongue and the laryngeal inlet is decreased (at the C6 level in adults)
- The larynx is funnel shaped and narrowest at the level of the cricoid ring (cylindrical and narrowest at the level of the vocal cords in adults)
- The trachea is shorter and an endotracheal tube may inadvertently slip into the bronchus
- The airway is much smaller and even relatively minor inflammation greatly increases resistance to airflow

Self-test 5: What clinical features might you expect in a toddler with an inhaled foreign body partially obstructing:
A The larynx?
B The right main bronchus?
How should each be managed?

Answers: History reveals sudden onset with choking and the circumstances surrounding inhalation of the foreign body. There is no fever or preceding illness. Other features will differ according to the site of airway obstruction.

The larynx	*The right middle lobe bronchus*
Symptoms	
Inspiratory ± expiratory stridor	Expiratory ± inspiratory wheezing
Persistent barking cough	Paroxysmal coughing
Hoarseness	
Examination	
	Unilateral focal signs: Wheeze on the right Reduced air entry on the right

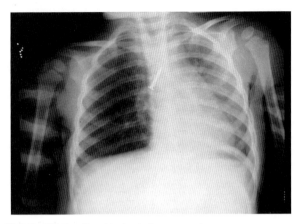

Figure 13.4   Foreign body in upper airway.

The larynx

Neck radiograph:
Foreign body
may be seen

The right middle lobe bronchus

Chest radiograph:
Foreign body may be
seen (Figure 13.4)
Inspiratory and
expiratory films of the
chest may show
mediastinal shift on
expiration (Figure 13.5)

Management:

A *Foreign body in the larynx*
- Five back blows with infant supported prone and head down on the rescuer's forearm or across the thighs
- If not successful, then five chest thrusts with infant's back on the rescuer's thigh and head down
- Direct laryngoscopic removal may be necessary

B *Foreign body in bronchus*
- Remove with bronchoscopy under general anaesthetic

Self-test 6: Figure 13.2a (p. 132) is the computed tomography (CT) scan of a 6-month-old baby with a cavernous haemangioma on the anterior chest (A) and also around the upper airway (B). The chest radiograph (Figure 13.2b) showed mediastinal widening which differed in appearance from a normal thymus (Figure 13.2c). How might this infant have presented?

Answer: With stridor starting within the first few weeks after birth and getting progressively worse and a soft skin lesion (cavernous haemangioma) also appearing within a few weeks after birth, and gradually getting bigger.

(a)

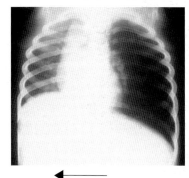

Chest radiograph in inspiration

Chest radiograph in expiration

Right lung normal

Left lung overinflated

– translucent
– sparse vessels

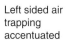

Mediastinum shifted to right

Left diaphragm depressed

Left sided air trapping accentuated

(b)

CT of chest with contrast in airway

Illustration of findings on expiration

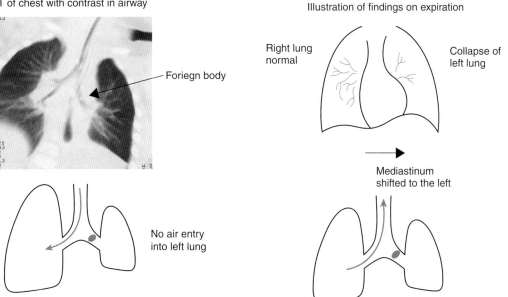

Foriegn body

Right lung normal

Collapse of left lung

Mediastinum shifted to the left

No air entry into left lung

Inspiration

Expiration

Figure 13.5 Radiological images and illustrations of inhaled foreing body producing (a) partial (check-valve) and (b) complete (stop-valve) obstruction of the left main bronchus. Images courtesy of Dr Julion Vyas.

Acute presentation

A preschool child with a fever and then a fit

Age: 15 months

LEENA PATEL

Presentation

The mother of 15-month-old Maya describes her condition to the staff in the accident and emergency department (A&E):

'I thought she was asleep as she curled up on my lap. Then her arms jerked. As I lifted her to face me, the jerk had stopped but I was horrified to see that her eyes had rolled back and her lips were blue. I went into a panic as I thought her limp body was dead or dying. My husband tried mouth-to-mouth while I rang for an ambulance. But within a minute or two, she just appeared to be sleepy. I hadn't known that a fever needed to be taken seriously.'

Self-test 1: When might you consider a child to have a fever?

Answer: As with other biological measurements, normal body temperature varies between individuals and at different times of the day (36.1–37.4°C).

Fever is a temperature higher than   37.8°C ear or oral
37.2°C axilla
38°C rectal

Initial considerations and action

Maya's presentation is of a typical simple febrile convulsion (Table 14.1) and illustrates that it can be a frightening experience for parents. The convulsion stopped spontaneously and she is now alert (see Chapter 22

Table 14.1   Simple febrile convulsions

Definition: benign generalized convulsion in otherwise normal children who are febrile secondary to an extracranial infection.

Incidence 2–4 per cent of children aged 6 months to 5 years (most common 9–22 months of age)

Brought on by fever and genetic predisposition when the brain is developmentally susceptible

Can be the first sign of illness in up to 40 per cent of the children

Most commonly associated with viral infections

Should be differentiated from complex convulsions (Table 14.2)

for management of a prolonged convulsion). Her ear temperature is 40.2°C and she is given a dose of paracetamol orally.

History

The clinical features in a child with a fever and convulsion help:

- To differentiate simple febrile convulsion from complex convulsion (Table 14.2)
- To rule out a convulsion from any other cause, especially meningitis (see Chapter 22)
- To determine the cause of the fever

The history of the convulsion should be obtained from the person who witnessed it.

Table 14.2 Differentiating features of simple febrile and complex convulsions

	Simple febrile convulsion	**Complex convulsion**
Age	6 months–5 years	Any age
Fever	Fever at the time of the convulsion, often abrupt rise in temperature	No fever or low-grade fever
Convulsion	Usually <5 minutes, not >15 minutes Generalized Usually single in a fever episode	>15 minutes Partial or focal In cluster or multiple within 24 hours
After the convulsion	Complete recovery within 1 hour	Altered consciousness persists, focal neurological signs
Other features	Child otherwise 'well'	Child unwell Neurodevelopmental abnormality
Risk of epilepsy (%)	1	5–10

Maya's history

Maya had been well until that morning when she felt hot. Mother comforted Maya and let her curl up on her lap because she was whingey. That was when she had the convulsion.

Maya has not had any convulsions or major illnesses in the past. Her birth history is unremarkable. She has had her first year vaccines without any problems. There are no concerns about her development. Father has only just learnt from his mother that he had a fit with a fever when he was little. No one in the family has epilepsy.

Mother is asked about specific symptoms and systemic upset which might indicate the cause of the fever. Maya has not had:

- A rash
- A cough, been pulling her ears or other respiratory symptoms
- Diarrhoea or vomiting
- Urinary symptoms – she has had a reasonable number of wet nappies, has not cried when passing urine and her urine has not been smelly or red. There is no family history of urinary tract infections

Interpretation of the history

Maya's history suggests a simple febrile convulsion and not a complex convulsion (see Table 14.2). The relevance of father's history is that it increases Maya's risk of having further febrile convulsions. Features associated with a fever include:

- Feeling unwell, lethargy – explains Maya being whingey
- Dehydration from excessive sweating and poor oral intake
- Loss of appetite

In the absence of specific symptoms and an obvious explanation for Maya's fever, the two possibilities are:

- A viral infection
- A urinary tract infection

Examination

The junior doctor in A&E notes the following:

- Alert, not miserable or irritable
- Does not look unwell
- Well-perfused, warm extremities, capillary refill time 2 seconds
- No dehydration
- No rash
- No lymphadenopathy
- Ear, nose and throat (ENT), chest and abdominal examination: no abnormality

- Neurological examination: normal tone and movements, no weakness
- No photophobia, anterior fontanelle closed, no neck stiffness

Interpretation of the examination

Maya does not have any clinical features of meningitis. About 15 per cent of children with meningitis have convulsions. They differ from children with simple febrile convulsions in that:

- The convulsions tend to be focal, prolonged or multiple
- Their history and examination are not normal: abnormal findings include:
  - petechiae
  - signs of circulatory failure
  - signs of meningism
  - level of consciousness remains disturbed after the convulsion has stopped

Self-test 2: What clinical features are suggestive of meningitis in an older child and adult, and how do these differ in infants and toddlers?

Answer:

Older child and adult	Infants and toddlers
Neck stiffness	Neck stiffness is unusual
Kernig's sign	Shrill high-pitched cry
Photophobia, phonophobia	Bulging fontanelle
Severe headache	
Irritability or drowsiness	
Persistent vomiting	

Investigations and results

For the febrile convulsion (see Chapter 22)

An EEG, neuroimaging and other investigations are not routinely indicated for a simple febrile convulsion.

For the cause of the fever

Investigations should be arranged according to clinical suspicion. A clean catch urine sample is obtained from

Table 14.3   Maya's urine microscopy

WBC	350×10^6/L
RBC	50×10^6/L
Protein	Trace
Glucose	Negative
Blood	+

RBC, red blood cell count; WBC, white blood cell count.

Maya for microscopy and culture. The microscopy result is available within an hour, but the culture result will not be ready for 24 hours (Table 14.3).

Self-test 3: How should a urine sample be obtained from young children who are not toilet trained when investigating for urinary tract infection (UTI)?

Answer: The three methods and their advantages and disadvantages are shown below. A bag sample should not be obtained for bacterial culture – it is non-invasive but there is a high probability (30–90 per cent) of it being contaminated (i.e. bacteria originating and multiplying outside rather than in the urinary tract).

	Advantage	Disadvantage
Suprapubic aspiration	Theoretically zero rate of contamination	Invasive Success rate variable
Catheterization	Almost 100% success rate	Invasive Potential iatrogenic UTI
Clean catch	Non-invasive	Time-consuming Requires patience and effort Small possibility of contamination

Self-test 4: Does Maya's urine microscopy result confirm a UTI?

Answer: No. Maya has pyuria – defined as white blood cell count (WBC) $> 10 \times 10^6$/L urine. Pyuria is seen in:

- UTI
- Up to 10% febrile children without a UTI

- UTI is confirmed by a culture result with a pure bacterial growth of any number from a suprapubic aspirate
- $>10^5$ colony-forming units (CFUs)/mL from clean catch or catheter samples

Diagnosis

Maya's diagnoses are:

- Simple febrile convulsion
- Suspected first UTI or viral infection

Management and follow-up

Maya is admitted to hospital for observation and requires management for the:

- Febrile convulsion
- Fever
- Cause of the fever

Management of the febrile convulsion

This involves giving parents information and advice about febrile convulsions (Table 14.4).

Fever management

The aim is to reduce discomfort and parental anxiety.

- External cooling measures (see Table 14.4)
- Antipyretic:
  - paracetamol:
    oral 10–15 mg/kg per dose $\left.\right\}$ 4- to 6-hourly
    rectal 20 mg/kg per dose (maximum 60 mg/kg per day)
  - ibuprofen if temperature $> 39.5°C$
  There is no evidence that antipyretics prevent first or recurrent febrile convulsions.
- Maintain hydration (see Table 14.4)
  Not recommended:
  - cold sponging, cold baths or showers, sponging with alcohol (can increase discomfort)
  - aspirin (associated with Reye's syndrome)

Management of suspected UTI

Aim of treatment is:

- To relieve symptoms
- To clear the infection
- To prevent recurrence, renal scarring and long-term complications

Antibiotic treatment

Maya is given:

- Trimethoprim orally twice a day pending the result of urine culture
- Fluids liberally

On the ward round the following morning, she is described by mother and the nurses as having remained well except for a fever. She has been taking fluids and tolerated them. The urine culture result is obtained by telephone and reveals:

- Culture $> 10^5$ organisms/mL
- *Escherichia coli*
- Sensitive to nitrofurantoin, nalidixic acid, cefadroxil
- Resistant to ampicillin, co-amoxiclav, trimethoprim

Maya is therefore given nitrofurantoin orally four times a day for 7 days and the trimethoprim is stopped. Mother feels that she will be able to manage Maya at home and she is allowed to go home. She is given appointments for further investigations and follow-up.

The standard duration of antibiotic treatment is 7–14 days. Short 2- to 4-day courses have a number of advantages (see Self-test 5), but the disadvantage is that infection may not clear, especially in those with recurrent UTI.

Further investigations

Maya has some more investigations:

- Urine re-tested 5 days later: no WBCs or red blood cells (RBCs) and no growth on culture
- Ultrasonography: normal size and appearance of both kidneys, normal bladder
- DMSA (^{99m}Tc-dimercaptosuccinic acid) scan: good symmetrical activity bilaterally with right kidney

Table 14.4   What information and advice to give to parents about a febrile convulsion

---

Reassurance about the febrile convulsion

It is common

Frightening for parents but:

- Usually brief, self-limited and not dangerous: does not cause death or brain damage
- Child does not suffer pain or discomfort during the convulsion
- Occur because growing brains of little children are more sensitive to fever and normal brain activity is disturbed

Child can have all the routine immunizations

Prognosis after a first febrile convulsion

Recurrent febrile convulsions – in about 40 per cent of children

Factors that increase the risk of a simple febrile convulsion recurring are:

- First-degree relative with a febrile convulsion
- First convulsion at age <12 months
- Age <2 years
- Within 6 months of the first convulsion

Epilepsy: 1 per cent in those with no neurodevelopmental abnormality; factors associated with a risk of afebrile or unprovoked convulsions and epilepsy are:

- Complex febrile convulsions
- Recurrent febrile convulsions
- Neurodevelopmental abnormalities
- Family history of afebrile convulsions

Management of fever

External cooling measures

Clothing: remove excess clothing and leave light underwear

Environment: allow air to circulate in room and turn down central heating but do not let child get too cold

Paracetamol 4- to 6-hourly regularly for 48 hours during the febrile illness

Maintain hydration: plenty of fluids given as small frequent sips

Consult GP

Management of a convulsion

Look at the watch to time the length of the convulsion

Turn child on side – recovery position (reduces risk of choking and inhaling secretions) and away from hard or sharp objects

(continued)

Table 14.4 (*continued*)

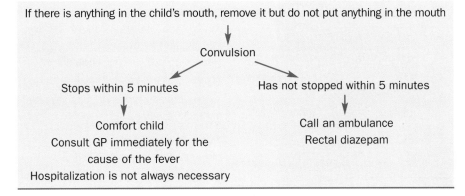

If there is anything in the child's mouth, remove it but do not put anything in the mouth

↓

Convulsion

↙ ↘

Stops within 5 minutes   Has not stopped within 5 minutes

↓   ↓

Comfort child   Call an ambulance
Consult GP immediately for the   Rectal diazepam
cause of the fever
Hospitalization is not always necessary

at 46 per cent and left kidney at 54 per cent (Figure 14.1(a)). No evidence of cortical scarring

Antibiotic prophylaxis

After completing the course of nitrofurantoin, Maya is advised to continue the medicine once a day to prevent reinfection until the results of the abdominal ultrasonography and DMSA scan are available. Maya is reviewed in the outpatient clinic with the results: because they do not show a urinary tract abnormality or renal scarring, the prophylactic antibiotic is discontinued and Maya is discharged.

Had urinary tract abnormalities or renal scarring been identified on investigation, the following would be required:

- Follow-up in hospital
- Long-term antibiotic prophylaxis
- Further investigations, including micturating cystourethrogram (MCUG), to look for vesicoureteric reflux (VUR) (Figure 14.1)
- Monitoring of growth, blood pressure (BP), urinary symptoms, urine culture, renal function

Information for parents and GP

Maya's parents and the GP are kept informed about:

- The diagnosis of UTI
- Rationale for antibiotic treatment, prophylaxis and investigations
- Results of investigations

Self-test 5: What might be the advantage of a short 2- to 4-day course of antibiotic compared with longer courses for treating UTIs?

Answer:
- Reduced antibiotic resistance
- Reduced adverse effects of antibiotics
- Improved compliance
- Reduced costs

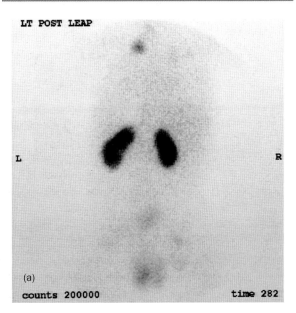

(a)
counts 200000   time 282

Figure 14.1 Radiological investigations in a child with UTI: (a) normal DMSA (^{99m}Tc-dimercaptosuccinic acid) scan; (b) micturating cystourethrogram (MCUG) of vesicoureteric reflux (VUR).

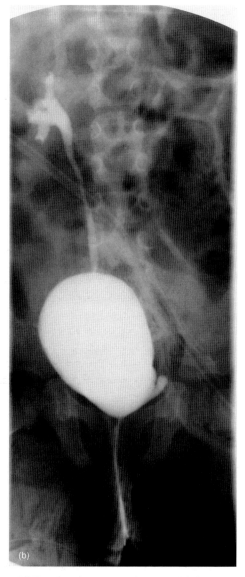

(b)

Figure 14.1 *Continued.*

Background information

Pathophysiology of febrile convulsions

This is not known but possible contributory factors are:

- Relative lack of myelination in the immature brain and increased oxygen consumption during a febrile illness (Table 14.5)

Table 14.5 Causes of fever

Infections

Viral, e.g. adenovirus, echovirus, Coxsackie virus, parainfluenzae, measles, cytomegalovirus, human herpes virus 6 (HHV6), hepatitis

Bacterial, e.g. upper or lower respiratory, urinary tract, meningitis, septicaemia, osteomyelitis,[a] endocarditis,[a] typhoid,[a] tuberculosis[a]

Not infectious

Immunization, e.g. MMR, DTP

Drugs

Dehydration: in infants, hypertonic

Chronic inflammation,[a] e.g. juvenile arthritis, inflammatory bowel disease

Malignancy, e.g. leukaemia, lymphoma, Ewing's tumour[a]

Other: sickle-cell crisis, Kawasaki's disease[a]

[a]Fever may be prolonged.
MMR, mumps/measles/rubella vaccine;
DTP, diphtheria/tetanus/polio vaccine.

- Immaturity of thermoregulatory mechanisms
- 'Neurotropic' viruses directly invade the central nervous system

Urinary tract infections – a snapshot

Incidence

- Two per cent of boys and 8 per cent of girls will have a UTI by 8 years of age
- Peak age is in the first 2 years
- More common in boys in the first 3 months of life and thereafter more common in girls
- Annual incidence of first symptomatic UTI is 3 per 1000 girls and 2 per 1000 boys aged 0–14 years
- Prevalence of UTI in febrile children <2 years age is 5 per cent

Definition

- Presence of a pure bacterial growth $>10^5$ CFU/mL urine

Pathogens that cause UTI

- *Escherichia coli* (most common – about 80 per cent of UTIs)
- *Proteus* species (more common in boys)
- *Klebsiella* species
- Enterococci
- Coagulase-negative staphylococci

Pathophysiology

The urinary tract is normally sterile. Infection is most commonly ascending (Figure 14.2), but can be haematogenous (especially in neonates and immunocompromised children) or from direct extension (e.g. from vesicointestinal or vesicovaginal fistula).

Factors that predispose to UTI and renal damage are:

- Vesicoureteric reflux
- Anatomical obstruction, e.g. posterior urethral valves, ureteric obstruction
- Functional abnormalities, e.g. neuropathic bladder associated with spina bifida

Clinical features of UTIs

- **Non-specific** (especially in preschool age children and therefore requires a high index of suspicion):
  - unexplained fever (prevalence of UTI is approximately 5 per cent)
  - rigors
  - unwell
  - irritability
  - vomiting
  - anorexia
- **Specific:**
  - dysuria (crying on urination), hesitancy, urgency, frequency (wetting in a toilet trained child)
  - smelly urine
  - abdominal or loin pain
  - haematuria
- **In neonates:**
  - prolonged jaundice
  - apnoea
  - poor weight gain

Radiological investigations after a first UTI

Age of child (years)	<1	1–5	>5
Initial investigation	Abdominal ultrasonography	Abdominal ultrasonography	Abdominal ultrasonography
	DMSA scan	DMSA scan	
	MCUG		
Further investigations	Necessary according to abnormality identified on initial investigation		

Outcome after first UTI

- **Further infection:**
  - in 50 per cent of girls within the first year and 75 per cent within 2 years of initial infection
  - in 18 per cent of boys with first UTI before age 1 year and 32 per cent of boys with initial infection at an older age

  The likelihood of further infection:
  - decreases with each infection-free year
  - increases with the number of previous infections
- **Renal scarring:** 5–15 per cent children; new scars are rare after 5 years of age
- **Permanent renal damage, especially if treatment is delayed (see Figure 14.2):**
  - impaired renal function
  - hypertension
  - renal failure

Vesicoureteric reflux – a snapshot

- A congenital abnormality associated with incompetence of the vesicoureteric junction and resulting in retrograde flow of urine from the bladder to the ureter (Figure 14.3)
- Associated with developmental abnormalities of the urinary tract, e.g. renal dysplasia
- Improves or disappears as the child gets older

Prevalence

- One to two per cent in asymptomatic children
- One-third children with UTI
- One-third siblings of patients with VUR

Autosomal dominant inheritance.

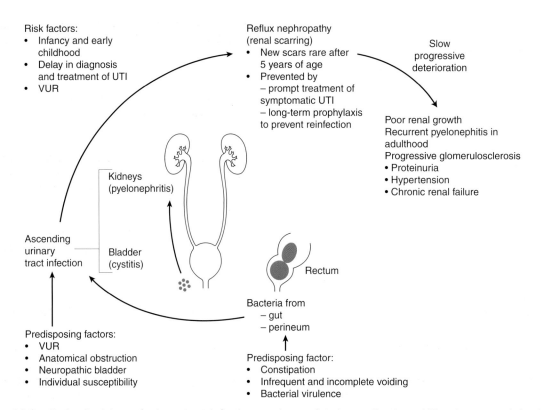

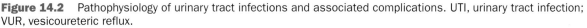

Figure 14.2   Pathophysiology of urinary tract infections and associated complications. UTI, urinary tract infection; VUR, vesicoureteric reflux.

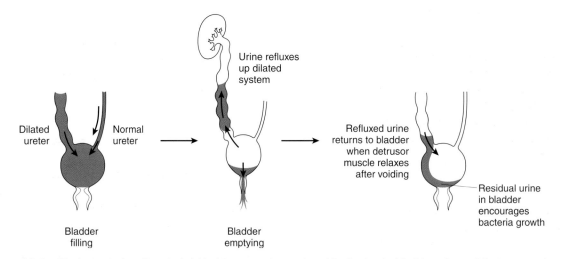

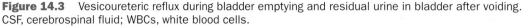

Figure 14.3   Vesicoureteric reflux during bladder emptying and residual urine in bladder after voiding. CSF, cerebrospinal fluid; WBCs, white blood cells.

Grades

- **Mild-to-moderate reflux:** reflux reaches kidney but does not dilate ureters or renal pelvis
- **Severe reflux:** ureteric, calyceal and/or renal pelvic dilatation of increasing severity

Presentation

- Silent or identified from MCUG after UTI
- Risk factor for reflux nephropathy (i.e. renal scarring)

Self-test 6: With regard to urinary tract infections, the following are true:

A Poor or interrupted urine stream is relevant in infant boys

B Remain localized to the urinary tract in children of all ages

C Double voiding should be encouraged in toilet-trained children

D Constipation is associated with recurrent UTI

E Absence of WBCs in the urine excludes UTI

F Chemical tests of urine are reliable and diagnostic

G Pyelonephritic scarring is the most common cause of hypertension in children

Answers: True:

A Suggests obstruction in the urethra – most common is posterior urethral valves

C It helps to reduce residual urine in the bladder (see Figure 14.3)

D Poor perineal muscle relaxation associated with detrusor instability impedes both bladder and rectal emptying

G

False:

B Often accompanied by septicaemia in neonates who cannot localize infections well

E UTI can be present in the absence of WBCs

F Chemical markers of infection, including urinary nitrites (nitrates are reduced to nitrites by certain bacteria) and leucocyte esterase (produced by activated WBCs), have a number of limitations

Further sources of information

Articles

Larcombe J. Urinary tract infection in children. Clinical evidence. *British Medical Journal* 1999; **319**: 1173–5

Offringa M, Moyer VA. Evidence based management of seizures associated with fever. Evidence based paediatrics. *British Medical Journal* 2001; **323**: 1111–14

Verrier Jones K. Prognosis for vesicoureteric reflux. *Archives of Disease in Childhood* 1999; **81**: 287–94

Self-test 7: For a previously healthy toddler with a fever and brief convulsion:

A A lumbar puncture is essential

B Antiepileptics will inevitably be required

C The risk of recurrence is greater if there is a first-degree relative with febrile convulsions

D The MMR vaccine is contraindicated

Answers: False:

A Probability of bacterial meningitis is low (<5 per cent)

B The risk of developing epilepsy is small (1 in 100)

D One in 1000 children may get a febrile convulsion 8–10 days after being given the MMR vaccine

True: C.

Self-test 8: The following are true for bacterial meningitis:

A The most common pathogen in neonates is *Listeria monocytogenes*

B The long-term outcome is worse with pneumococcal than with meningococcal meningitis

C WBCs, protein, glucose and lactate are raised in the cerebrospinal fluid (CSF)

D Dexamethasone just before the first dose of intravenous antibiotic reduces hearing and neurological impairment

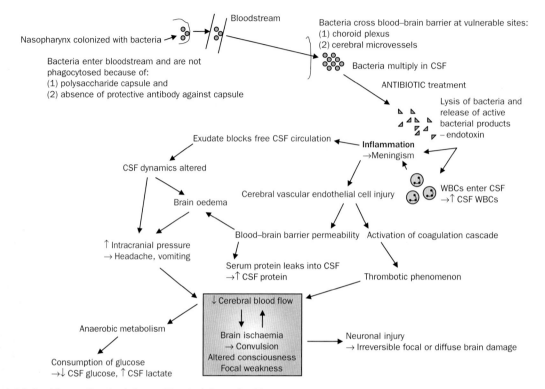

Figure 14.4 The pathophysiology of bacterial meningitis.

Answers: False:

A Group B β-haemolytic streptococci and Gram-negative organisms are common

C Glucose is reduced

True: B,D.

Self-test 9: Explain the pathophysiology that results in the clinical features of bacterial meningitis.

Answer: See Figure 14.4.

Self-test 10. There is good evidence that the MMR vaccine is associated with:

A Febrile convulsion

B Crohn's disease

C Autism

D Thrombocytopenic purpura

Answer: True: A, D.

A young boy who wakes with a puffy face one morning

Age: 4 years

STEVEN RYAN

Presentation

Four-year-old Robert Jones was taken to see his family doctor for morning surgery. When he had woken up that morning, it was noted by his mother that both his eyelids were swollen and his face was a little bit puffy. The previous morning she thought that he had looked tired and his face was then, in hindsight, also a little bit puffy. The GP noted the concerns and briefly examined Robert confirming that his eyelids and face were swollen. He telephoned the hospital and spoke to the paediatrician who arranged for Robert and his mother to be seen in the ambulatory clinic that afternoon.

Self-test 1: What are the causes of facial swelling (Figure 15.1)?

Answers:

A Fluid	Leaky blood vessels	Anaphylaxis
		Septic shock
	Raised venous pressure	Heart failure
	Low blood albumin	Renal or gut losses
		Liver failure
	Fluid overload	
	Tissue inflammation	Infection including viral infection
	Blocked lymphatic vessels	Primary lymphoedema
B Air	Subcutaneous emphysema	Asthma

Initial considerations and action

Tissue swelling is one of the core pathophysiological events that can occur as the result of a disease or disorder. The likely causes may be determined by a number of features (Table 15.1).

At this stage it is not possible to make a definitive diagnosis but anaphylactic reaction can be ruled out, though a milder allergy is possible. Henoch–Schoenlein purpura also seems unlikely because the family doctor does not report any purpura.

History

The following history is obtained.

Presenting complaint

- Puffy face yesterday morning and puffy face with swollen eyelids this morning – his face had seemed fine when he went to bed the previous evening
- Eyes somewhat less swollen this afternoon
- Has been lethargic over the last few days
- Passing less urine than usual
- Recently had a cold with fever and was off nursery for 3 days

Past history and health

- Robert has been a healthy boy other than having had a fever convulsion at 2 years

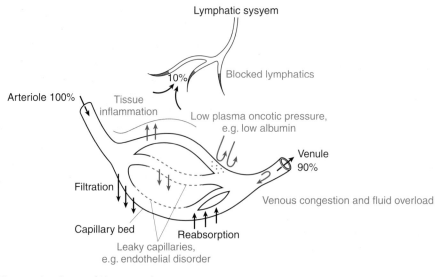

Figure 15.1   The mechanisms of tissue oedema.

Table 15.1   Causes of facial swelling: key features in the history

Feature	Example
Age of patient	
Newborn baby	Hydrops fetalis
Teenager	Glandular fever
Speed of onset	
Very rapid (seconds)	Anaphylactic reaction
Several days	Acute renal disorder
Distribution over	
Ankles	Henoch–Schoenlein purpura
Eyes	Glandular fever
Widespread	Capillary leak
Other features in history	
Reduced urine production	Renal disorder
Wheezing	Allergic reaction
Other features on examination	
Purpura	Henoch–Schoenlein purpura
Palpitations	Cardiac failure

- He has mild eczema that is controlled currently by emollients
- Robert has been thriving and developing normally; his most recent weight was 16.8 kg (2 weeks ago)

Self test 2: What is a quick way of estimating a child's weight? Give Robert's weight.

Answer: Add 4 to age then double that sum. For Robert $(4 + 4) \times 2 = 16$ kg

Family history

- His father and mother are in good health as is his 9-month-old sister
- There is no family history of chronic illness

Immunizations

These are up to date.

Interpretation of the history

The history suggests that Robert has been well until recently and makes it likely that a new, acute problem has arisen rather than a complication of a chronic underlying disorder. Of note in the history:

- The swelling has improved slightly, meaning that either the process is resolving or change in posture might allow the swelling to go down (it was worst first thing in the morning)
- Lethargy might be caused by an intercurrent infection (such as glandular fever) or hypovolaemia (fluid redistribution from the intravascular to the extravascular compartment)
- The history of eczema implies atopy and children with atopy are at increased risk of allergic reactions to foods that frequently cause facial swelling
- The reduction in the amount of urine produced could indicate a renal problem, but it might also indicate that his fluid intake has reduced because he feels unwell
- A recent infection can predispose to:
  - an allergic-type reaction with swelling but usually accompanied by an urticarial rash
  - a glomerulonephritis resulting in disturbance of renal function such as fluid retention or albumin loss

Examination

When Robert was examined, these were the findings:

- Swelling of both eyelids and mild swelling of the face
- Swelling over both shins and on to ankles – pits on pressure
- Abdomen soft and non-distended
- No oedema over sacrum
- Pulse rate 125/minute; blood pressure 88/56 mmHg
- Heart sounds: normal I and II, no added sounds or murmurs
- Weight 18.4 kg
- Height 105.2 cm
- Respiratory rate 22/minute, chest clear on auscultation, no dullness to percussion
- Healthy tonsils and no cervical lymphadenopathy

Interpretation of the examination

The finding of generalized oedema suggests a generalized disease process. Glandular fever (which generally causes only periorbital swelling) or an allergic reaction now looks unlikely. It is important to note the sudden weight gain (1.6 kg) in a short time. This makes fluid retention related to low serum albumin levels the most likely explanation for the swelling. When such oedema occurs, it can be associated with sacral oedema (best seen first thing in the morning, as the sacrum's been dependent all night) and also transudation of fluid from serosal surfaces into body cavities. Here, there is no evidence of the former or of ascites or pleural effusions. There is nothing to suggest heart failure as the cause.

Investigations

Robert's urine was tested with a proprietary reagent strip (Table 15.2).

This simple test shows the presence of large quantities of albumin in the urine and suggests nephrotic syndrome as a result of a primary kidney disorder. In this situation, it is important to check blood pressure, because hypertension can also arise from kidney diseases. The elevated heart rate could indicate a cardiac response to hypovolaemia. Blood pressure is normal, but remember that blood pressure is maintained in children until they are on the verge of severe shock.

The absence of blood in urine is reassuring because this is associated with a more aggressive type of glomerulonephritis. The high specific gravity (normal 1.005–1.010) is also an indicator of the large amount of protein leaking into the urine. The negative leucocyte test makes a coincident urine infection very unlikely.

Table 15.2 Investigations for Robert

Investigation	Result
Albumin	++++
Blood	Negative
Ketones	Negative
pH	6
Specific gravity	1.030
Leucocyte test	Negative

A urine sample is sent to the laboratory for analysis and a blood test is done. Here are the results:

Biochemistry

Urea	6.8 mmol/L (slightly elevated)
Creatinine	58 µmol/L (normal)
Sodium	140 mmol/L (normal)
Potassium	4.5 mmol/L (normal)
Albumin	15 g/dL (low)
Cholesterol	6.9 mmol/L (high)

Immunology

Complement C3 and C4	Normal

Haematology

Haemoglobin	16.6 g/dL (high)
White cell count and differential count	Normal

Microbiology

Hepatitis B serology	Negative
Blood bacterial culture	Negative

Urine

Protein loss is highly selective

The nephrotic syndrome is now completely confirmed by the low level of serum albumin. Importantly, a number of features suggest that the underlying disorder is most likely to be minimal change glomerulonephritis, rather than a more aggressive condition:

- The normal creatinine suggests normal creatinine clearance and hence glomerular filtration rate (GFR)
- There is no evidence of complement activation (with diminished levels of C3 and C4) – in keeping with a more aggressive inflammatory process
- A highly selective protein loss (large amounts of albumin – less of other larger proteins); more disruptive glomerular damage allows larger molecules to leak through

Other features of note are the raised cholesterol (a typical feature of nephrotic syndrome) the high haemoglobin level caused by haemoconcentration and the negative test for hepatitis B, which, although unlikely here, is a common worldwide cause of nephrotic syndrome.

As it is very likely to be minimal change nephrotic syndrome, a renal biopsy is not undertaken.

Self-test 3: For each of the conditions listed, which clinical information matches best?

A Nephrotic syndrome
B Nephritic syndrome
C Haemolytic–uraemic syndrome
D Chronic pyelonephritis
E Henoch–Schoenlein glomerulonephritis

1 A 17-year-old girl with recurrent urinary tract infections in early infancy and vesicoureteric reflux
2 A 9-year-old boy who had a purpuric rash on his buttocks and arms with abdominal pain over several months at age 1 year. He has had persistent blood in his urine ever since
3 A 2-year-old girl who has had diarrhoea and vomiting for 3 days and now has stopped passing urine and is very pale with anaemia
4 A 6-year-old girl who had a sore throat 1 week previously. She has a headache, is passing smoky urine, is hypertensive and has slight facial oedema
5 A 5-year-old girl in Malawi who has *falciparum* malaria and now has developed low blood albumin level with generalized severe oedema

Answers: A5/B4/C3/D1/E2.

Diagnosis

Minimal change nephrotic syndrome.

Self-test 4: What are the chances of relapse after successful treatment of the presenting episode?

A 0
B 5–10 per cent
C 20–33 per cent
D 50–75 per cent
E 100 per cent

Answer: D.

Treatment and progress

Robert is admitted to the ward and the following treatment is undertaken:

- Specific treatment: a course of prednisolone is started and within a few days the albumin loss in the urine starts to diminish
- Fluid management: fluid intake is restricted until urine production increases with normalizing albumin levels. Salt intake is also restricted during this time. Robert is weighed daily and his fluid intake and output measured. He does not require diuretics or albumin infusions
- Anti-infective treatment: he is started on penicillin and given pneumococcal immunization – this is because pneumococcal infection is common with nephrotic syndrome

Robert goes into remission and is discharged home on a reducing course of prednisolone. His parents are warned that there is a significant risk of relapse and that viral infections might act as a trigger. They are given a supply of reagent strips to monitor albumin loss in his urine.

Background information

The glomerulus: structure and function

By birth the kidneys have developed their full complement of their glomeruli and renal tubules (around 1 million for each kidney). The glomerulus essentially acts as a filter and the filtrate is then subject to the processes of the renal tubule with the ultimate production of urine. The glomeruli are found in the cortex of the kidney. Figure 15.2 shows schematically the structure of the glomerulus. Arterial blood arrives via the afferent arteriole and then circulates though the glomerular capillaries before exiting through the efferent arteriole. The hydrostatic pressure within the glomerulus forces filtrate to leak out through the capillary walls into the Bowman's capsule. The filtrate then passes through the tubule for further processing.

The filtrate passes through fenestrations in the endothelial layer of the capillary, through the glomerular basement membrane, and then through filtration slits – gaps between the foot processes of the epithelial

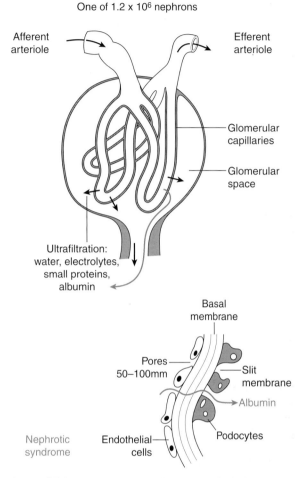

One of 1.2×10^6 nephrons

Figure 15.2 The structure of a glomerulus with changes seen in nephrotic syndrome.

cells of the renal surface (Figure 15.2). Mesangial cells lie within the knot of capillaries in the glomerulus and act to support the structure of the glomerulus, but also probably have an important immunological scavenging function.

This filtration mechanism allows the production of an ultrafiltrate containing solutes, peptides and some low-molecular-weight proteins, but not larger ones such as albumin and globulins. Erythrocytes do not cross the filter under normal circumstances. Glomerular filtration rate, as measured by creatinine clearance, is around 40 mL/min per 1.73 m² body surface area at birth, increasing to around 120 mL/min per 1.73 m² by age 4 years.

Damage to the glomerular filtration apparatus allows the passage of larger protein molecules into the urinary space and this includes albumin. When enough is lost the serum albumin concentration falls, as liver production fails to keep up, and the reduction in plasma oncotic pressure allows tissue fluid accumulation to occur. Generally, the more severe the glomerular insult, the larger the proteins that are lost and the less 'selective' the proteinuria. Coincident haematuria is also seen when there is inflammation of the glomerulus. In minimal change glomerular disease (which accounts for 80 per cent of childhood nephrotic syndrome) light microscopy reveals no abnormality, but high power electron microscopy may reveal thinning of the foot processes of the podocytes.

Other renal pathologies that can cause nephrotic syndrome include:

- Membranous glomerulonephritis
- Mesangiocapillary glomerulonephritis
- Malaria
- Adult diabetes mellitus

How to understand urine microscopy

Figure 15.3 shows the items that may appear under high power when microscopy of urine is undertaken.

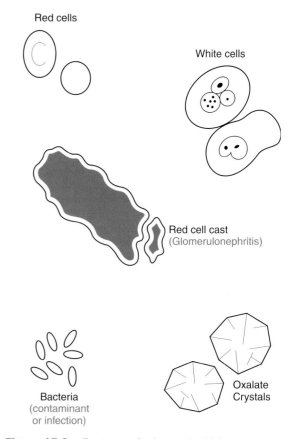

Figure 15.3   Features of urine under high-power microscopy.

Further sources of information

Book

Postlethwaite RJ. *Clinical Paediatric Nephrology*, 2nd edn. Oxford: Butterworth–Heinemann, 1994

Articles

Chesney RW. The idiopathic nephrotic syndrome. *Current Opinion in Paediatrics* 1999; **11**: 158–61

Orth SR, Ritz E. The nephrotic syndrome. *New England Journal of Medicine* 1998; **338**: 1202–11

Websites

www.niddk.nih.gov/health/kidney/pubs/cns/cns.htm

National Kidney and Urologic Diseases Information Clearinghouse – a good review.

www.nlm.nih.gov/medlineplus/ency/article/000503.htm

Medline Plus (NLM USA) – information on post-streptococcal glomerulonephritis.

Self-test 5: A 7-year-old developed a sore throat and, 10 days later, he was noted to have puffy eyes and reduced urine output. During the original illness, the GP took a throat swab and subsequently prescribed penicillin, based on the result. His urine looked 'smoky'. His GP noted that his blood pressure was 140/102 and there was blood on reagent-stick testing of his urine. At hospital it was noted that his serum albumin level was normal and his serum complement 3 level reduced.

A Why did his urine look smoky?

B What organism most probably caused the sore throat?

C Why is this not nephrotic syndrome?

D What renal disorder is it most likely to be?

E What are the most important principles of management in this case?

Answers:

A Because it contained blood

B α-Haemolytic streptococci

C He has a normal serum albumin value

D Post-streptococcal glomerulonephritis

E Fluid balance and control of hypertension

16

Acute presentation

A child with a black eye

Age: 13 months

JACKIE GREGG

Presentation

Referral from the accident and emergency department (A&E):

Callum, aged 13 months, had been taken to A&E at 7.30 pm by his parents. He had been walking independently for 2 weeks. Callum had fallen and hit his head earlier in the day and seemed fine immediately afterwards. However, the swelling and bruising alarmed his mother when she returned from work. She telephoned the GP who advised taking Callum to the hospital.

On examination, Callum was alert and playful and examination of the neurological system was normal. He had swelling and bruising to the right orbit and upper eyelid. The examining doctor also noted an area of bruising on Callum's left upper arm and buttocks. Callum's father said that he seemed to bruise easily.

The A&E doctor is concerned that the bruising is non-accidental.

Initial considerations and action

Many children have bruises. The pattern and distribution of the bruising will depend on the age and activities of the child, e.g. an active schoolboy is likely to have bruising to his shins, particularly if he plays football. Toddlers who tend to fall frequently often have bruises to prominent parts of the body, such as the forehead. The extent of the bruising to Callum is more than one would expect such a young child to have sustained accidentally, but if accidental this would indicate inadequate supervision.

A bleeding disorder needs to be considered, in particular:

- Idiopathic thrombocytopenic purpura
- Haemophilia
- Leukaemia

Self-test 1: Which points in the history would help to identify a possible bleeding disorder?

Answer: History or family history of easy bruising, prolonged bleeding after dental extractions, excessive blood loss during or after surgery, heavy menstruation, frequent nose bleeds.

Bruising may be confused with:

- Paint/ink/dirt
- Mongolian blue spot
- Capillary haemangioma

Mongolian blue spots (Figure 16.1) may be mistaken for bruises. They are large blue–grey areas most common over the sacrum and buttocks, but they may also occur over the shoulders. They are seen in young children of Oriental, Asian or African–Caribbean origin. They gradually fade by the age of 5 years.

Assessment of a child who may have been abused takes time. A detailed history, including developmental and social history as well as explanations of the cause of the injuries, is required. The paediatrician arranges to see Callum and his parents in a quiet consulting room in A&E to take a detailed history. Parents and

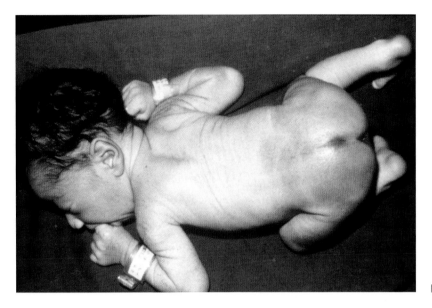

Figure 16.1 Mongolian blue spot.

child may become distressed and it is helpful to have an experienced nurse present.

History

Callum is the son of 20-year-old Joanne and 22-year-old John. They are not married, but have been living together in a council flat for the last 6 months. Before that, Joanne and Callum lived with Joanne's parents.

Callum was born at term after an uneventful, unplanned pregnancy. Callum was described as a healthy boy with a good appetite. He had been crawling from 10 months of age and started walking about 2 weeks ago. He is still very unsteady and falls frequently but seems 'fearless'. Callum likes a lot of attention, and he sleeps well at night and for an hour during the day.

John cares for Callum while Joanne is at work and has done so since they moved into their flat. Before that he had been unemployed. He enjoys looking after Callum, although he admits that it gets a bit boring at times. Joanne's mother occasionally baby-sits.

John explained that Callum had been playing in the living room at lunchtime while he was in the adjoining kitchen preparing lunch. John heard a scream followed by crying, and found Callum lying on the floor next to the coffee table. He noted reddening to the right eye and presumed that Callum had fallen against the corner of the coffee table. As Callum stopped crying fairly quickly and ate his lunch, John didn't think he needed to bother the doctor, even though the eye started to swell.

The couple were asked how and when the bruising to the arm and buttock had occurred. Joanne explained that she hadn't seen much of Callum for 4 days, other than putting him to bed after John had bathed and changed him. She works long hours in a local supermarket and had been doing some overtime. There hadn't been bruising 4 days ago. John thought that the bruising to the buttock had been there the previous day, but that he couldn't think of a particular incident when Callum had fallen and hurt himself, because he falls so frequently.

There was no family history of easy bruising, bleeding disorders, prolonged bleeding after tooth extraction or surgery, prolonged nose bleeds or a history of very heavy periods in Joanne or other female relatives.

Interpretation of the history

There are a number of important areas that need to be covered when a child presents with bruising or any other injury:

- Details of how and when the injury occurred and whether the history given by the carers is consistent

- Does the explanation fit with the pattern of bruising or injury?
- Are the injuries consistent with the child's stage of development?
- Has there been delay in presentation for medical attention and, if so, why?
- Behaviour problems or any specific worries about the child
- Previous injuries
- Social history
- Possible medical cause for the bruising

Self-test 2: Is the explanation satisfactory in this case?

Answer: Yes and no. The fall against the coffee table could account for the black eye, but it is of concern that there is no explanation for the other bruising.

Meaning of the history in Callum

Details of how the injury occurred and consistency of the history

Falling against the corner of the coffee table could account for the bruising and swelling to the eye. The history from the A&E doctor was brief, so assessing consistency is not possible – discrepancy in the accounts of the incident given by the carers raises considerable concern about what actually happened. Neither John nor Joanne can give an explanation for the bruising to the buttock and arm. Nappies offer a lot of protection to the buttocks. It is possible that Callum could have hurt himself while toddling around without his nappy on. Most parents watch their children closely in such circumstances in case they wee or pooh! One would have expected a child's carers to have been aware of a significant injury such as this.

Adequate explanation

The bruising to the eye could have happened as described. No explanation is given for the other bruising and, in view of the age of the child and level of supervision required, this is of concern.

Developmental history

Callum has just started to walk. Children at this stage of their development fall frequently and often have bruising to prominent parts of the body. It is hard to imagine how a child of such limited mobility could sustain two areas of bruising to different parts of their body without an adult knowing about it.

Delay in presentation

Joanne appears to have responded promptly when she returned home and saw the bruising, whereas John seemed very sanguine. Most parents would have sought urgent medical attention, even though the child seemed all right in himself.

Behaviour problems or specific worries about the child

All children are demanding, but there may be a difficulty with a particular child that is causing the carers increased stress.

The factors predisposing to abuse are:

- Factors in the child:
  - disability
  - low birthweight
  - unwanted child or sex
  - demanding child
- Factors in the carer:
  - drug and alcohol abuse
  - poverty and unemployment
  - poor educational achievement
  - poor parenting experiences, including periods in care
  - experience of abuse
  - mental health problems
  - domestic violence

Previous injuries

Repeated injuries suggest neglect or previous deliberate injury. Recurrent bruising may indicate a bleeding disorder or repeated abuse.

Social history

More information is required, including possible previous involvement with Social Services in relation to

Callum, whether John or Joanne has been in care, and if there is a history of domestic violence. The last is associated with emotional harm and physical abuse. There may be other elements in the carer, which is an influencing factor in physical abuse.

Bleeding disorder

A bleeding disorder seems unlikely, because the history of bruising is very recent. It could be argued that Callum wasn't active enough to cause even minor trauma; however, he has been crawling for 3 months. Note that children with bleeding disorders can also be physically abused.

Examination

Joanne gives consent for Callum to be examined.

Self-test 3: Who can legally give consent on behalf of a child?

Answer: Anyone with parental responsibility (PR). This is:
- Usually the mother
- The local authority if the child is subject to a care order, although in this case PR may be shared with the parents
- The father if he was married to the mother at the time of the child's birth or has obtained a Court Order giving him PR
- Another relative or carer who has obtained PR by a Court Order

A young person is a child up to the age of 16 years. Children should be involved in the consent process once they have the ability to understand the issues (Gillick competent).

The purpose of the examination is:

- To document and describe any injuries
- To assess the general health, development and well-being of the child
- To note any signs of neglect or emotional disturbance
- To assess the interaction between child and carers

- Height, weight and head circumference on the 25th centile
- Appropriately clothed, but grubby, dirty finger nails
- Normal examination of systems, including CNS (fundi visualized – no retinal haemorrhages seen)
- Nappy rash
- Frenulum intact
- Red/purple bruising to right orbit, with swelling of upper eyelid
- Green/black bruising with some yellowing to outer aspect of the left upper arm, approximately 2 cm horizontally by 4 cm vertically, 3 cm above olecranon process
- Four parallel linear bruises, green/black in colour, 1 cm × 8 cm and 1 cm apart, lying horizontally across the left buttock
- Walking with unsteady toddler gait, fell twice during examination
- Relates well to Joanne, but takes less of an interest in John

Careful documentation of injuries is essential. The site, size, shape and colour of the bruise must be recorded, and the presence of swelling or tenderness noted. Using a body map to document bruising and other injuries is often easier than freehand drawings (Figure 16.2). Photographs are extremely helpful. It is important to palpate the scalp and part the hair to look for bruising to the head. It is essential to check the mouth and frenulum. A tear to the frenulum (Figure 16.3) can occur accidentally by a child falling on his mouth, but it can also occur by a punch or a spoon being forcefully shoved into the mouth.

Self-test 4: How accurately will the paediatrician be able to date the bruising?

Answer: Bruising can't be dated accurately.

Distribution of bruising is an indicator of abuse:

- Buttocks, lower back and outer thighs – often related to punishment

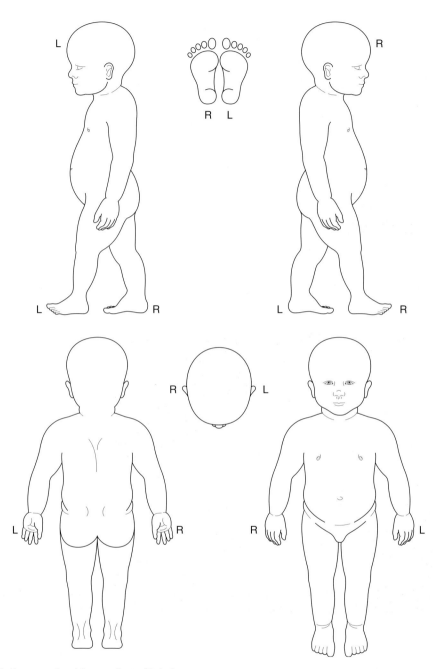

Figure 16.2   Body maps to aid recording of injuries.

- Inner thigh and genital area – suggests sexual abuse or punishment for wetting
- Head, neck and face – common in abuse
- External ear – rarely accidental
- Distal to elbow and knees – commonly accidental

Pattern of bruising may suggest particular injuries:

- Finger-tip bruising where a child has been gripped with excessive force, on the face which may result from a child being force-fed, or on the arms and chest in a baby who has been shaken

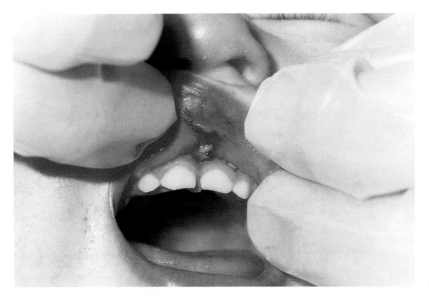

Figure 16.3 Torn frenulum.

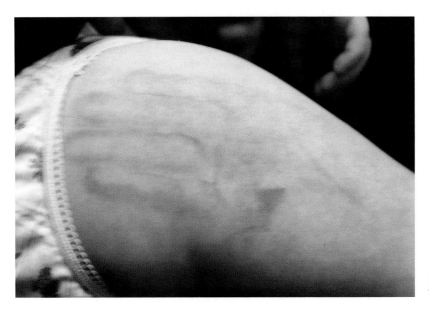

Figure 16.4 Slap mark on upper thigh.

- Slap marks may leave a hand print (Figure 16.4)
- Imprint from an implement, e.g. belt or stick

Self-test 5: What does Figure 16.5 show?

Answer: Bruising to the lower half of the back, buttocks and thigh. The pattern of bruising on the left buttock is compatible with a slap mark. The bruising is of varying colour and therefore of different ages. The extent of the bruising is far in excess of that seen in a normal healthy child, and therefore is highly likely to be non-accidental.

Interpretation of the examination

Callum appears to be a healthy child whose growth and development are age appropriate. The grubby clothes,

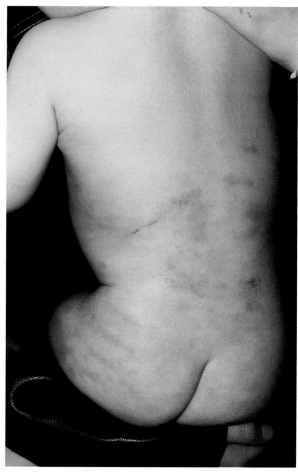

Figure 16.5   Self-test 5. Bruising to a 14-month-old child.

extensive nappy rash and dirty fingernails suggest an element of neglect.

The outline of the bruising to the arm is nondescript and therefore it is difficult for the doctor to suggest how it might have been caused. The pattern of bruising to the buttock is compatible with a handprint.

Accurately ageing bruising is not possible. There are various different schemes that highlight the caution doctors should adopt when discussing the ages of bruises in court. The red/purple discoloration to the orbit, plus swelling and tenderness, indicates recent trauma, probably less than 48 hours, whereas the bruising to the buttock and arm is likely to be older.

Differential diagnosis

Although a bleeding disorder cannot be ruled out, the paediatrician considers that the bruising is likely to be non-accidental in nature:

- The alleged accident causing the bruising to the eye was unwitnessed
- There isn't an explanation for the bruising to the arm and the child's developmental level is such that it is highly unlikely to have occurred without a carer being aware of it
- The pattern of bruising to the buttock is compatible with Callum being slapped forcefully

Investigations

- **Clotting studies** (see Chapter 23)
- **Skeletal survey:** in view of the significant bruising, it is important to look for an underlying bony injury, old or new
- **Computed tomography (CT) of the brain:** if there are concerns about possible shaking injury, to look for subdural haemorrhage
- **Examination of the fundi by an ophthalmologist:** to detect retinal haemorrhages, which are associated with a shaking injury

Results

Callum had normal clotting studies and the skeletal survey was negative.

Diagnosis

Non-accidental injury.

Management and follow-up plan

The paediatrician explains to the parents that he is concerned about the extent of bruising to Callum, particularly as it isn't clear how it happened. He points out the hand print on the buttocks and asks how it happened – the parents reply that they don't know. The paediatrician informs the parents that the clotting studies are normal and therefore Callum must have sustained significant trauma to result in the bruising. He explains that he has a duty to inform Social Services, because there is no explanation. He explains the need for a skeletal survey and obtains consent for the bruising to be photographed. The paediatrician needs to be prepared for many possible different responses from the parents. This may range from passive acceptance to anger and denial, with threats to remove the child from the ward. Should the parents try to remove the child, health professionals should try to dissuade them and stall them while the police are summoned.

Callum's father storms off but his mother stays. By this stage it is 10 pm and the paediatrician arranges for Callum to be admitted to the ward. He contacts Social Services. The social worker assesses the immediate level of risk to the child based on the medical information available, and decides that Callum will be safe overnight in the hospital because his mother is cooperating. He arranges for a social worker from the local team to contact the paediatrician next morning. Consideration needs to be given to the safety of any other children in the household, if there are any.

The social worker contacts the paediatrician the next morning and discusses the medical findings. A strategy meeting is arranged for the police, social worker and paediatrician to exchange information and plan a joint investigation (Table 16.1).

In the short term it is important to ensure the child's safety. It is not appropriate for Callum to spend any length of time in an acute hospital ward. Possible options are for Callum to go home to his parents, to another family member or to foster carers. The social worker considers that the potential risks of Callum returning home to his parents are too high. After further checks it is agreed that Callum will go with his mother to his grandparents' house and that they will take responsibility for supervising the care at all times. Callum's mother agrees to this plan and it is unnecessary for the social worker to obtain an Emergency Protection Order. Such an order can be obtained from a magistrate and lasts up to 8 days with a possible extension of up to 7 days. Callum is discharged from hospital.

Table 16.1   Role of social services and the police in child protection

Social services

Social Services have a duty to investigate cases of suspected abuse and will carry out an assessment of the family. The Framework for the Assessment of Children in Need is a new approach to the assessment of children and families. It provides a systematic way of analysing, understanding and recording what is happening to children and young people within their families and the community within which they live (Figure 16.6)

The police

The police have a duty to investigate criminal offences committed against any individual, including children. All police forces have child protection units (CPUs), which normally take primary responsibility for investigating child abuse cases. The police officers in such units have received specialist training, much of it jointly with social workers. It is usual policy for Social Services to discuss all referrals regarding possible child abuse with the police CPU. In more serious and certain abuse, the police usually decide on early involvement and often a strategy meeting involving the police, Social Services and the paediatrician is held to plan a joint investigation

The child protection conference is held 3 days later (Table 16.2). The paediatrician attends and provides a medical report. The professionals at the case conference decide that Callum is at ongoing risk and therefore his name is placed on the child protection register.

Self-test 6: What is the child protection register?

Answer: It is a list of children in the locality who have been subjected to abuse or to likely abuse, which is held by Social Services. The benefits are that the child becomes the subject of an interagency child protection plan with automatic review at least every 6 months.

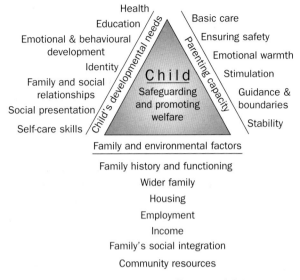

Health
Education
Emotional & behavioural development
Identity
Family and social relationships
Social presentation
Self-care skills

Child's developmental needs

Basic care
Ensuring safety
Emotional warmth
Stimulation
Guidance & boundaries
Stability

Parenting capacity

Child
Safeguarding and promoting welfare

Family and environmental factors

Family history and functioning
Wider family
Housing
Employment
Income
Family's social integration
Community resources

Figure 16.6   The Assessment Framework Triangle used by Social Services to assess children in need. (From Department of Health, Department of Education and Employment. *Framework for the Assessment of Children in Need and their Families*. London: The Stationery Office, 2000.)

Table 16.2   Child protection conference

Aims:	exchange of information
	Decide if child's name to be included on child protection register
Chair:	senior social worker
Present:	social workers, police, health visitor or school nurse, child's (and siblings) teacher, parents, paediatrician, GP

Callum is to continue to live at his grandparents' house while Social Services carry out a full assessment. Whether or not Callum returns to the care of his parents will depend on their willingness to acknowledge concerns and work with the different agencies. If they do not, Social Services may consider applying for a Care Order through the Family Court. This would give them the authority to determine where Callum lives and who cares for him.

The police interview both parents and other possible witnesses. They will then decide if they have enough evidence to prosecute. They will require a statement from the paediatrician and, if the case goes to court, the paediatrician may be required to attend to give evidence in the Criminal Court.

How to write a report/statement

Points to note:

● Notes must be clear, legible, full and contemporaneous. They are the basis from which a medical report will be written
● Avoid jargon, explain any medical terms
● Ensure that the thinking process in the report is clear and well reasoned
● Make it clear in the report that you have considered all the possible alternatives
● Stay within your level of expertise – to stray is dangerous and will get you into trouble in Court

Report

Initial paragraph

Name	Give full name
Age	Over 21
Qualifications	
Address	Use professional address
Occupation	e.g. full registered medical practitioner
Present employment	
Experience	e.g. 5 years' experience in acute paediatrics

Main introductory paragraph

Set the examination in context:

On Sunday 1 September 2002 I was asked to exam Callum ... (d.o.b) ... by the A&E doctor at ABC District General Hospital, because of unexplained bruising. Callum was accompanied by his parents, Joanne ... and John ..., who gave consent for the examination. They told me that ... .

Relevant medical history

● State positives and negatives – in unexplained bruising it is important to show that you have considered all the possible causes of bruising, both accidental and non-accidental, and medical

- Comment on the developmental level of the child if this is going to be of importance in your conclusions

Social history
Examination
- State that consent has been obtained from the carer with parental responsibility
- Record findings, positive and negative
- Record details of injuries

Investigations
- State whether normal or abnormal, no need to give actual results

Opinions/conclusions
- Be clear, concise and honest – if there is doubt say so, for example:

In my opinion my findings are consistent with Callum having been slapped on the buttock with excessive force.

Statement of truth
I believe that the facts I have stated in this report are true and that the opinions I have expressed are correct.

Signature and date
- Do not forget to sign and date your report. It is also useful to keep a personal copy of the report

Background information

Incidence and prevalence

The concept that carers may abuse their children was first recognized as a medical problem in the 1950s, although children have been physically harmed, neglected and subjected to sexual abuse throughout history. The different categories of abuse are:

- Physical: bruises, burns, lacerations, fractures and internal injuries, poisoning, fabricated and induced illness
- Neglect
- Emotional

- Sexual: includes the involvement of children in pornography

It is estimated that 1.5–2 per cent of all children have been physically abused by the age of 17 years. Nearly half are aged 0–4 years and boys slightly outnumber girls. Of serious head injuries 70 per cent occurred to children less than 1 year old. Disabled children are seen to be at increased risk and in some instances the abuse may be the cause of the disability.

It is common for children to suffer from more than one form of abuse. A degree of emotional abuse is usually associated with other forms of abuse. It is estimated that one in six physically abused children has also been sexually abused.

The sustained abuse or neglect of children physically, emotionally or sexually can have major long-term effects on all aspects of a child's health, development and well-being. Problems may extend into adulthood and lead to difficulties in forming or maintaining close relationships, and in the development of the attitudes and skills needed to be an effective parent.

Further sources of information

Books

Meadow R (ed.) *ABC of Child Abuse*. London: BMJ Books, 1989

Department of Health, Home Office, Department for Education and Employment. *Working Together to Safeguard Children*. London: The Stationery Office, 1999

Article

Stephenson T. Bruising in children. *Current Pediatrics* 1999; **5**: 225–9

Self-test 7: The orthopaedic surgeons ask the medical registrar to assess as possible non-accidental injury a 4-month-old girl who has just been admitted with a fractured right femur. Her mother had explained that she had rolled off the couch 2 days ago and that she had seemed fine. However, she had suddenly become unsettled today. When granny had visited she had noticed that the baby didn't move her right leg and seemed to be in pain when her nappy was changed. Granny advised her daughter to seek medical advice:

A What are the most important features in the history?

B What should the medical registrar do next?

C What are the developmental issues that need to be considered in this case?

D What investigation should be carried out next?

E Who should the medical registrar involve at this point?

Answers:

A The timing of the injury doesn't fit with the presentation of the symptoms; another adult, not the mother, noted the signs; falling off a couch is unlikely to produce enough force to result in a fracture to the femur

B Take a detailed medical and social history and carry out a physical examination

C Most children don't start to roll over until 5 months. Has this baby advanced motor skills?

D Skeletal survey

E The registrar should discuss the case with his or her consultant, who will make a referral to Social Services

A chronic rash

Age: 13 months

LEENA PATEL

Presentation

When Tom is 13 months of age, Tom's mother asks the health visitor about the rash on his face, arms and legs. She had been told it was a 'baby rash' when it appeared a few weeks after Tom was born. Recently, the rash appears to have spread more, looks rather angry and Tom scratches almost constantly. The health visitor thinks it might be eczema but asks the clinic doctor to see Tom.

Self-test 1: Would you agree with the health visitor's diagnosis?

Answer: Although the health visitor may be right, it is the doctor's duty to assess Tom and ascertain whether he has:

1 Atopic eczema or some other condition such as scabies

2 An acute-on-chronic condition; acute rashes, such as impetigo and chickenpox, are common in childhood (Table 17.1) and Tom has a history of recent worsening

Initial considerations and action

A rash since early infancy in this toddler suggests a chronic condition. The presence of itching (pruritus) helps differentiate it from some common skin conditions that are non-itchy (Table 17.1). The most common cause of a chronic itchy rash in childhood is atopic eczema.

Table 17.1 Acute and chronic rashes

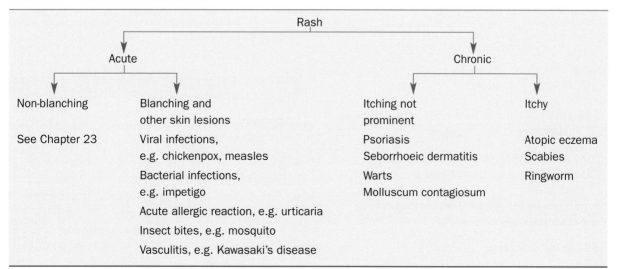

	Rash		
Acute		**Chronic**	
Non-blanching	Blanching and other skin lesions	Itching not prominent	Itchy
See Chapter 23	Viral infections, e.g. chickenpox, measles	Psoriasis	Atopic eczema
	Bacterial infections, e.g. impetigo	Seborrhoeic dermatitis	Scabies
	Acute allergic reaction, e.g. urticaria	Warts	Ringworm
	Insect bites, e.g. mosquito	Molluscum contagiosum	
	Vasculitis, e.g. Kawasaki's disease		

History

Important points in the history and examination of a child with a chronic itchy rash

To diagnose whether it is atopic eczema or another itchy skin condition (e.g. scabies)

- Rash:
  - how it started
  - type of lesions: redness, scaling, thickening with accentuation of skin creases (lichenification) from chronic rubbing, excoriation, fissuring, changes in pigmentation
  - distribution
  - change over time
- Dryness
- Itching, scratching
- Specific signs: linear infraorbital fold (called Dennie–Morgan crease), hyperlinearity of palms
- Any coexisting conditions:
  - asthma, hayfever, rhinitis
  - allergic reactions
  - skin infections
- Anyone in the family with:
  - asthma, hayfever
  - itchy lesions of scabies
- Any pets

To determine the cause of the recent deterioration (e.g. bacterial infection)

- Any known aggravating factors, e.g. woollen clothes, foods, contact with animal
- Signs of infection: pustules, crusting, weeping, redness, oedema, lymphadenopathy

To identify current and past treatment, including diet changes, and effectiveness

- Details of treatment and whether it helped
- Dietary restrictions and response

To understand the physical and emotional impact on the child and family

- Sleep disturbance
- School, work
- Teasing/bullying
- Abnormal body image

To explore parents' concerns and expectations about treatment

Tom has had dry skin since he was a baby. When he was a few weeks old, red dry blotches appeared on his cheeks and later he had blotches all over. His mother was told not to worry about them because they would soon clear. The rash has seemed better at times but has never really cleared. His mother intermittently applied baby oil to Tom's skin but it did not help much. As Tom appeared healthy in every other way, his mother did not want to bother the GP. However, Tom's rash has been awful for the past few weeks, becoming more red and raw on the hands and face. His mother asks why Tom's skin has got worse instead of getting better. It seemed to flare up 'out of the blue'. His 6-year-old sister has named him 'pickle face'. Tom scratches almost constantly, even at night. It makes him miserable. The Piriton the chemist recommended hasn't touched him. Bath time is a battle. The sheets are a mess from blood and scales. Mother is exhausted from trying to stop Tom from scratching, lack of sleep and the housework.

Tom was not unwell with a fever or runny nose when his skin flared up. He does not suffer from any other illness and does not have any medicines regularly. He does not have asthma or hayfever and is not allergic to any foods or medicines. He had cows' milk formula as a baby. Father has asthma and mother gets cold sores. They do not smoke and do not have any pets. Tom is the only one in the family with itchy skin.

Examination

Observation and examination, while the mother related Tom's history, revealed:

- A bright and responsive child who scratched his face despite the mittens on his hands
- Severe redness with excoriation, scaling and some oozing on the face, hands, wrists, arms and legs (especially around the elbows and knees)
- A few dry slightly red patches on the chest and back but the nappy area was spared

- Visibly enlarged lymph nodes in the axillae and groins and palpably enlarged nodes in the anterior triangles of the neck – soft, not tender and not hot
- No pallor of mucous membranes, jaundice, petechiae or enlarged liver or spleen

Interpretation of the history and examination

Features of atopic eczema compared with other diagnoses (Table 17.2)

Atopic eczema is suggested by the:

- **Age of onset:** first 12 months of life in up to 60 per cent of children
- **Nature of the rash:** extent and severity varies from the odd, mildly inflamed patch to extremely distressing severe inflammation affecting almost the whole of the body surface area (Figure 17.1)
- **Itching:** except for the first few months of life, the sensation of itch and the resultant scratching are universal
- **Chronic fluctuating course:** usually most troublesome in the first few years and becomes less severe as the child gets older

Table 17.2 The UK diagnostic criteria for atopic eczema

The child must have:
An itchy skin condition in the last 12 months + three or more of the following:

1 Onset below the age of 2 years in a child older than 4 years
2 History of flexural involvement (front of elbows, behind knees, front of ankles, neck)
3 History of a generally dry skin
4 Personal history of asthma or hayfever or in a child under 4 years of age, history of atopic disease in a first-degree relative
5 Visible flexural dermatitis or in a child under 4 years of age, dermatitis involving the cheeks, forehead and outer limbs

Adapted with permission from Blackwell Publishers (Williams HC et al. The UK Working Party's diagnostic criteria for atopic dermatitis III. Independent hospital validation. *British Journal of Dermatology* 1994; **131**: 406–16).

Asthma occurs at some time in up to 40 per cent of children with atopic eczema. Although eczematous skin lesions may be a feature of an immunodeficiency state, Tom does not have any clinical features suggestive of this:

- Serious systemic infections
- Persistent systemic infections
- Unusual infections
- Recurrent systemic infections
- Malabsorption
- Failure to thrive
- Petechiae

The cause of the recent deterioration

Explanations for Tom's recent deterioration that may be considered and excluded are:

- Exacerbation of atopic eczema caused by a specific trigger, e.g. contact with cat – Tom has no such history
- Associated secondary skin infection – the lesions on Tom's face and limbs have the appearance of a bacterial infection (Table 17.3 and see Figure 17.1)
- Another common skin condition:
  - scabies: no family history and Tom does not have papules or blisters on the palms, interdigital spaces or soles (Figure 17.2, p. 174)
  - chickenpox: Tom's rash does not have the characteristic appearance, distribution and evolution (see Figure 17.1)
  - acute allergic reactions or insect bites: no history

Current and past treatment and its effectiveness

Details about current and past treatment and the response to treatment are helpful in planning future treatment. Often parents will have tried other treatments (including alternative therapies such as Chinese herbal teas and homoeopathy). Reasons why baby oil was not helpful for Tom may be:

- The intermittent application – frequent applications daily are necessary to moisturize dry skin in atopic eczema
- Lack of anti-inflammatory effect
- Diagnosis other than atopic eczema

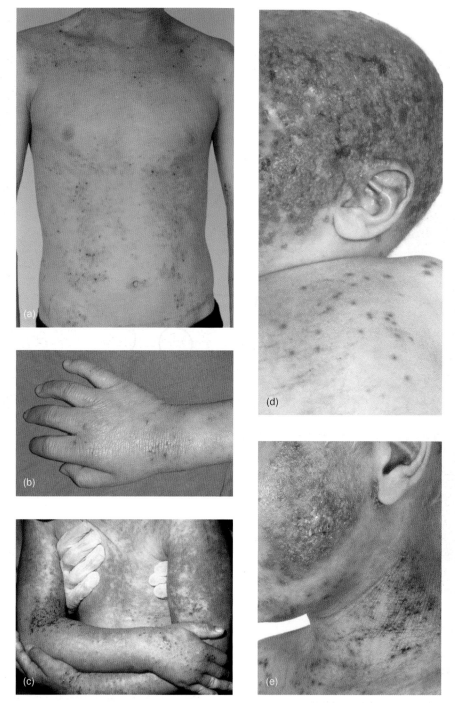

Figure 17.1 Examination findings in children with atopic eczema: (a) the trunk of a boy with extensive atopic eczema; (b) thickening of the skin and lichenification are signs of chronic atopic eczema; (c) scratching results in excoriation and skin inflammation may be followed by areas of hyper- or hypopigmentation; (d) an infant and (e) a teenager with secondary bacterial infection (pustules, crusting and weeping) on the face;

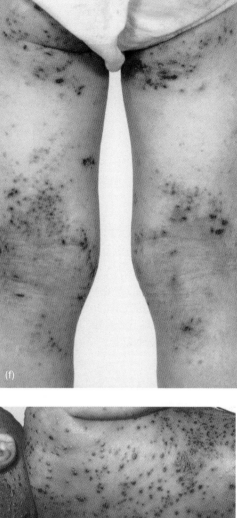

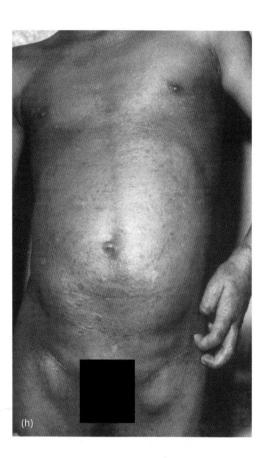

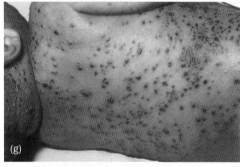

Figure 17.1 (*continued*) (f) inflamed ectopic eczema with recurrent herpes simplex infection; (g) exacerbation of atopic eczema associated with chicken pox; (h) gross lymphadenopathy is common in children with troublesome atopic eczema.

Piriton (chlorpheniramine) is:

- An antihistamine
- Available over the counter
- Of benefit in histamine-induced acute allergic rashes (e.g. bee sting or drug reaction) but not atopic eczema

A sedative may assist sleep in a child with troublesome itching. The sedating effect of chlorpheniramine is not effective enough or comparable to trimeprazine (Vallergan). The itching in atopic eczema is the result of numerous mediators in addition to histamine, and is therefore not relieved by antihistamines.

Tom's history does not suggest a specific food allergy. Many parents wrongly believe that their child is allergic to a food. A child should not unquestioningly be labelled as being 'allergic' to a particular food simply because a carer mentions this. A detailed history and

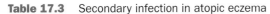

Table 17.3   Secondary infection in atopic eczema

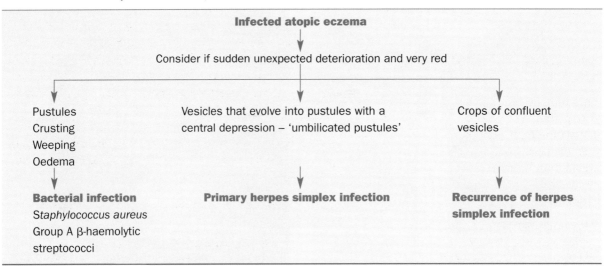

Infected atopic eczema		
Consider if sudden unexpected deterioration and very red		
Pustules Crusting Weeping Oedema	Vesicles that evolve into pustules with a central depression – 'umbilicated pustules'	Crops of confluent vesicles
Bacterial infection *Staphylococcus aureus* Group A β-haemolytic streptococci	**Primary herpes simplex infection**	**Recurrence of herpes simplex infection**

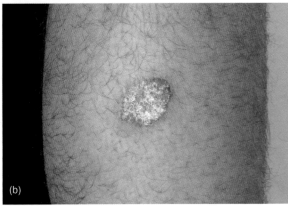

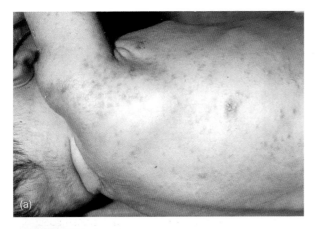

Figure 17.2   The typical rash of (a) scabies and (b) psoriasis.

careful assessment of the information obtained is required to ascertain whether the food does indeed trigger the child's eczema. If any foods are being avoided, it is important to clarify:

- Which foods are avoided
- Why these foods are avoided
- How carefully the diet is adhered to
- If the eczema has improved

Impact on the child and family

Tom's condition is distressing for him and the family as a result of:

- Intense itching, which leads to scratching and then to excoriation and bleeding, and finally sleep disturbance for Tom and mother
- The time, effort and cooperation needed for cleaning and bathing Tom
- The time and effort needed to wash Tom's clothes and bedlinen

Physical, psychological and social suffering in children older than Tom is the result of:

- Restrictions in daytime activities, schooling, work and social life
- Physical disfigurement, embarrassment, bullying
- Mess and nuisance of topical treatment

Even the simple task of holding a pencil and writing is difficult with sore greasy hands, which make the paper greasy.

Exploring parents' expectations about treatment

Tom's mother had not expected his skin to get worse. Most parents expect treatment to be curative rather than symptomatic and this will need to be addressed when management is discussed.

Had Tom been seen before for his skin condition, the medical records may have provided useful information about:

- Previous management and whether it was effective
- Skin swab results and whether he had MRSA (methicillin-resistant *Staphylococcus aureus*)
- Specific concerns

Self-test 2: Explain Tom's lymphadenopathy.

Answer: When there is infection in any area, the draining lymph nodes are inflamed and enlarged (see Figure 17.1, p. 172–173), and may rarely be complicated by abscess formation. Tom's extensive infected eczema explains the generalized lymphadenopathy. Reassuringly, the enlarged lymph nodes do not have any features of abscess formation (no redness, warmth, tenderness or fluctuation). The absence of systemic symptoms, hepatosplenomegaly, pallor and petechiae excludes sinister pathology such as acute lymphoblastic leukaemia.

Self-test 3: Why is the itching in atopic eczema not relieved by an antihistamine?

Answer: Because the itching in atopic eczema is mediated not only by histamine but also by many other factors. Table 17.4 differentiates atopic eczema from other common skin conditions.

Table 17.4 Atopic eczema differentiated from other common skin conditions

Typical features	Atopic eczema	Scabies	Psoriasis	Seborrhoeic dermatitis	Tinea corporis
Onset	<2 years	Recent	Any age but rare in neonates	Infancy, adulthood	
Itching	Very itchy	Very itchy	Uncommon	Unusual	Yes
Mood	Restless	Placid			
Appearance	Dry, erythematous Maculopapular rash	Papules, vesicles Moth-eaten eczema	Well-demarcated pink plaques with thick silvery scale	Dry, scaly, erythematous papular rash; diffuse scaling and crusting on scalp	Macular, papular or annular erythema with raised scaly edge and central clearing
Distribution	Symmetrical flexure surfaces	Symmetrical	Extensor surfaces, lumbosacral	Focal and patchy or symmetrical	Asymmetrical
Face	Common	Uncommon	Uncommon	Common in adults	
Scalp	Common	Uncommon	Common	Common (cradle cap)	
Nappy area	Spared			Common	
Specific signs		Burrows on hands and feet	Nail dystrophy, Koebner's response		Nail dystrophy
Acute exacerbations	Bacterial or viral infections		Streptococcal infections		

Investigations

Serum IgE levels are above the reference ranges in 80–85 per cent of patients with atopic eczema. However, it is not essential because the diagnosis of atopic eczema is clinical.

As Tom's eczema is thought to be infected, skin swabs are taken for bacteriology and virology (Table 17.5). Allergy tests are not reliable and fail to predict those who will benefit from avoidance measures.

Diagnosis

Tom's most likely diagnosis is atopic eczema with an acute-on-chronic exacerbation secondary to bacterial infection.

Almost one in seven children (15 per cent) suffer from atopic eczema at some time. Secondary bacterial infection is commonly associated with exacerbation of atopic eczema.

Table 17.5   How to take skin swabs in atopic eczema

Skin swabs for bacteriology

Method: as lesions are often dry, the end of a sterile swab is moistened with sterile water before swabbing the skin

Usefulness: in identifying common pathogens and their sensitivity to antibiotics
- *Staphylococcus aureus*
- Multi-resistant strains of *Staph. aureus* and methicillin-resistant *Staph. aureus* (MRSA)
- Group A β-haemolytic streptococci

Note: as *Staph. aureus* colonizes the skin of most patients with atopic eczema, identification of the organism is not in itself an indication for antibiotic treatment

Skin swabs for virology

Method: the end of a sterile swab is dipped in the virology transport medium before swabbing the skin

Indications:
Herpes simplex infection is suspected
An acute exacerbation of atopic eczema because herpes simplex infection may not be clinically obvious

Management

The principles of management are:

- Providing information to the family about the natural history of atopic eczema and rationale for treatment
- Providing support to the family for the burden of a chronic disorder
- Controlling the acute exacerbation by treating secondary infection with topical antiseptics and systemic antibiotics
- Preventing and treating skin dryness with emollients
- Reducing skin inflammation with topical corticosteroids
- Helping the child sleep at night with a sedative
- Avoiding known triggers

Explanation and education for carers and patients

Treatment should be tailored for each patient depending on previous treatment. The doctor explains to Tom's mother:

- The natural history of atopic eczema: it is most troublesome in the first few years and usually causes less suffering as the child gets older
- The treatment recommended (see below)
- The role of eczema/dermatology nurse specialists and community nurses in providing additional information and support

Providing support

Support is provided by nurse specialists, community nurses, organizations such as the National Eczema Society and other parents.

Oral antibiotics

As secondary bacterial infection is suspected, Tom is recommended oral antibiotics (Table 17.6) because:

- The lesions are widespread
- The risk of sensitization and resistance is greater with topical antibiotics

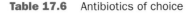

Table 17.6   Antibiotics of choice

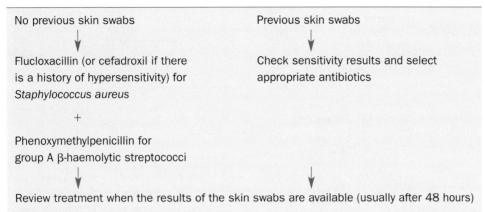

No previous skin swabs	Previous skin swabs
↓	↓
Flucloxacillin (or cefadroxil if there is a history of hypersensitivity) for *Staphylococcus aureus*	Check sensitivity results and select appropriate antibiotics
+	
Phenoxymethylpenicillin for group A β-haemolytic streptococci	
↓	↓
Review treatment when the results of the skin swabs are available (usually after 48 hours)	

Primary herpes simplex infection: eczema herpeticum

The following are the features of a primary (initial) herpes simplex infection in a child with atopic eczema:

- Systemically unwell, a high fever
- Scattered, thin-walled vesicles with clear or turbid fluid initially
- Lesions with a characteristic central depression later

Tom does not have these features. Primary herpes simplex lesions are invariably complicated by secondary bacterial skin infection. Management therefore includes preventing and treating secondary bacterial infection. Severe cases require hospital admission, intravenous aciclovir, intravenous antibiotics and close monitoring of fluid balance.

Recurrent herpes simplex skin infection

This is common in children with atopic eczema. The vesicles appear confluent and quickly rupture, leaving a patch of inflamed skin that may be difficult to distinguish from ordinary eczematous lesions (see Figure 17.1). The child is not likely to be systemically unwell. As with primary infection, it is important to prevent and treat secondary bacterial infection. There is no proven benefit of aciclovir.

Emollients

- Emollients improve hydration of the skin by reducing evaporation and may act as a protective barrier.
- Emulsifying ointment or white soft paraffin needs to be applied liberally as often as necessary to keep the skin moisturized
- Ointments are preferable to creams, lotions and oils as:
  - they are greasier and therefore better and longer-lasting emollients for dry skin
  - the absence of preservatives or stabilizers in an ointment reduces the risk of irritation or contact sensitization
- An interval of at least 1 hour is recommended in between application of emollient and that of topical corticosteroid, and vice versa, so as not to dilute the effect of the corticosteroid
- Emollients are safe even if applied frequently

Topical corticosteroids

Topical corticosteroids control the inflammation and relieve symptoms but treatment is not curative. The basic principles are to use:

- Ointments rather than creams
- The least potent preparation as sparingly as possible to affected areas only (Table 17.7)

Table 17.7 Topical corticosteroid preparations of choice

| Site | Potency and preparation | |
	First line	Second line
Scalp	*Mild potency* One per cent hydrocortisone scalp lotion once daily	Seek advice
Face and neck	*Mild potency*: twice daily, e.g. One per cent hydrocortisone ointment Vioform–Hydrocortisone ointment	Seek advice
Trunk and limbs	*Mild potency*: twice daily, e.g. One per cent hydrocortisone ointment Vioform–Hydrocortisone ointment	*Moderate potency* – twice daily, e.g. Synalar 1 in 4 dilution (fluocinolone acetonide 0.00625%) ointment Betnovate-RD (betamethasone valerate 0.025%) ointment Eumovate (clobetasone butyrate 0.05%) ointment

As most parents think topical steroids are dangerous, it is explained to Tom's mother that:

● Topical steroids come in four strengths: mild, moderate, potent and very potent
● Mild and moderate potency corticosteroids used sensibly provide symptomatic benefit and are relatively safe. Potent corticosteroid preparations should not be used unless recommended by a specialist

As Tom's eczema is infected, topical treatment with Vioform–Hydrocortisone ointment (containing 1 per cent hydrocortisone and an antiseptic clioquinol) to all eczema lesions twice a day is recommended until the exacerbation is controlled. An improvement is expected in most patients within 7–14 days. Tom will need to be reviewed after 14 days with a view to revising and reinforcing treatment (Figure 17.3).

Side-to-side comparison of topical treatment

● The aim is to find the most suitable topical corticosteroid for continuing use
● The face and neck are treated separately from the rest of the body, dividing it into right and left sides
● The rest of the body is divided into two halves or four quadrants, and one 1/2 or quadrant is treated as a control with emollient only and no topical corticosteroid
● The patient's current topical corticosteroid preparation may be compared with one or more new ones, usually from a different potency category or including an antibacterial agent if there is a history of recurrent secondary bacterial infection

---

Self-test 4: (1) What are the adverse effects of topical corticosteroids and (2) when are they more likely to occur?

Answer:

1 *Local effects* *Potential systemic effects*
   Skin atrophy   Hypothalamic–pituitary–adrenal suppression
                  Impaired growth
                  Cushing's syndrome
                  Reduced bone mineral density

2 Risk of adverse effects is greater:
   ● In infants and those with extensive involvement
   ● With severe inflammation
   ● With prolonged treatment with potent and very potent preparations (and failure to step down to less potent treatment)
   ● With application of occlusive dressings

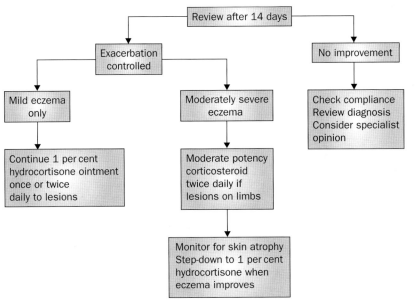

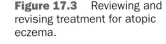

Figure 17.3 Reviewing and revising treatment for atopic eczema.

Self-test 5: Why are oral corticosteroids not routinely recommended for atopic eczema in childhood?

Answer: Because
1. Prolonged treatment for a chronic condition is associated with a significant risk of adverse effects
2. Short courses bring temporary relief and rebound worsening when treatment is discontinued

Night-time sedative

Tom is recommended a sedative because he has difficulty getting to sleep and the itching disturbs his sleep. The drug of choice is trimeprazine tartrate (2–3 mg/kg before bedtime) in children over 6 months of age (its sedative effect is stronger than that of chlorpheniramine). Mother is reassured that it is not addictive. Daytime use of sedating antihistamines should be avoided.

Avoiding known triggers

The following should be avoided:

- Foods if there is a clear history of food triggers with the diet supervised by a paediatric dietician – this is not the case for Tom
- Irritant clothing such as woollens
- Soap and detergents

Washing and bathing

The frequency of bathing depends on what best suits Tom and whether he prefers a shower. Soap should be avoided and emulsifying ointment or a dispersible bath oil should be used instead. Cetrimide shampoo may help infected eczema affecting the scalp and face.

Tom's progress

A considerable improvement in Tom's eczema is noticeable within 2 days. *Staphylococcus aureus* (sensitive to flucloxacillin) and group A β-haemolytic streptococci (sensitive to penicillin) are isolated from the skin swabs. He is advised to complete the 2-week course of oral flucloxacillin and phenoxymethylpenicillin, and to continue the topical treatment until he is reviewed in the outpatient clinic in 2–3 months. A summary of the management of atopic eczema is as follows (Figure 17.4):

- First-line treatment:
  - explanation and discussion

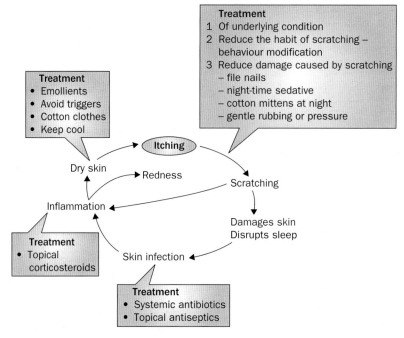

Figure 17.4 Management of atopic eczema.

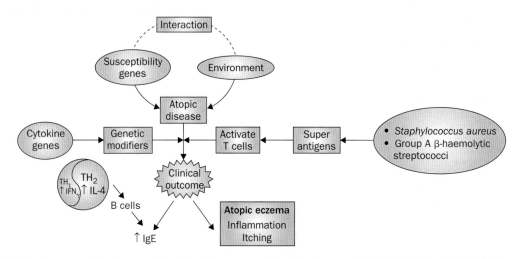

Figure 17.5 A proposed pathogenesis of atopic eczema. IFNγ, interferon-γ; IL-4, interleukin 4; TH, T-helper cells.

- – avoidance of known triggers
- – emollients
- – topical corticosteroids
- – systemic antibiotics for bacterial infections
- – night-time sedatives
- Second- and third-line treatments:
  - – topical tacrolimus ointment
- – elimination diets
- – oral corticosteroids
- – cyclosporin
- – phototherapy and photochemotherapy
- – no proven benefit
- – wet wraps to the whole body
- – evening primrose oil

Background information

Pathogenesis of atopic eczema

Atopic disease results from complex, and as yet poorly defined, interactions between susceptibility genes and the environment (see Chapter 26). These interactions modified by other factors such as cytokine genes, T lymphocytes and superantigens (e.g. from *Staphylococcus aureus)* are likely to influence whether an atopic individual manifests any clinical features of atopic eczema (Figure 17.5).

Further sources of information

Articles

Barnetson R St C, Rogers M. Childhood atopic eczema. *British Medical Journal* 2002; **324**: 137–9

Charman C. Clinical evidence: atopic eczema. *British Medical Journal* 1999; **318**: 1600–4

McHenry PM, Williams HC, Bingham EA. Fortnightly review: Management of atopic eczema. *British Medical Journal* 1995; **310**: 843–7

Williams H. New treatments for atopic dermatitis. *British Medical Journal* 2002; **324**: 1533–4

Self-test 6: The following is report of the skin swab from a child with an exacerbation of atopic eczema:

Organisms isolated	Sensitivity to:		
	Penicillin	Ampicillin	Methicillin
Staphylococcus aureus	Resistant	Resistant	Resistant
Group A β-haemolytic streptococci	Sensitive	Sensitive	Resistant

A What *three* conclusions can you draw from this bacteriology report?

B If the child is admitted to hospital for treatment, what is the single most important precaution that must be taken?

Answers:

A

1 Two organisms have been isolated

2 The *Staphylococcus aureus* is methicillin resistant

3 The group A β-haemolytic streptococci are sensitive to penicillin

B Isolation in a cubicle.

Self-test 7: When might you consider referring a child with atopic eczema to hospital?

Answers: Indications for referral to hospital and possible admission to hospital are:

1 Severe acute flare-ups, often caused by infection, which cannot be controlled at home

2 Eczema herpeticum

3 Troublesome atopic eczema poorly controlled with first-line treatment

CHAPTER 18

Chronic disorder

A pale picky eater who drinks too much milk and will not sleep

Age: 3 years

JACKIE GREGG

Presentation

Referral letter from GP:
Please see this 3-year-old boy who doesn't eat. His mother is worried that he is underweight and looks pale. In addition he doesn't sleep and his mum is exhausted.

Initial considerations and action

The information in the referral letter is very limited:

- A 3 year old who doesn't eat – a common problem. What parents usually mean is that the child doesn't eat what they think he should eat. A detailed dietary history is needed. A child who truly doesn't eat is more likely to have an organic problem
- Underweight: is the child actually underweight and failing to thrive and, if so, why? (see Chapter 6)
- Looks pale: is this the result of anaemia and, if so, what is the cause of the anaemia? He may be pale because he is short of sleep or because has a chronic disorder

---

Self-test 1: What is the most common cause of anaemia in children?

Answer: Dietary iron deficiency.

Sleep problems are extremely common. Usually the child does sleep, but only in short bursts or at the wrong time, causing more distress for the parents than the child. The three most common problems are:

- Frequent waking in the night
- Refusing to go to bed
- Getting into the parents' bed

The paediatrician arranges to see the child in his clinic in 3 weeks' time.

History

The child, Peter, attends the clinic with his mother and grandmother.

Feeding and dietary history

Peter's mother is very concerned because she says he doesn't eat. On further questioning it is apparent that Peter does eat, but he is fussy and picks at his food. He has about two spoonfuls of breakfast cereal in the morning, which his mum feels is not enough, so she gives him a bar of chocolate on the way to nursery. Peter has a drink of juice and a biscuit mid-morning, he eats a slice of bread with butter at lunchtime, followed by crisps, and may have a few chicken nuggets at teatime. Mum is worried that he will be hungry in the night and gives him chocolate biscuits before bed. Peter doesn't eat anything unusual, such as soil or sand (pica).

Self-test 2: What is pica?

Self-test 2: What is pica?

Answer: Pica is persistent ingestion of non-food substances. Children with iron deficiency often have pica and may eat soil, stones, chalk, sand, foam, rubber and carpet.

Peter's mum is asked what he likes to drink and how much he has over a 24-hour period. Peter likes milk. He has a nine-ounce bottle of milk on waking, another bottle at lunch, a bottle of milky tea mid-afternoon and at teatime, a bottle of milk before bed and several drinks in the night.

Mealtimes can be a bit variable. If mum is out and there is going to be some delay, she offers Peter crisps 'to keep him going'. His mum says that she is on a constant diet and doesn't sit down with Peter while he eats, because she may be tempted to eat his food and break her diet.

Peter was born at term and weighed 3.7 kg. He fed well as a baby and gained weight at a satisfactory rate. Weaning wasn't a problem. He started to become a bit fussy at 18 months. When he refused food his mum tried to coax him and at times to force him. Meal times became a battle, with his mum becoming more and more anxious. He enjoyed milk and his mum was relieved that he was getting some protein.

Review of systems

Peter is otherwise in good health. He doesn't have any respiratory symptoms; he tends to be constipated, but isn't on any treatment. Peter is lively, but his mum feels that he tires easily. Mum is worried about his weight because she can see his ribs. She has noticed him to be pale over the past few months.

Sleep history

Sleep is a major concern. Peter settles into bed quite happily. However, he wakes three to four times each night. He won't settle back to sleep unless he has a drink of milk. Mum has tried to leave him to cry, but hasn't managed to leave him longer than 15 minutes. He gets very upset and she is worried that he will make himself sick.

Family history

Peter is an only child. His mother is a single parent and his grandmother helps out with his care. Granny feels that

Peter needs to put a bit of weight on and should have knock-out drops to make him sleep.

Self-test 3: What is the significance of Peter's milk intake? Which of the following are relevant?
A The milk intake is excessive
B Milk doesn't provide enough calories
C Too much milk reduces solid food intake
D Milk is low in iron
E Too much milk promotes allergies

Answer: A/C/D.

Interpretation of the history

Areas to consider are:

- Diet
- Calorie intake
- Growth
- General well-being and symptoms of organic disease
- Sleep pattern

Meaning of the history in Peter

Diet

Peter's diet is very poor and is mainly limited to milk and chocolate. His iron intake will therefore be very poor. In addition iron absorption from food is inhibited by tannin in tea. Mum's constant dieting means that he is having limited experience of a normal eating pattern.

Calorie intake

Peter is having a considerable amount of milk, and probably therefore has an adequate calorie and protein intake.

Growth

Parental concerns about their child's weight are very common. With so many fat children around, parents often don't know what a child of appropriate weight should look like – you should be able to see the ribs.

General well-being and symptoms of organic disease

Peter's family have no concerns other than him being a bit tired. The pallor would suggest anaemia, probably as a result of iron deficiency in view of his poor diet. Peter doesn't have any symptoms to suggest any other organic disease. His diet is poor but he isn't anorexic. Leukaemia is the most common malignancy at this age, but this usually presents with abnormal bruising, malaise and infections as well as pallor caused by anaemia. The constipation is likely to result from lack of fibre and roughage in the diet.

Sleep pattern

The problem is frequent night waking, which is reinforced by the drinks of milk.

Examination

- Height: 25th centile
- Weight: 25th centile
- Mucous membranes pale
- Cardiovascular system (CVS): normal examination
- Respiratory system (RS): normal examination
- Abdomen: normal examination, no hepatosplenomegaly
- Skin: no bruising or petechiae

Interpretation of the examination

Peter's height and weight are in proportion. When the paediatrician checks previous weights in the parent-held record, there has been no fall off in weight gain. Peter is not therefore failing to thrive, so his calorie intake must be adequate. There are no findings to suggest a chronic disorder.

The pallor may be caused by iron deficiency anaemia. β-Thalassaemia trait (the heterozygous form) may be confused with mild iron deficiency (Table 18.1). In Britain, thalassaemia is seen predominantly in those of Greek Cypriot or Bangladeshi origin.

Peter doesn't have any findings that would indicate leukaemia.

Table 18.1 Thalassaemia

Thalassaemia syndromes result from inherited defects of globin chain synthesis. There are two main types, α-thalassaemia in which there is reduced rate of α chain synthesis and β-thalassaemias, which are associated with a deficiency of β chains. The latter is the more common. Individuals have an increased proportion of HbF and HbA_2

Clinical symptoms

Thalassaemia major (homozygous for abnormal β genes)

- Failure to thrive
- Severe anaemia and jaundice from 6 months of age
- Extramedullary erythropoiesis leading to thickened skull bones and brittle long bones
- Marked hepatosplenomegaly

Thalassaemia minor (heterozygous for abnormal β gene)

- Usually asymptomatic
- Anaemia mild or absent
- Red cells may be hypochromic and microcytic

Investigations

- Haemoglobin: 9.2 g/dL (low)
- Red blood cell count: reduced
- Mean cell volume: reduced
- White cell count: normal
- Platelets: normal
- Blood film: hypochromic/microcytic
- Serum ferritin: reduced

Peter is anaemic and the blood film is indicative of iron deficiency (Figure 18.1). The low ferritin is diagnostic of iron deficiency. (Note that serum ferritin is an acute phase reactant and will be elevated in acute inflammatory states and liver disease – it will therefore be a less reliable indicator of iron stores in these conditions.)

Serum iron (reduced) and iron-binding capacity (increased) do not add anything to the diagnosis in straightforward cases.

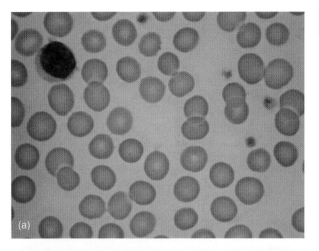

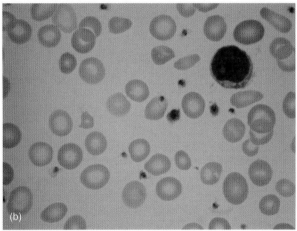

Figure 18.1 (a) Normal blood film; (b) blood film of a child with iron deficiency anaemia.

Investigation in suspected thalassaemia traits: haemoglobin electrophoresis detects which haemoglobins are present, but not their amounts so quantitative measurements of HbA_2 and HbF would need to be carried out.

Diagnosis

Iron deficiency anaemia caused by poor diet.

Self-test 4: Which foods are good dietary sources of iron?

Answer: Red meat, liver, oily fish, poultry.

Treatment and follow-up plan

Management consists of reassuring mum, improving the diet, and replenishing the iron stores by giving iron supplements.

The paediatrician reassures Peter's mother that Peter is well and that his growth is satisfactory. He shows her Peter's growth chart and demonstrates that he is putting on weight at a steady rate and that his height and weight are in proportion. He explains that Peter has anaemia resulting from a diet deficient in iron. As Peter is drinking so much milk, which has a low iron content, he feels full up, so his appetite will be poor for other foods.

Improving Peter's diet

Peter's mum is advised to reduce the amount of milk he is drinking to no more than a pint a day. Rather than give Peter a full bottle when he wakes in the morning, it is preferable to offer a small amount to satisfy his immediate needs and then offer him breakfast while he is hungry. The same applies to other mealtimes.

Snacks between meals need to be carefully monitored and not given too close to the next meal. Dilute fruit juices can be given instead of milk at mealtimes and as snacks. However, intake must be watched, because large quantities of juice can also decrease appetite.

Regular mealtimes are important for a child. Mum is asked to join him for meals and set an example by eating a healthy meal – she is reassured that this can be done as part of a calorie-controlled diet.

The issue of the bottle needs to be tackled, but it's probably easier for Peter's mum to deal with one thing at a time. For children, getting most of their calories from a bottle is easy and they become lazy – eating proper food takes more effort!

Peter should be changed to a cup as soon as possible. Some parents like to continue offering a bottle at bedtime because they feel that it helps their child to settle. Offering drinks in the middle of the night when a child wakes up helps to maintain night waking.

Peter is prescribed a 3-month course of oral iron. His mum is advised that it will turn his stools black.

To achieve good compliance, prescribe a once-daily dose and a 'child-friendly' oral iron preparation. Iron is available as iron salts and iron chelates. The latter is much more acceptable to the child and family because:

- It doesn't stain the teeth
- It can be mixed with milk or juice without altering absorption
- It has fewer gastrointestinal side effects
- It is a sugar-free preparation
- Children like the taste

The paediatrician arranges for Peter's mum to see the dietician before she leaves the clinic. The dietician provides advice on foods high in iron, foods and quantities suitable for a child of this age (Figure 18.2 and see below), and dietary measures to treat constipation. She recommends encouraging Peter to eat foods rich in vitamin C, which increases iron absorption. She also provides written information and arranges to see Peter's mum when she comes back to clinic.

Dietary sources of iron and improving absorption

- Dietary iron occurs in two forms:
  - haem and non-haem
- Haem iron is well absorbed and its bioavailability is not affected by other dietary factors. It is present in:
  - red meat
  - liver
  - oily fish
  - poultry
- Non-haem iron is less well absorbed because its bioavailability is affected by dietary factors as a result of the way it is bound in foods. It is present in:
  - egg yolk
  - fortified breakfast cereals and baby foods
  - green leafy vegetables
  - peanut butter
  - dried fruit
  - pulses
  - bread
  - wholegrain pasta
- Absorption enhanced by:
  - vitamin C and protein

- Absorption inhibited by:
  - tannins – in tea
  - phytates – in unrefined cereal
  - phosphates – in eggs
  - oxalates – in rhubarb and spinach
  - polyphenols – in spinach, coffee

Dietary management of constipation

- Give plenty of water or fruit juice
- Give wholemeal bread instead of white or brown
- Encourage high-fibre breakfast cereals, e.g. Weetabix, Shreddies, Shredded Wheat
- Give plenty of vegetables, particularly baked beans and peas
- Encourage fresh fruit; eat the skin if edible

How to promote healthy eating in a young child

Do:

- Start weaning at 4 months by slowly introducing different tastes and textures of food
- Let the child 'help' to feed him- or herself as soon as he or she wants to
- Eat together as a family when the child is old enough – children learn by example
- Expect the child to sit at the table for meals, but set a time limit. Let the child get down from the table once it is clear that he or she isn't going to eat any more
- Offer different tastes, but remember that children have likes and dislikes too. It doesn't matter that the diet is repetitive, provided it is nutritious
- Make food fun and appealing. Vary texture and colour, cut food up into interesting shapes and bite-size pieces

Don't:

- Let the child snack shortly before a meal
- 'Reward' the child for not eating by giving crisps or sweets
- Give more than a pint of milk a day or lots of fizzy drinks or juice
- Force feed a child or let mealtimes turn into a battle
- Put too much food on the plate and overfeed the child

Milk and Dairy Foods

Try to give a pint of full fat milk daily. Try cheese, yogurts, fromage frais, custard and milk puddings as good alternatives to some of the milk.

Meat and Alternatives

All types of meat and fish are suitable. Many children enjoy minced meat, sausages, chicken, fish fingers, and fish in sauces. Plus vegetables like chick peas and lentils make good casseroles. Eggs and baked beans are good too.

Starchy Foods

Give these foods at each meal. Most children enjoy eating breakfast cereals and porridge. Other starchy foods to encourage include bread, potatoes, chapati, yam and green banana, pasta, tinned spaghetti and rice.

Breakfast

Small bowl of breakfast cereal and milk or toast fingers with butter/margarine and jam/honey. Beaker of milk to drink.

Snack Meal

Sandwich in bite size shapes e.g ham, cheese, peanut butter. or baked beans or cheese on toast. Small pot of yogurt/fromage frais. Beaker of water or fruit juice.

Main Meal

Pasta dishes e.g. macaroni cheese, spaghetti bolognese. Chapati/rice and curry. Fish in white, cheese or parsley sauce. Roast meat or mince e.g shepherds pie. Fish fingers/chicken nuggets. Serve with fingers of carrots, swede etc or peas and a scoop of mashed potato. Fruit segments/slices/shapes Beaker of water or fruit juice.

Bedtime

Beaker of milk and a biscuit.

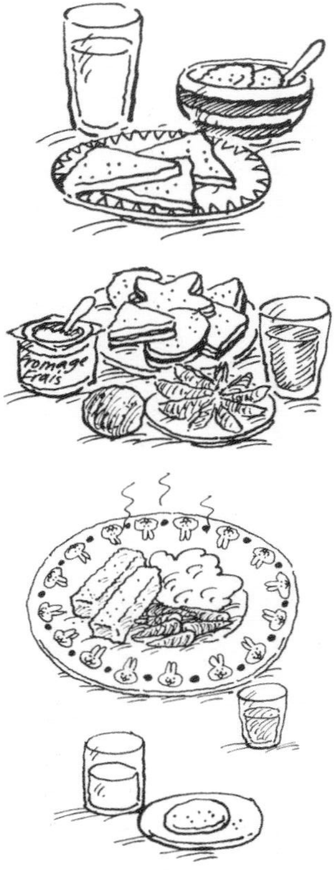

Fruit and vegetables

Give 2 portions a day - cooked or raw. All types fresh, frozen or tinned are good.

Fats and Oils

Growing children still need margarine/butter and oils.

Sugary Foods

Foods containing sugar are often part of a child's diet. Try not to give them between meals. Look after your child's teeth.

Vitamins

A vitamin supplement, containing vitamins A, C and D, is recommended for all children from six months up to at least two years and preferably five years. Ask your health visitor about this.

Figure 18.2 Sensible eating for age 1–5 years: suggestions and advice for a well-balanced diet. (From leaflet 'Help, my child won't eat', © Paediatric Group of the British Dietetic Association, www.bda.uk.com, with kind permission.)

- Get upset by the mess – it's better to put clean clothes on after eating than before
- Rush the child when eating
- Let the child become distracted by noises such as the TV
- Make a fuss if the child refuses to eat – this is normal and part of growing up

Tackling the sleep problem

Sleep problems need to be tackled by behavioural measures and parents have to be determined to stick to the programme. Sedatives can be used in an emergency as a short-term measure.

Most programmes use a graded approach and the following is one example that could be used in a child waking in the night.

- **Explain normal sleep patterns to parents:** children and adults have periods of deep sleep interspersed by shorter periods of light sleep when they are more active and dream (rapid eye movement or REM sleep). This cycle lasts about 90 minutes and is repeated during the period of sleep. During REM sleep, children and adults may wake, but learn to turn over and go back to sleep – a skill that the child who wakes in the night has to learn!
- **'Educate' the child:** when the child wakes and cries for attention, he should be left to cry for 3–10 minutes (depending on how long the parents can hold out) before being comforted. If the child cries for too long he may become hysterical, when some children may vomit, which heightens the parent's anxiety. A child who is very upset won't be aware of what's happening around him or her and will take much longer to settle
- **Give minimal comfort:** the parent should give just enough comfort to settle the child, and then leave. No drinks, playing, watching TV or anything that is worth waking up for!
- **Building up the time:** the duration of crying should be increased by 5 minutes each time before comforting the child, without letting the child become too anxious. The child learns that mum is around and eventually learns to go back off to sleep without needing her physical presence

Something that needs to be tackled alongside this programme are the drinks of milk when Peter wakes. Mum is asked to give minimum comfort without giving him a drink, which some children may accept. If he doesn't settle after 5 minutes mum can offer him a small amount of half-strength milk, but only on the first occasion he wakes. Each night the milk should be more and more dilute until it's not worth having. By this stage it should be relatively easy to stop letting him have a drink.

It is important to support Peter's mum in carrying out the behavioural measures. The paediatrician involves granny in the management strategies so that she can support her daughter rather than undermining her. The health visitor is asked to see mum to offer advice and support. The paediatrician arranges to see Peter again in 6 weeks.

Clinic review

When Peter returns to the clinic, it is apparent that his mum has made considerable progress with improving his diet. Mum is congratulated on how well she has done so far. The dietician makes some further suggestions about offering Peter different tastes.

Peter is reviewed again in 6 weeks. His haemoglobin is within the normal range, but the iron stores are still slightly low and a further course of oral iron is prescribed. Peter's diet is improving, although he's still quite fussy. He still has a bottle of milk at bedtime, but mum says that she is going to tackle that before he starts school.

Peter responded readily to the measures to decrease fluids in the night. After a fortnight he was waking once in the night, but mum felt that he still needed a drink. She is advised to offer Peter a small drink of juice in the night only if he asks for it, rather than assuming that that is what he wants. Mum was feeling much better about the whole matter because she was less tired.

Peter is discharged from follow-up and the health visitor is asked to continue to monitor Peter and support his mum.

Background information

Causes of anaemia

- **Deficiency:** inadequate dietary intake of iron or folate, low birthweight, low haemoglobin at birth, malabsorption syndromes

- **Haemolysis:** red cell enzyme deficiency, haemoglobinopathies, red cell membrane defects, blood group incompatibility, autoimmune haemolytic anaemia
- **Increased blood loss:** gastrointestinal, parasites, menstruation, bleeding disorders
- **Bone marrow disturbance:** aplastic anaemia, red cell aplasia, chronic inflammatory disorders, renal failure, chronic infection, malignant infiltration

Iron deficiency anaemia

Epidemiology

The most common cause of anaemia after the neonatal period is iron deficiency. This is found in a large percentage of young children in all communities but particularly among immigrant populations in poor inner city areas. Probably 10–18 per cent of white children and 17–31 per cent of children from ethnic minorities have iron deficiency anaemia with haemoglobin less than 11 g/dL. Many other children will be iron deficient (serum ferritin < 12 µg/L) without anaemia. As most iron deficiency is dietary, it is likely that other young children in the same household will also be deficient. It is also seen in low-birthweight infants because of their reduced iron stores, combined with their greater expansion of blood volume accompanying rapid growth.

Changes in the blood

Serum ferritin is reduced before there are any abnormalities in the red blood cells. Eventually a microcytic/hypochromic anaemia results. Usually the mean cell volume and mean cell haemoglobin fall before the haemoglobin, but the changes can occur together.

Treatment

The aims are to build up iron stores with iron medication, and then to maintain them with an iron-rich diet. Education is therefore a key element in management and prevention.

Iron transport and metabolism (Figure 18.3)

Seventy-five per cent of iron stores are circulating in the blood and the remainder is stored as ferritin (bound to apoferritin) and haemosiderin in the liver, spleen, bone marrow and kidney. Iron absorption is an active process and most absorption occurs in the upper part of the small intestine. Iron must be in the ferrous state, but most dietary iron is in the ferric form. Little iron is absorbed in the stomach, but gastric secretions dissolve the iron and facilitate its reduction to the ferrous form, as does ascorbic acid (vitamin C) and other reducing substances. Other dietary factors affect the availability of iron for absorption, e.g. the phytic acid found in cereals reacts with iron to form insoluble compounds in the intestine.

Iron is transported in plasma in the ferric state bound to transferrin. When iron in the plasma is low, iron is removed from ferritin and transported by transferrin to the parts of the body where it is needed. Transferrin can bind strongly to receptors in the cell

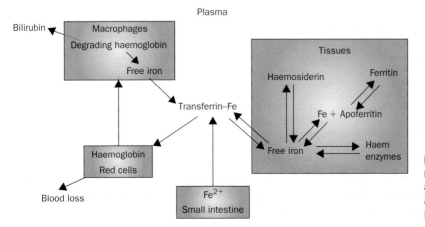

Figure 18.3 Iron transport and metabolism. Reprinted from Guyton and Hall, *Textbook of Medical Physiology*, 9th edn, © 1996, with permission from Elsevier.

membrane of erythroblasts in the bone marrow, where it is ingested and delivers iron directly to the mitochondria, where haem is synthesized. Free iron released from degraded red cells is either stored in the ferritin pool or reused to form new haemoglobin.

When body iron stores are high and apoferritin is saturated, plasma transferrin cannot release iron to the tissues; it remains fully bound with iron and cannot accept iron from the intestinal mucosal cells. The rate of absorption from the gastrointestinal tract is therefore reduced.

The term infant has adequate reserves for the first 4 months of life. However, an average of 0.8 mg iron must be absorbed each day during childhood to build up to the required adult stores. As less than 10 per cent of iron in the diet is absorbed, a diet containing 8–15 mg iron is necessary for optimal nutrition. During the first years of life, because relatively small quantities of iron-rich foods are taken, it is often difficult to attain these amounts. Milk has a low iron content; although absorption from breast milk is 50 per cent, only 10 per cent is absorbed from cows' milk. This is one of the main reasons why cows' milk is not recommended until 12 months of age – infant formulas are supplemented with iron. Children are therefore at risk of developing iron deficiency if weaning is unduly delayed beyond 4 months or the diet is inadequate.

Sleep problems

Many first-time parents are unprepared for the normal pattern of sleep. Newborn babies may sleep most of the day and be wakeful at night. By week 3 sleep is usually more evenly distributed throughout the 24-hour period. By 6 weeks, sleep is more often at night and, by 3 months, most sleep takes place between 7 pm and 7 am, with most wakefulness being in the afternoon and early evening. Table 18.2 shows the number of hours that an infant is likely to sleep.

Sleep problems are common and can be a great stress to parents. Studies on sleep problems in children never tend to show exactly the same results – so much depends on the question that is asked and the study population. However, all do agree that there is a high prevalence of problems (Table 18.3).

Table 18.2 Average number of hours sleep each 24-hour period

Age	Birth	4 months	14 months
Hours of sleep	14–18	14–15	13–14

Table 18.3 Sleeping behaviour in young children

Problems	Percentage of age group in years				
	1	2	3	4	5
Wakes once or more every night	29	28	33	29	19
Wakes at least one night each week	57	57	66	65	61
Takes >30 minutes to fall asleep	26	43	61	69	66
Gets out of bed at least once	14	26	42	49	50
Needs comforting object in bed	18	46	50	42	20
Goes to sleep with light on	7	13	20	30	23

Further sources of information

Books

Green C. *Toddler Taming*. London: Century, 1984

Lilleyman JS, Hann IM (eds). *Paediatric Haematology*. London: Churchill Livingstone, 1992

Leaflets for parents on feeding

Food for the Growing Years

Food for the School Years

Help My Child Won't Eat

Following a Vegetarian Diet

Available from the British Dietetic Association Paediatric Group, Unit 21, Goldthorpe Industrial Estate, Goldthorpe, Rotherham, S. Yorks S63 9BL.

Articles

James J, Laing C. Iron deficiency anaemia. *Current Paediatrics* 1994; **4**: 33–7

Beltramini AU, Hertzig ME. Sleep and bedtime behavior in preschool-aged children. *Pediatrics* 1983; **71**: 153–8

Self-test 5: Eighteen-month-old Jason is taken to the doctor because he is pale and listless. He was born at 32 weeks' gestation, but didn't have any complications apart from being slow to suck. He is the youngest of seven children and, for convenience, he was changed to doorstep milk at about 9 months of age. He isn't a particularly fussy eater, but doesn't eat any fruit and drinks mainly tea. He is found to have iron deficiency anaemia.

A What is the cause of the iron deficiency?

B Why?

C What alterations would you make to his diet and why?

D Which other professionals would you involve?

Answers:

A A combination of prematurity and poor diet

B Pre-term babies have low iron stores, because most iron is transferred in the third trimester; early introduction of doorstep milk, which is low in iron

C Decrease the tea intake because tannin inhibits absorption of iron; replace with fruit juices rich in vitamin C, which will enhance iron absorption

D Dietician: assesses dietary intake and offers advice on how to correct any deficiencies; health visitor: provides advice and support within the home setting

Presentation

Referral letter from the school doctor to a paediatrician:

I should be most grateful if you would see Layla who is now 6 years old. She is short with her height (98 cm) below the 0.4th centile. Her weight at 15.5 kg is between the 0.4th and 2nd centiles.

Self-test 1: Does height below the 0.4th centile imply poor growth?

Answer: No. It has to be compared with:
- Previous measurements, if any are available, to assess the growth rate (height velocity)
- Parents' heights to appreciate the child's genetic potential

Initial considerations and action

Growth is a sensitive index of health in childhood and variations from normal help in the:

- Diagnosis of disease
- Monitoring of disease activity and response to treatment

Poor growth implies a poor growth rate irrespective of whether a child is 'short' or 'tall' from a height measurement.

Short stature is defined as height below the 2nd centile. This implies that 2 per cent of the population are short. Short stature may be perfectly normal for some children, but a feature of disease in others (Figure 19.1). A healthy child may be short:

- Simply because the parents are short (familial short stature)
- As a result of delayed skeletal and physical maturation (constitutional delay)

Short stature picked up by a school doctor involved with screening and surveillance in schools, as opposed to presentation to a general practitioner, might suggest that:

- The child is an otherwise healthy girl
- Her parents have either not noticed the short stature or are not terribly concerned about it

These will need to be explored in the history and examination. A routine outpatient clinic appointment is made when a history and examination can be undertaken (Table 19.1) to:

- Identify parents' concerns, if any, about her growth
- Assess Layla's present height in comparison to previous measurements and her parents' heights
- Obtain clues that might explain her short stature

Self-test 2: Layla's height and weight centiles are not significantly different. This means that her weight is appropriate for her height. The differential diagnoses for her short stature includes:

A Familial short stature

B Hypothyroidism

C Growth hormone deficiency

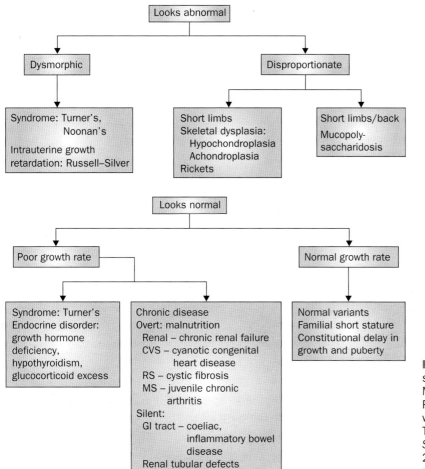

Figure 19.1 Classification of short stature. CVS, cardiovascular system; MS, musculoskeletal system; RS, respiratory system. Redrawn with modifications from Besser M, Thorner MO, Styne DM, Brook CGD, *Slide Atlas of Clinical Endocrinology*, 2nd edn, Copyright 1994, with permission from Elsevier.

D **Coeliac disease**

E **Turner's syndrome**

Answers: A and E are true. Short stature with relative overweight or underweight is seen in the following conditions:

Relative overweight
Endocrine conditions:
  Hypothyroidism
  Growth hormone deficiency
  Glucocorticoid excess
Chromosomal defects:
  Turner's syndrome
  Down's syndrome

Relative underweight
Chronic or systemic condition, e.g. coeliac disease
Intrauterine growth retardation (IUGR), e.g. Russell–Silver syndrome

History (see Table 19.1)

Layla is seen with her mother in the outpatient clinic when she is aged 6 years and 3 months.

The mother has been concerned about Layla's height but has not sought medical advice because the family moved 2 years ago from Canada to Libya before coming to the UK. Layla has not always been short and her mother first became concerned when Layla started school over a year ago. She is the smallest in her class. Although she has settled in well at school and seems happy, her mother is worried that Layla might get picked on and teased because she is so small, tends to be very shy and is not a 'local kid'. The teacher has mentioned talking to an

Table 19.1 Important aspects of the history and examination in a child with short stature

History

Reason for referral

History of growth problem:

- Time of first concerns about stature, change in stature over time
- Birth size in relation to gestation: weight, length, head circumference
- Pubertal development: delayed (constitutional delay in growth and puberty [CDGP], Turner's syndrome)

Perinatal events:

- Pregnancy: clues to growth retardation *in utero* from infections, drugs, smoking, alcohol
- Delivery: premature, asphyxia, breech (hypopituitarism)
- Postnatal period: hypoglycaemia (congenital hypopituitarism), jaundice (congenital hypothyroidism or hypopituitarism), floppiness and feeding difficulty (Prader–Willi syndrome), puffy hands and feet (Turner's syndrome)

Medical history:

- Symptoms of problems associated with specific syndromes such as Turner's syndrome: recurrent ear infections, impaired hearing, urinary tract infections, cardiac defect, learning difficulty with maths
- Symptoms of tumour around the pituitary gland: morning headaches, visual field defect
- Symptoms of systemic illness
- Medications: treatment with corticosteroids
- Developmental problems in specific areas such as speech, hearing, learning, vision

Psychosocial history to determine the impact of short stature on the child:

- Teasing
- Emotional problems
- School adjustment

Family history:

- Parents' heights: short (familial short stature, inherited condition, e.g. skeletal dysplasia)
- Height of siblings
- Delayed puberty: age of menarche in mother, growth spurt or shaving in father (CDGP)
- Consanguinity, inherited conditions

Examination

Measurements: weight, standing height, sitting height, head circumference

Height in relation to:

- Previous heights (height velocity)
- Parents' heights
- Stage of puberty
- Weight

(continued)

Table 19.1 (continued)

Pubertal development

Subcutaneous fat and muscle bulk

Unusual or dysmorphic features in face, eyes, nose, ears, mouth, hairline, neck, upper limbs, hands, palms, fingers, nails, feet or skin

Signs of specific syndromes such as Turner's or Noonan's syndrome

Signs of specific endocrine disorders such as hypothyroidism, growth hormone deficiency or corticosteroid excess

Signs of a congenital (e.g. septo-optic dysplasia) or acquired (e.g. craniopharyngioma) lesion affecting the hypothalamus, pituitary (and growth hormone secretion) and the optic chiasma: visual fields, fundi, pupils, squint, nystagmus, acuity

Signs of chronic systemic disease: cardiovascular respiratory system, gastrointestinal tract, genitourinary tract, musculoskeletal system, central nervous system

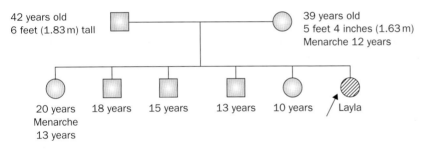

42 years old
6 feet (1.83 m) tall

39 years old
5 feet 4 inches (1.63 m)
Menarche 12 years

20 years
Menarche
13 years

18 years

15 years

13 years

10 years

Layla

Figure 19.2   The family tree.

educational psychologist because Layla struggles with addition and subtraction. Mother wonders whether Layla is neglected at school because of her size.

Layla was born after a normal pregnancy and delivery with a birth weight of 3.09 kg. She was fine soon after birth. Except for being slow with talking, her mother had no concerns about her development. She suffered from ear infections and tonsillitis until her tonsils and adenoids were removed at 3½ years of age. She has not had urinary tract infections or any other serious illnesses.

Layla is the youngest of a large family, with five older siblings varying in age from 10 to 20 years (Figure 19.2). Her siblings and parents are of normal stature. Mother is 5 feet 4 inches (1.63 m) and father 6 feet (1.83 m). There are no exceptionally short individuals in the family.

Interpretation of the history

Although the referral came from the school doctor, the history reveals that mother is quite concerned about:

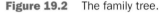

- Layla's size
- The possibility that she might suffer at school from teasing or being neglected

If Layla had always been short, intrauterine growth retardation (IUGR) and conditions associated with it would need to be considered. Normal stature initially and short stature by school age indicate a poor growth rate. It raises the possibility of Turner's syndrome, endocrine conditions or a systemic illness.

There is no history of treatment with inhaled or oral glucocorticoids and no specific features to suggest acquired hypothyroidism, growth hormone (GH) deficiency or systemic disease.

The most likely condition is Turner's syndrome as a result of the history of recurrent ear infections, delay in speech (which may have been the result of impaired hearing from the ear infections) and difficulty with maths. Typically the growth rate of girls with Turner's syndrome is normal in the first 2–3 years and slows thereafter. Short stature is usually obvious by school age.

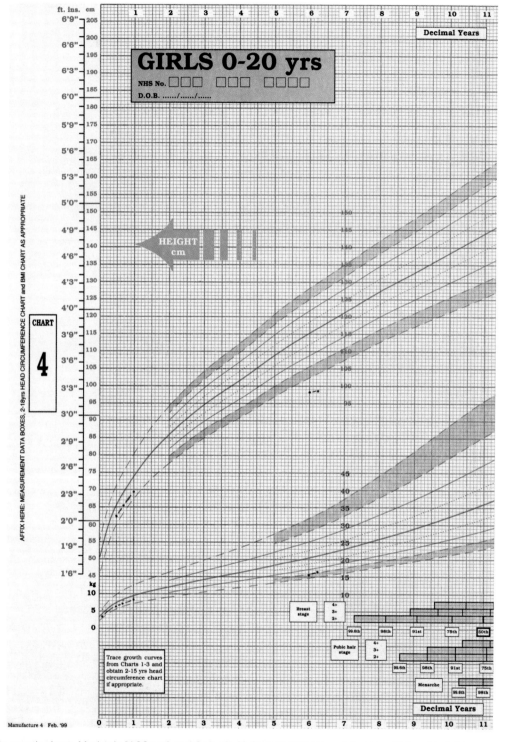

Figure 19.3 Layla's growth chart. Mother's [163 cm] and father's [6 feet or 183 cm − 14 cm = 169 cm] heights and the mid-parental height [(183 cm + 163 cm)/2 − 7 cm = 166 cm] are plotted on the right side of the chart.

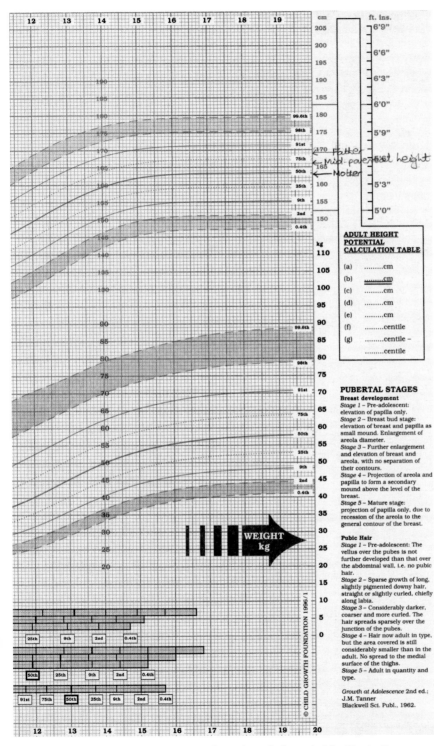

ADULT HEIGHT POTENTIAL CALCULATION TABLE

(a) ....cm
(b) ....cm
(c) ....cm
(d) ....cm
(e) ....cm
(f) ....centile
(g) ....centile –
   ....centile

PUBERTAL STAGES

Breast development
Stage 1 – Pre-adolescent: elevation of papilla only.
Stage 2 – Breast bud stage: elevation of breast and papilla as small mound. Enlargement of areola diameter.
Stage 3 – Further enlargement and elevation of breast and areola, with no separation of their contours.
Stage 4 – Projection of areola and papilla to form a secondary mound above the level of the breast.
Stage 5 – Mature stage: projection of papilla only, due to recession of the areola to the general contour of the breast.

Pubic Hair
Stage 1 – Pre-adolescent: The vellus over the pubes is not further developed than that over the abdominal wall, i.e. no pubic hair.
Stage 2 – Sparse growth of long, slightly pigmented downy hair, straight or slightly curled, chiefly along labia.
Stage 3 – Considerably darker, coarser and more curled. The hair spreads sparsely over the junction of the pubes.
Stage 4 – Hair now adult in type, but the area covered is still considerably smaller than in the adult. No spread to the medial surface of the thighs.
Stage 5 – Adult in quantity and type.

Growth at Adolescence 2nd ed.;
J.M. Tanner
Blackwell Sci. Publ., 1962.

© CHILD GROWTH FOUNDATION 1996/1

Examination (see Table 19.1)

When Layla walked into the consulting room the paediatrician noted that she appeared well and there was no obvious disproportion between her limbs and trunk.

Layla's growth measurements are noted and plotted on charts (Figure 19.3):

- Standing height: 98.5 cm (<0.4th centile)
- Sitting height: 56.2 cm
- Weight: 16.1 kg (2nd centile)
- Head circumference: 49.8 cm (10th centile)

Mother's height is measured at 163 cm. She has an excellent parent-held baby record which shows that Layla's length and weight were around the 9th centile during the first year of life.

Examination also reveals:

- Pulse 90/min, regular and normal volume
- No goitre
- No unusual or abnormal features in face, neck, upper limbs, hands or skin
- Visual fields and fundus examination normal
- Nipples are normally placed and no breast development
- Chest shape normal
- No cardiovascular abnormality
- No truncal obesity or dimpling of fat over the anterior abdomen

---

Self-test 3: Interpret Layla's growth chart (Figure 19.3).

Answer: Layla's growth chart shows:

- Her height was around the 9th centile in her first year but is now well below it – this confirms the poor growth rate suggested by the history
- Her present height is below the 0.4th centile and also well below her parental target, indicating that she is exceptionally short for an offspring of her parents
- Her weight is on a higher centile than her height.

Interpretation of the examination

Height velocity (rate of growth) rather than height is a better indicator of health because it can demonstrate

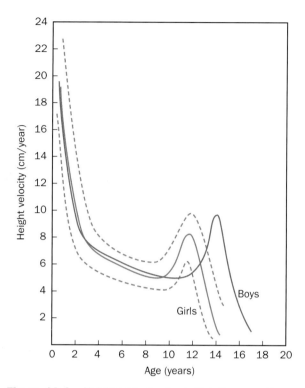

Figure 19.4 Height velocity chart. Pink lines are the 3rd, 50th and 97th centiles for girls. The blue line is the 50th centile for boys.

abnormal growth irrespective of a child's height on a centile chart. At least two height measurements separated by 3 or more months are needed to estimate height velocity. Although gender-specific height velocity charts are available (Figure 19.4), it is easier to interpret the height velocity of a child from the height distance chart because every child seen by a paediatrician will have height plotted on one (Figure 19.5). For a healthy child who has normal height velocity, successive heights plotted on a height chart will be seen to follow the same centile line, with only minor deviations either way (i.e. the child's personal centile). Deviation below the personal centile line suggests poor growth and loss of height. Deviation above the personal centile line indicates rapid growth and gain in height.

Disproportion between the trunk and limbs is obvious in certain conditions such as achondroplasia, but may be more subtle in other skeletal dysplasias (e.g. hypochondroplasia). Body proportions can be assessed objectively from the sitting height and subischial leg

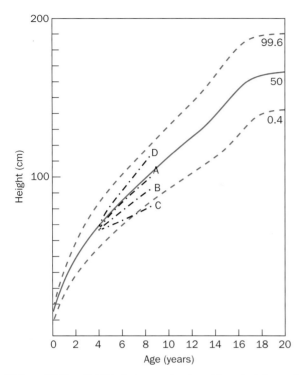

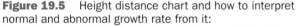

Figure 19.5 Height distance chart and how to interpret normal and abnormal growth rate from it:
Growth rate (or height velocity) can be interpreted without a height velocity chart from a height distance chart.
Serial height measurements of four children are illustrated:
A has a normal growth rate – the trajectory is parallel to the 50th centile line.
B and C have poor growth rates – their trajectories are deviating downwards (e.g. endocrine causes of short stature, Turner's syndrome, chronic systemic disease).
D has a rapid growth rate – the trajectory is deviating upwards (e.g. precocious puberty).

length (calculated from standing height minus the sitting height) ratios and measurements plotted on gender-specific charts. Layla's measurements do not reveal any disproportion.

Layla is a schoolgirl with:

- Short stature, height <0.4th centile and below parental target (Table 19.2)
- Poor growth rate
- A history of recurrent ear infections and difficulty with maths
- No disproportion
- No features of endocrine deficiency

Table 19.2 How to plot parents' heights on a growth chart, and calculate mid-parental height and predicted adult height target for a child

---

Plotting parents' heights on the right side (adult range) of the growth chart

Corrections are required before a father's height (cm) can be plotted on a girl's chart and mother's height (cm) plotted on a boy's chart:

	Value in cm that should be plotted	
	For mother	*For father*
For a girl	Mother's height	Father's height −14 cm
For a boy	Mother's height +14 cm	Father's height

Calculating mid-parental height (cm)

Mid-parental height = [(Father's height + Mother's height)/2] −7 for a girl and +7 for a boy

Predicted adult height target of the child

The range in centimetres is the mid-parental height ± 8.5 cm for a girl and ±10 cm for a boy

---

Although Layla does not have any dysmorphic features of Turner's syndrome, it cannot be excluded because the only consistent feature of the condition is short stature.

Neither the history nor the examination reveals features of acquired hypothyroidism or growth hormone deficiency.

Investigations

Chromosome analysis for Turner's syndrome should be considered in girls with short stature and poor growth rate (and delayed puberty). This is explained to Layla's mother and a blood sample is taken from Layla. The result is available after a few weeks and her karyotype is 45XO. This confirms Turner's syndrome.

A number of other investigations are essential for associated cardiac, renal, audiological, gastrointestinal and endocrine abnormalities. As Layla will be referred to a paediatric endocrinologist for further management, the paediatrician explains to her mother that it is most appropriate for these investigations to be undertaken by the specialist.

Diagnosis

Layla has short stature as a result of Turner's syndrome.

Management

Layla has Turner's syndrome but no on-going ear, nose and throat (ENT), major cardiac or renal problems that need immediate management. She requires management for:

- The Turner's syndrome
- The potential emotional and psychological problems associated with:
  – being short and
  – having Turner's syndrome (especially infertility)

After receiving the karyotype result, the paediatrician sees Layla again with her parents. He explains the diagnosis and its implications, mentioning:

- The blood test result
- The need to refer Layla to a specialist
- That Turner's syndrome is caused by a lack of or abnormality of one female sex chromosome
- It affects girls
- Girls with the condition are short but growth hormone treatment has the potential to improve adult height
- The ovaries do not work and oestrogen treatment will be required to take Layla through puberty
- Infertility
- Treatment should be supervised by a specialist in paediatric endocrinology
- The problems Layla has with addition and subtraction are characteristic of the condition, and discussing this with her teacher may help to plan her future educational needs

Management of potential emotional and psychological problems

Associated with short stature

The paediatrician discusses with the mother her concerns that Layla may be teased or neglected as a result of her small size. Feeling different or rejected by others can have a negative effect on a short child. It is possible that Layla is treated like a much younger child because she is the 'baby' in the family (the youngest of six children) and there is a tendency for strangers to judge the age of a child by their height (at 6 years and 3 months, Layla is the same height as an average 3½ year old). This can lead to immature behaviour in a short child and may interfere with social maturation (and may explain Layla's shyness) because the child behaves in a way that is consistent with what others expect. The paediatrician advises her mother to:

- Build positive self-esteem and a strong positive self-image by praising and encouraging Layla
- Stay in touch with Layla's teacher about her school work and any signs of social or behaviour problems

Associated with Turner's syndrome

The prospect of infertility can be very distressing for parents and girls with Turner's syndrome. They need to be informed about the potential for *in vitro* fertilization with a donated egg. The specialist paediatrician, nurse specialist and parent support groups will be able to provide detailed information and support for the family.

Background information

Normal growth

Growth is a dynamic process that starts at conception and ends after full pubertal development. Postnatal growth is regulated by genetic, nutritional and endocrine factors (Table 19.3).

The centile lines on a distance chart show the normal pattern of growth in height and weight. Serial

Table 19.3 The three endocrine phases of postnatal growth and key hormones involved in regulating it

Growth phase	Growth pattern	Key hormones
Infancy	Rapid growth in the first year (23–25 cm/year), then rapid deceleration until age 2–3	Fetal growth factors
Childhood	Relatively slow but steady growth until the onset of puberty (5–7 cm/year)	Growth hormone (thyroxine)
Puberty	Growth accelerates to produce the pubertal growth spurt (mean peak height velocity 10 cm/year in boys and 8 cm/year in girls) and then decelerates until growth ceases	Sex hormones (testosterone in boys, oestrogens in girls) Growth hormone

height measurements of a child over a considerable time span plotted on a distance chart:

- Yield more information than isolated height measurements
- Show the child's pattern of growth in relation to the centile lines
- Help estimate height velocity (increment in height divided by the time elapsed)

Growth centile charts

Growth charts are derived from measurements of numerous healthy children. For every variable measured, such as height, the values at each age are ranked into 100 equal parts using statistical methods. A select number of these ranks or centiles (e.g. 0.4th, 2nd, 9th, 50th, 75th, 91st, 98th and 99.6th) are plotted as curves against age to produce growth centile charts. Such centile charts help to describe the position of a measurement from a child like Layla in relation to healthy children.

A histogram of the measurements from healthy children for a variable such as height will reveal a symmetrical bell-shaped normal distribution (Figure 19.6). According to the empirical rule, approximately 95 per cent of the measurements are within 2 standard deviations of the mean. In other words:

- Only 5 per cent of measurements from healthy children fall outside the range between −2 and +2 standard deviations
- The measurement of a particular child is more likely to be abnormal than normal if it falls below −2 standard deviations (i.e. below about the 2nd centile) or above +2 standard deviations (i.e. above about the 98th centile).

There is no strict division between normal and abnormal but this way of interpreting a measurement gives a probability of whether it is normal or abnormal.

Familial short stature – a snapshot

History

- Small birth size but normal for the family
- Parents are short but healthy
- Healthy child

Examination

- Short stature with height <2nd centile
- Normal growth rate: child's personal centile line follows parallel to the centile lines on the growth chart

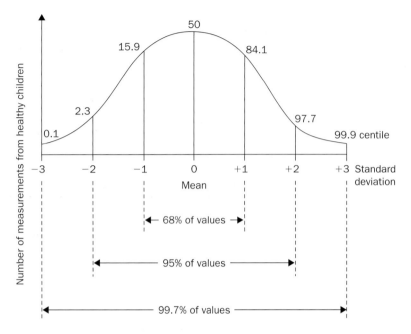

Figure 19.6 Symmetrical bell-shaped normal distribution of a variable such as height. The relationship between centiles and standard deviations is shown.

- Child is not inappropriately short compared with parents – child's projected adult height falls within 8.5 cm of the mid-parental height

Investigations

- Bone age is not delayed

Constitutional delay in growth and puberty – a snapshot

Definition

Temporary short stature associated with delayed skeletal and pubertal development in otherwise healthy children. Onset of puberty and therefore the pubertal growth spurt are delayed. Final adult height falls within the target predicted from parent's heights.

This is more common in boys than in girls and the most common reason for boys presenting with short stature, delayed puberty or both (see Chapter 31).

History

- Birth size normal
- History of delayed puberty in one or both parents
- Healthy child

Examination

- Inappropriately short compared with parents
- Normal growth rate
- Weight appropriate for height or lean

Investigations

- Bone age delayed – height is normal for bone age

Turner's syndrome – a snapshot

Incidence

- One in 2500 live female births

Presentation

- Neonatal period: puffy hands and feet, coarctation of the aorta
- During childhood: short stature, recurrent ear infections
- During adolescence: delayed puberty

Clinical features

- Short stature and poor growth rate after the first few years of life

- Oestrogen deficiency: lack of sexual maturation, amenorrhoea, infertility, osteoporosis
- Face and neck:
  - short neck, neck webbing, low posterior hairline
  - rotated ears
  - high arched palate
- Ears: recurrent middle-ear infections, impaired hearing
- Eyes: squint, ptosis
- Skin: naevi
- Limbs:
  - puffy hands and feet from lymphoedema
  - nails hyperconvex
  - short fourth and fifth metacarpals
  - increased carrying angles, Madelung's deformity
- Chest: broad shield chest, wide spaced nipples
- Cardiac: coarctation or aortic stenosis, hypertension
- Renal: congenital anomalies
- Autoimmune: thyroid: autoimmune thyroiditis, hypothyroidism
- Gastrointestinal tract: chronic inflammatory bowel disease
- Carbohydrate: glucose intolerance, insulin-resistant diabetes
- Learning:
  - difficulties with arithmetic and geometry
  - difficulty with visuospatial coordination
  - lower social competence
  - normal intelligence except when karyotype contains ring X chromosome
- Gonadoblastoma when karyotype contains Y chromosome

Investigations

- Karyotype (Figure 19.7):
  - monosomy: 45X
  - mosaicism: 45X/46,XX 45X/46,X,I(Xq) 45X/47,XXX 45X/46,XY
  - various structural defects: isochromosome X, ring X
- Ultrasonography of the pelvis: ovaries not seen or small, uterus may be small

- Ultrasonography of the abdomen to identify kidney abnormalities such as horseshoe kidney
- Cardiology assessment including echocardiogram to identify any abnormality
- Luteinizing-hormone-releasing hormone (LHRH) test: high follicle-stimulating hormone (FSH) and LH levels caused by non-functioning ovaries and lack of oestrogen-mediated negative feedback on the anterior pituitary

Noonan's syndrome – a snapshot

- Incidence: 1 in 1000–2500 live births
- Normal karyotype but phenotypic features similar to Turner's syndrome
- Autosomal dominant or sporadic

Features

- Normal or delayed puberty
- Testes normal, small or undescended
- Short stature
- Mild learning disability
- Characteristic facies: hypertelorism, epicanthic folds, anti-mongoloid palpebral slant, ptosis, micrognathia, low-set posteriorly rotated ears, broad nasal tip, deeply grooved philtrum
- Webbing of neck, pectus carinatum or excavatum, cubitus valgus
- Congenital heart defects: right-sided congenital heart defects especially pulmonary valve stenosis, atrial septal defect (ASD), hypertrophic cardiomyopathy

Acquired hypothyroidism – a snapshot

Cause

- Autoimmune thyroiditis is most common; occurs in 1–2 per cent of school-age children and is more common in girls than in boys

History

- Sleepy
- Tired, lazy, 'slow'
- Constipation

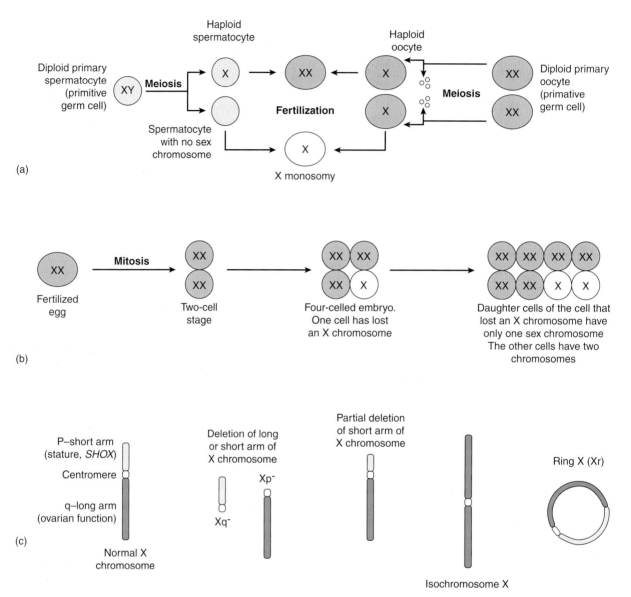

Figure 19.7 X-chromosome abnormalities in Turner's syndrome: (a) X-chromosome monsomy – sex chromosome is lost during formation of the gametocytes; (b) X-chromosome mosaicism – sex chromosome is lost during early embryonic development; and (c) X-chromosome defects – the X chromosome is structurally defective but not lost. (Modified with permission from: http://tuners.nichd.nin.gov/)

- Intolerance to cold weather
- Poor school work

Examination findings

- Short stature and poor growth rate
- Relatively overweight

- Coarse facial features
- Sallow complexion
- Goitre is rare
- Dry, rough skin
- Cold skin
- Deep hoarse voice

- Slow pulse
- Slowly relaxing deep tendon reflexes

Investigations

- Bone age – markedly delayed
- Thyroid function tests – low thyroxine and high thyroid-stimulating hormone (TSH) levels (if primary hypothyroidism)

Growth hormone deficiency – a snapshot

Incidence

- One in 4000–10 000 live births

Aetiology

Isolated or associated with deficiencies of other pituitary hormones.

Primary pituitary defect
- Sporadic: environmental insult, developmental abnormality
- Genetic: autosomal recessive, dominant and X linked

Secondary involvement of pituitary gland
- Tumour: craniopharyngioma
- Langerhans' cell histiocytosis
- Trauma
- Cranial radiotherapy

Associated with other congenital malformation
- Septo-optic dysplasia

History

- Breech delivery, birth asphyxia
- Hypoglycaemia, jaundice in neonatal period (congenital hypopituitarism)

Typical examination findings of growth hormone deficiency

- Short stature (well below 0.4th centile) and poor growth rate
- Relatively overweight
- Podgy, truncal obesity and dimpling over anterior abdomen
- Thin, under-muscled limbs
- Mid-facial crowding because of undergrowth of the maxillae
- Delayed teeth eruption
- High-pitched voice owing to laryngeal hypoplasia
- Normal body proportions
- Head relatively large because brain growth normal
- Associated with midline defects such as cleft lip and palate
- Micropenis

Investigations

- Bone age – markedly delayed
- GH stimulation tests (e.g. stimulation with arginine, glucagon) – low peak growth hormone levels
- Serum insulin-like growth factor I (IGF-I) level low
- To define cause: magnetic resonance imaging (MRI) of the brain

Further sources of information

Articles

Committee on Genetics. Health supervision for children with Turner syndrome. *Pediatrics* 1995; **96**: 1166–73

Voss LD. Short stature: does it matter? A review of the evidence. *Journal of Medical Screening* 1995; **2**: 130–32

Voss LD, Mulligan J. Bullying in school: are short pupils at risk? Questionnaire study in a cohort. *British Medical Journal* 2000; **320**: 612–13.

Website

www.cgf.org.uk

The Child Growth Foundation Information Booklets.

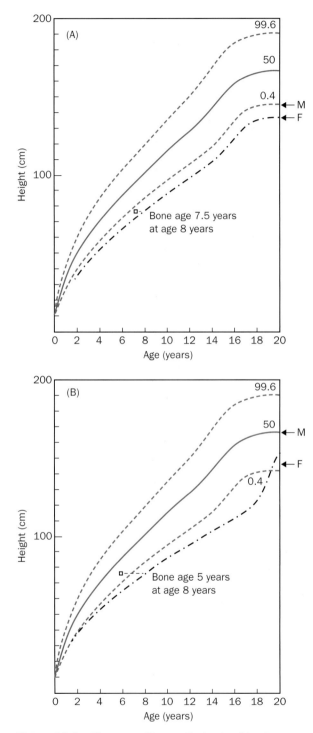

Figure 19.8   These are the growth charts of two boys who had been seen in early childhood because of short stature. (See Self-test 4)

Self-test 4: These are the growth charts of two boys who had been seen in early childhood because of short stature (Figure 19.8). Neither required any treatment. What is the most likely diagnosis?

Answers:

A Familial short stature: height in keeping with parental target, normal growth rate, bone age not delayed

B Constitutional delay in growth and puberty: height in childhood below parental target, normal growth rate, bone age delayed

Self-test 5: List the hormones produced by the anterior pituitary, the hypothalamic hormones that regulate their secretion and their target tissues. Can short stature result from deficiency of each of the pituitary hormones?

Answer: Table 19.4 shows the hormones secreted by the anterior pituitary (Figure 19.9), their regulating hypothalamic hormones, their target tissues and the effects of deficiency.

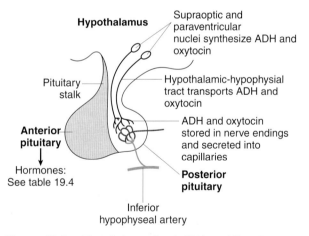

Figure 19.9   The pituitary gland. ADH, antidiuretic hormone.

Self-test 6: Explain why a tumour affecting the pituitary, such as a craniopharyngioma, will cause visual field defects. What other clinical features would you expect with such a tumour?

Table 19.4 Hormones secreted by the anterior pituitary, their regulating hypothalamic hormones, target tissues and effects of deficiency

Hypothalamus					
Inhibitory hormone	Somatostatin	Dopamine			Somatostatin, dopamine
Releasing hormone	GHRH	TRH, VIP	GnRH	TRH	CRH, ADH
Pituitary secretory cells	Acidophils		Gonadotrophs	Basophils	Corticotrophs
	Somatotrophs	Lactotrophs		Thyrotrophs	
Pituitary hormone	Growth hormone (GH)	Prolactin	Gonadotrophins LH FSH	TSH	ACTH
Target gland	Direct effects on tissues not glands	Direct effects on tissues not glands	Gonads	Thyroid gland	Adrenal cortex
Main physiological effects	Promotes growth Promotes protein synthesis Mobilizes fatty acid from adipose tissue Decreases glucose use	None in children	Stimulates production of sex hormones Stimulates development of germ cells	Stimulates synthesis and secretion of thyroid hormones	Stimulates synthesis and secretion of glucocorticoids and androgens
Major effects of deficiency	Extreme short stature Poor growth rate Overweight for height		Secondary hypogonadism Lack of pubertal development	Secondary hypothyroidism Short stature Poor growth rate Overweight for height	Secondary adrenal insufficiency Underweight, weight loss Tiredness Poor growth rate

ACTH, adrenocorticotrophin; ADH, antidiuretic hormone; CRH, corticotrophin-releasing hormone; FSH, follicle-stimulating hormone; GH, growth hormone; GHRH, growth hormone-releasing hormone; GnRH, gonadotrophin-releasing hormone; LH, luteinizing hormone; TRH, thyroid hormone-releasing hormone; TSH, thyroid-stimulating hormone; VIP, vasointestinal peptide.

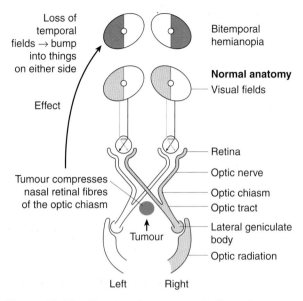

Figure 19.10   The visual pathway and effect of a tumour compressing the optic chiasma.

Answer: Craniopharyngioma arises from the remnants (squamous cell rests) of the hypophyseal recess/ Rathke's pouch between the tuber cinereum and pituitary. Extension upwards compresses the central nasal fibres of the optic chiasma (Figure 19.10). The clinical features that would be expected from an intracranial tumour
close to the pituitary and hypothalamus are those caused by:

- Raised intracranial pressure: morning headache or nausea/vomiting
- Compression of the optic chiasma: visual field defect, bitemporal hemianopia or loss of acuity, blindness
- Compression of the pituitary: endocrine deficiency – short stature, delayed/arrested puberty, diabetes insipidus
- Compression of the hypothalamus: appetite disturbance or obesity

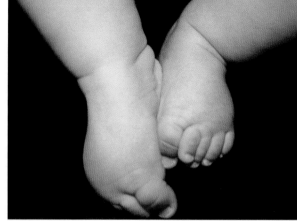

Figure 19.11

Self-test 7: The doctor observes these feet of a baby girl who attends for her first dose of primary immunization (Figure 19.11). Her feet have been like this since birth but she is otherwise healthy. Is any action required?

Answer: The feet are puffy, raising the possibility of Turner's syndrome. Without unduly alarming the mother, the doctor should inform the mother that this feature is unusual and should:

- Examine the baby thoroughly with special attention to:
  - other physical features of Turner's syndrome
  - any asymmetry between brachial and femoral pulses and heart murmur for coarctation of the aorta
- Explain the findings to the parent(s)
- Explain the need to do a blood test to check the chromosomes and arrange them
- Make arrangements to inform the parents as soon as the result of the karyotype is available

A heart murmur heard on routine check

Age: 4 years

JACKIE GREGG

Presentation

Four-year-old Henry is referred to the local paediatric department by his GP.

Henry had been taken to the GP immunization clinic for his preschool booster. He had had a slight temperature earlier in the week, but seemed fine in himself. The nurse immunizer, however, thought that he looked somewhat flushed. His temperature was 38.0°C and she decided to defer the immunization and asked the GP to see him. On examination, a systolic murmur was detected. Henry had a viral upper respiratory tract infection, but was otherwise well. The GP examined Henry a week later when he was apyrexial and fully recovered from the viral infection. The murmur was still present.

Self-test 1: What is the likely cause of the murmur?

Answer: An innocent murmur.

Initial considerations and action

Heart murmurs are caused by transmitted sound waves resulting from turbulent blood flow through the heart and blood vessels. Turbulence may occur under the following conditions:

- Normal blood flow: this is known as a functional or innocent murmur
- Acceleration of blood flow, e.g. blood flowing through a stenosed valve or increased blood flow

though a normal valve as a result of a pathological lesion re-routeing the blood
- Blood flowing by an abnormal route, e.g. ventricular septal defect (VSD) or patent ductus arteriosus (PDA)

Murmurs are often picked up incidentally when a child is being examined for another reason. Many newborn infants with potential shunts have no symptoms or murmur at birth because the pulmonary vascular resistance is still high. There is no pressure gradient across the shunt, so there is no flow of blood and therefore no murmur. Conditions such as VSD or PDA may therefore become apparent only at several weeks of age when the pulmonary vascular resistance falls. They may be picked up when a murmur is detected at the routine 8-week check.

During a febrile illness, innocent murmurs are often heard because of increased cardiac output – all that is necessary is a follow-up examination to see if the murmur persists when the child is well.

Innocent murmurs are extremely common in children – in one reported series, a cardiologist detected a heart murmur in most healthy schoolchildren on routine examination. Cardiac disease is relatively rare. In a child of this age, the chances are high that this is an innocent murmur, but it is important not to miss a cardiac defect.

History

Henry is seen in the paediatric outpatient by the consultant paediatrician with an interest in cardiology.

Henry's parents report him to be a lively and active child who has lots of energy. He hasn't had any respiratory symptoms, he eats well and his parents are happy with his growth.

He hasn't had any previous illnesses apart from an occasional upper respiratory tract infection and isn't on any medication

Henry was born at term, by normal delivery and weighed 3.7 kg. The pregnancy had been problem free, and his mother hadn't taken any medication and only occasional alcohol. There were no neonatal problems.

Henry's parents do not have any concerns about his development and his milestones have been achieved at the normal time.

There is no family history of congenital heart disease or sudden unexplained deaths.

Self-test 2: What is the significance of developmental delay in a child with a murmur?

Answer: The developmental delay may be a feature of a syndrome that is also associated with congenital cardiac defects.

Interpretation of the history

Factors in the history that may indicate a pathological cause for the murmur:

- **Age of the child:** most murmurs in neonates and a significant proportion in young infants are pathological
- **Prematurity:** there is a higher incidence of PDA
- **Maternal diabetes:** increased incidence of cardiac defects
- **Intrauterine exposure to drugs:** the teratogenic effects of prescribed medication as well as drugs of abuse need to be considered
- **Chromosomal, congenital abnormalities and dysmorphic syndromes:** e.g. Down's, Turner's, DiGeorge's and Noonan's syndromes
- **Past medical history:** rheumatic fever
- **Family history:** congenital heart disease, sudden unexplained death, hypertrophic cardiomyopathy
- Symptoms that would give a very high index of suspicion, e.g. cyanosis, breathlessness, recurrent chest infections

Self-test 3: Which of the following are features of rheumatic fever?

A **Polyarthralgia**

B **Fever**

C **Chorea**

D **Rash**

E **Subcutaneous nodules**

F **Seizures**

Answer: All except seizures.

Meaning of the history in Henry

The history hasn't highlighted any factors to indicate that Henry has an underlying cardiac defect.

Examination

The aim of the examination is to detect any symptoms or signs that indicate an underlying cardiac abnormality:

- **Growth:** height and weight on 25th centile
- **Appearance:** no cyanosis or clubbing, no dysmorphic features
- **Cardiovascular system (CVS):** grade 2 systolic murmur heard at left sternal edge, no radiation. Femoral and radial pulses readily palpable with no radiofemoral delay. Blood pressure (BP) normal
- **Respiratory system:** normal respiratory rate, chest clear
- **Gastrointestinal (GI) tract:** no hepatomegaly
- **Development:** age appropriate

Self-test 4: What is radiofemoral delay?

Answer: This sign is found in coarctation of the aorta. Blood bypasses the blockage in the aorta, by flowing through collateral vessels. This results in the femoral pulse being palpable (if present) after the radial pulse – radiofemoral delay.

Self-test 5: How is central cyanosis detected on examination?

Answer: By examination of the tongue.

Interpretation of the examination

- **Growth:** heart disease is a recognized cause of failure to thrive
- **Cyanosis:** peripheral cyanosis (blueness of the hands, feet, or lips) may occur when a child is cold or crying or unwell from any cause. Central cyanosis, seen on the tongue, is associated with a fall in arterial oxygen tension. It can be recognized clinically if the concentration of reduced haemoglobin in the blood exceeds 5 g/dL. It is present when unsaturated venous blood bypasses the lung. There are two causes of cyanosis in congenital heart disease:
  (1) decreased pulmonary blood flow with a right-to-left shunt, e.g. tetralogy of Fallot
  (2) normal or increased pulmonary blood flow with abnormal mixing of systemic and pulmonary venous return, e.g. transposition of the great arteries
- **Heart murmur:** features of the different types of innocent murmur are shown in Table 20.1. These murmurs may be confused with pathological murmurs. A murmur is not innocent if it is:
  - diastolic
  - loud – usually grade 2 and above (Table 20.2)
  - associated with a thrill
  - accompanied by symptoms
- **Heart failure:** signs are shown in Table 20.3
- **Dysmorphism and developmental delay:** important because many syndromes are associated with congenital cardiac anomalies

Apart from the murmur, Henry doesn't have any signs of cardiac disease.

Investigations

What the paediatrician does next will depend on how confident he is that this is an innocent murmur and whether or not he has ready access to echocardiography. Henry's parents are very anxious and so echocardiography is performed and is normal (Figure 20.1). (Chest radiograph and ECG are of little help in determining whether or not an asymptomatic murmur in a child other than a young infant is pathological. These tests weren't therefore ordered.)

Table 20.1 Types and qualities of innocent murmurs

- **Venous hum:**
  - caused by turbulent blood flow in head and neck veins
  - heard above or below clavicles
  - continuous, low-pitched rumble
  - disappears on lying flat or with compression of jugular vein
  - may be confused with patent ductus arteriosus (PDA)
- **Vibratory:**
  - lower left sternal edge
  - short, buzzing
  - changes with posture
  - may be confused with ventricular septal defect (VSD)
- **Ejection murmurs:** generated in the outflow tracts and great vessels on either side of the heart. Especially prominent when cardiac output is high, e.g. after exercise, in febrile children, anaemia
- **Pulmonary flow murmur:**
  - upper left sternal edge
  - short, ejection systolic
  - accentuated by inspiration and lying flat
  - may be confused with atrial septal defect (ASD) or pulmonary stenosis (PS)
- **Aortic flow murmur:**
  - upper right sternal edge, supraclavicular area
  - short, ejection systolic
  - may be confused with aortic stenosis

Table 20.2 Classification of murmurs by intensity

Grade	Intensity
1	Barely audible
2	Soft, but easily audible
3	Loud, no thrill
4	Loud, +thrill
5	Audible with stethoscope barely on chest
6	Audible with stethoscope off chest

If echocardiography is not available, factors that would prompt referral to a paediatric cardiologist for an asymptomatic murmur are:

- Presence of risk factors such as family history of congenital heart disease (CHD) or dysmorphic syndrome associated with CHD

- Clinical findings raising suspicion of a pathological lesion
- Uncertainty about the nature of the murmur
- Murmur in a child involved in strenuous competitive sports
- Parental anxiety
- All infants with a murmur, even if asymptomatic

Diagnosis

Innocent murmur.

Treatment and follow-up plan

None, apart from advising that Henry complete his immunizations.

Self-test 6: What is the routine immunization schedule?

Answer: See Table 20.4.

Table 20.3   Heart failure

Symptoms:

- Breathlessness, particularly on feeding and crying or on exertion
- Sweating
- Poor feeding
- Recurrent chest infections

Signs:

- Slow weight gain or failure to thrive
- Cool peripheries
- Tachypnoea
- Tachycardia
- Enlarged heart
- Heart murmur, gallop
- Hepatomegaly

How to give an immunization

- Check the child's immunization record to ascertain which vaccines are due
- Ensure that there is written consent
- Make sure that there are no contraindications: acute illness, history of severe local or general reaction to a preceding dose. Be aware that live vaccines are contraindicated in special risk groups: children being treated for malignant disease; a bone marrow transplant recipient in previous 6 months; high-dose steroids; impaired cell-mediated immunity, e.g. HIV. If in doubt, seek specialist advice
- Anaphylactic reactions to vaccines are very rare but cannot be predicted – be aware of the signs and how to manage them
- Check the expiry date on the label – vaccines should not be used after that date
- Check that the vaccine has been stored properly, otherwise it becomes less effective

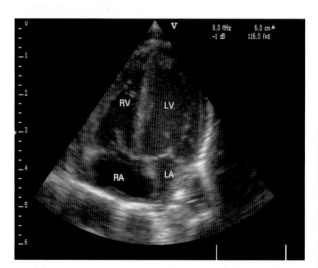

Figure 20.1   Echocardiogram of a normal heart. RV, right ventricle; LV, left ventricle; RA, right atrium; LA, left atrium. (Courtesy of Dr Ladusans, Royal Liverpool Children's NHS Trust.)

- Check the identity of the vaccine to ensure that the right product is to be used in the right way
- With the exception of BCG and oral polio, all vaccines should be given by intramuscular or deep subcutaneous injection.
- Give the vaccine into the anterolateral aspect of the thigh or upper arm
- Record the site where the vaccine has been given (this is important if more than one vaccine was given to allow any local reaction to be related to the causative vaccine)
- Record the date of immunization, the name of the vaccine and batch number in the child's records
- Complete documentation for the district database – essential, so that accurate population coverage figures are available (see answer to Self-test 6)

Table 20.4 Answer to Self-test 6

Vaccine	Age	Notes
BCG	Birth	If at risk
DTP-Hib, Men C, Polio	First dose (2 months)	Primary course
	Second dose (3 months)	
	Third dose (4 months)	
MMR	12–15 months	Can be given at any age >12 months
Booster DTaP, Polio	3–5 years	3 years after completion of primary course
Booster MMR	3–5 years	
BCG	10–14 years	
Td, Polio	13–18 years	
Men C	1–24 years	One dose to be given if not previously immunized

DTP, diphtheria/tetanus/pertussis; DTaP, diphtheria/tetanus/acellular pertussis; Hib, *Haemophilus influenzae* type b; Men C, meningococcal meningitis type C; MMR, measles/mumps/rubella; Td, tetanus/low-dose diphtheria.

Background information

Cardiac disease in children

The main cause is congenital heart disease. Rheumatic heart disease is now rare in developed countries, but is still a major cause of heart disease in some developing countries.

Congenital heart disease

Congenital heart disease may involve the heart, the great vessels or both. Most defects arise as a consequence of normal embryological processes becoming either arrested before completion, or deviated from the normal course. This results in either abnormal communication between the systemic and pulmonary circulations or obstruction to normal blood flow or a combination of the two.

Incidence

Seven to eight per 1000 live births.

Aetiology

Major chromosomal abnormalities account for 8 per cent of defects. More subtle chromosomal abnormalities are increasingly being shown to play a part, e.g. an abnormality of chromosome 22 is detected in many patients with aortic arch abnormalities. External teratogens such as rubella, systemic lupus erythematosus (SLE), alcohol and diabetes account for a small proportion. There is increased incidence in dysmorphic syndromes:

- Infants with the eight most common anomalies account for over 80 per cent of all lesions (Table 20.5)
- 10–15 per cent have complex lesions with more than one cardiac abnormality
- 10–15 per cent have a non-cardiac abnormality

Presentation

- Antenatal detection on ultrasonography
- Cyanosis
- Heart murmur
- Heart failure
- Shock

Table 20.5 Most common congenital heart lesions

Acyanotic	Cyanotic
Ventricular septal defect 32%	Tetralogy of Fallot 6%
Patent ductus arteriosus 12%	Transposition of the great arteries 5%
Pulmonary stenosis 8%	
Atrial septal defect 6%	
Coarctation of the aorta 6%	
Aortic stenosis 5%	

Subacute bacterial endocarditis

Children of all ages with congenital and rheumatic heart disease are at risk. The risk is greatest with those lesions that result in a turbulent jet of blood (e.g. VSD, coarctation of the aorta, PDA, aortic valve stenosis). The endocardium becomes infected in the presence of a bacteraemia or septicaemia. *Streptococcus viridans* is the usual infecting organism, the most common source of infection being the teeth.

Echocardiography may identify vegetations, which are composed of fibrin, platelets and bacteria. Small bits may break off, resulting in embolism in many organs, e.g. lungs, brain, kidneys, spleen, skin.

The child presents with fever, malaise, anorexia and splenomegaly. Cardiac signs change as the endocarditis produces damage.

Repeated blood cultures may be necessary to identify the organism. Intravenous antibiotics are required for at least 6 weeks to clear the infection; however, infected prosthetic material such as valves or shunts may need to be removed.

Prevention is important. Good dental hygiene is essential. Antibiotic prophylaxis is required for all dental treatment and any surgery likely to be associated with bacteraemia.

Rheumatic fever

This is the result of an abnormal immune response to a preceding infection with group A β-haemolytic streptococci which mainly affects children aged 5–15 years. Rheumatic involvement of the heart causes a pancarditis with infiltration by lymphocytes and plasma cells. This inflammation may heal with scarring, leading in later life to valvular heart disease, usually of the aortic and mitral valves.

Clinical features

Several weeks after a throat infection, the child develops:

- Acute migratory polyarthritis, involving the ankles, knees and wrists
- Fever
- Malaise
- Skin rash – erythema marginatum
- Rheumatic nodules – small, hard, painless lesions over extensor surfaces
- Pericarditis – may be associated with a pericardial friction rub, pericardial effusion and tamponade
- Myocarditis – may lead to severe heart failure
- Endocarditis – suggested by a heart murmur; can lead to significant valvular incompetence
- Chorea – develops 2–6 months after the initial infection

Management

- Bed rest
- Anti-inflammatory agents (high-dose aspirin)
- Antibiotics if there is persisting infection
- Steroids may be required if the inflammation doesn't settle
- Symptomatic treatment of cardiac complications
- Prophylactic antibiotics to prevent recurrence – recurrent episodes increase the severity of valvular disease

Further sources of information

Articles

Morris G, Wilson DG. Management of asymptomatic heart murmurs. *Current Paediatrics* 2000; **10**: 242–7

Dhillon R. Interpreting Paediatric ECGs. *Current Paediatrics* 1996; **6**: 162–7

Addendum

Abbreviations used for Figures 20.2–20.18 are as follows: ECG, electrocardiogram; LVH, left ventricular hypertrophy; PA, pulmonary artery; RA, right atrium; SVC, superior vena cava; Ao, aorta; LAA, left atrial appendage; RV, right ventricle; LV, left ventricle; RAD, right axis deviation; RAH, right atrial hypertrophy; RBBB, right bundle-branch block; RVH, right ventricular hypertrophy; V1–V6 apply to chest leads for the ECG and VR, VF and VL are the leads attached to the limbs.

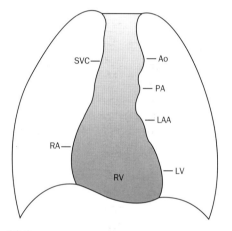

Figure 20.2

Ventricular septal defect (VSD)

Two types: perimembranous (close to tricuspid valve) and muscular.

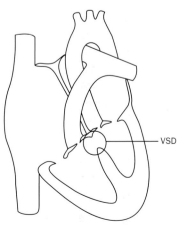

Figure 20.3

Symptoms

Depends on size:
– asymptomatic
– heart failure
– failure to thrive
– recurrent chest infections
– endocarditis

Signs

– parasternal thrill
– murmur heard at lower left sternal edge – if small/moderate defect, loud pansystolic murmur, if small defect, harsh systolic murmur

Chest radiograph

Normal if small defect
– cardiomegaly
– large pulmonary arteries (PA)

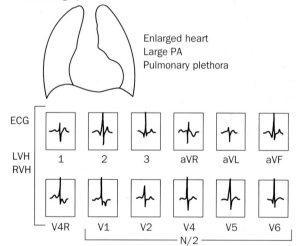

Figure 20.4

ECG

- Normal if a small defect
- Left and right ventricular hypertrophy

Management

– most close spontaneously in first few years of life
– 10 per cent require surgical closure

Patent ductus arteriosus (PDA)

The ductus arteriosus connects the pulmonary artery to the descending aorta. Failure to close shortly after birth frequently occurs in pre-term or sick neonates. In other children it is the result of a defect in the muscle of the duct.

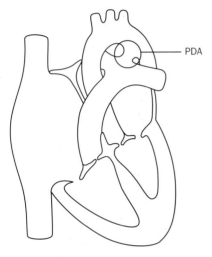

Figure 20.5

Symptoms

- Preterm – difficulties weaning from artificial ventilation if a large defect
- Other children – symptoms rare, but if a large defect may develop heart failure, failure to thrive, recurrent chest infections

Signs

- Murmur heard throughout cardiac cycle
- Machinery in quality
- Best heard below left clavicle

Chest radiograph

- Normal or enlarged heart
- Enlarged pulmonary arteries
- Pulmonary plethora

ECG

- Usually normal
- Left ventricular hypertrophy (LVH)

Chest radiograph

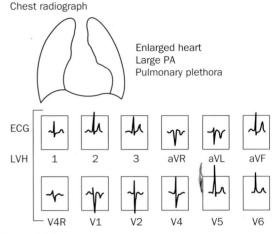

Enlarged heart
Large PA
Pulmonary plethora

Figure 20.6

Management

- Pre-term if symptomatic – indomethacin and fluid restriction, surgical ligation
- Child – closure by transvenous umbrella occlusion

Atrial septal defect (ASD)

Two types:

1. Ostium secundum (more common, see diagram): defect of foramen ovale and surrounding septum
2. Ostium primum: defect in the atrial septum just above the atrioventricular valves, with abnormality of the latter

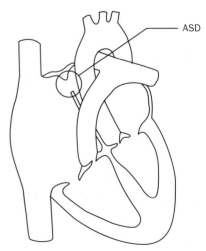

Figure 20.7

Symptoms

- Usually none
- May have recurrent chest infections, shortness of breath, tiredness on exertion, heart failure

Signs

- Systolic murmur at second left interspace (as a result of high blood flow through pulmonary valve)
- Mid-diastolic murmur at lower left sternal edge (caused by increased blood flow across tricuspid valve)
- Fixed and widely split second heart sound (excessive filling of the right ventricle delays closure of the pulmonary valve)

Chest radiograph

- Cardiomegaly
- Prominent right atrium and pulmonary artery
- Pulmonary plethora

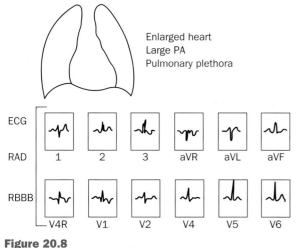

Chest radiograph

Enlarged heart
Large PA
Pulmonary plethora

Figure 20.8

ECG

- Secundum:
  - right axis deviation (RAD)
  - right ventricular hypertrophy (uncommon)
  - right bundle-branch block (RBBB)
- Primum:
  - left axis deviation
  - RBBB

Management

- Surgical repair at 4–5 years of age

Aortic valve stenosis

May occur in isolation, or in combination with other heart defects.

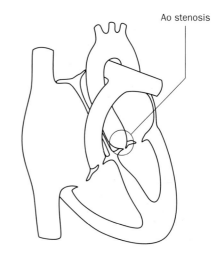

Ao stenosis

Figure 20.9

Symptoms

- Severe stenosis in the neonate may develop heart failure
- Severe stenosis in children may develop reduced exercise tolerance, dizziness or fainting on exertion, chest pain

Signs

- Pulses small in volume, slow rising, plateau type
- Systolic BP may be low
- Thrill in suprasternal notch or over carotid artery
- Systolic ejection murmur left sternal edge, radiating to neck
- Ejection click before murmur
- Aortic second sound soft and delayed

Chest radiograph

- May be normal
- Prominent left ventricle
- Poststenotic dilatation of ascending aorta

Chest radiograph

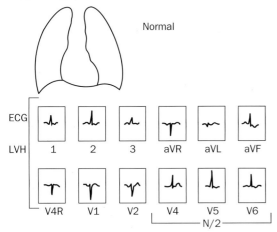

Normal

Figure 20.10

ECG

- Varying LVH

Management

Balloon or surgical valvotomy for those who are symptomatic. Regular surveillance is required to get the timing right. Those requiring treatment in the first few years of life will eventually need valve replacement.

Pulmonary valve stenosis (PS)

The valve is congenitally deformed, thickened and narrowed.

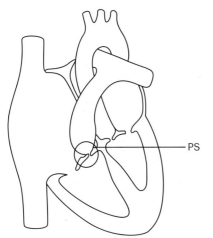

PS

Figure 20.11

Symptoms

- Usually asymptomatic
- Right-sided heart failure in severe stenosis

Signs

- Ejection systolic murmur second and third left intercostal space, radiating to the back
- Ejection click
- If severe, right ventricular heave, pulmonary component of second heart sound becomes softer and more delayed

Chest radiograph

- Poststenotic dilatation of pulmonary artery
- Enlarged right atrium and ventricle in severe defect

Chest radiograph

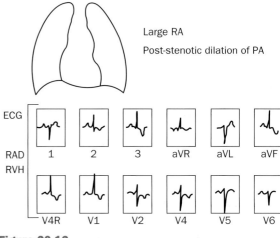

Large RA

Post-stenotic dilation of PA

Figure 20.12

ECG

- RVH

Management

Transvenous balloon dilatation if the gradient across the valve exceeds 50 mmHg.

Coarctation of the aorta

Localized narrowing of the descending aorta close to the site of the ductus arteriosus and usually distal to the left subclavian artery. Arterial blood bypasses the obstruction to reach the lower body through collateral vessels, which become enlarged. Often associated with bicuspid aortic valve and VSD.

Chest radiograph

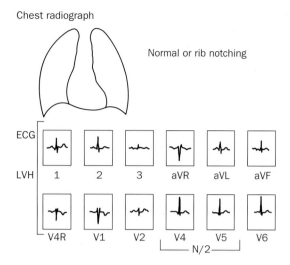

Normal or rib notching

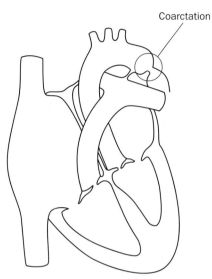

Figure 20.13

Symptoms

- Heart failure in the neonatal period if severe obstruction
- Hypertension in adults and older children

Signs

- Femoral pulses absent or weak and delayed
- High BP in arms
- Ejection systolic murmur heard between shoulder blades
- Collateral arteries palpable over scapulae

Chest radiograph

- Normal
- Rib notching from collateral vessels

ECG

- LVH

Management

- Majority require surgery

Figure 20.14

Tetralogy of Fallot (ToF)

Anatomical features

- Large VSD
- Aorta overrides the ventricular septum
- Infundibular and pulmonary valve stenosis, leading to RVH. This results in blood being shunted from the right to the left ventricle and into the aorta

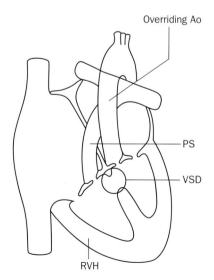

Figure 20.15

Symptoms

- Most babies are pink in the newborn period, so usually presents when a murmur is detected on routine check
- Cyanosis develops over the first few weeks of life
- Hypercyanotic spells – rapid increase in cyanosis as a result of spasm of infundibular muscle, leading to irritability, breathlessness and pallor

Signs

- Cyanosed at rest
- Clubbing of fingers and toes may develop
- Ejection systolic murmur third left intercostal space
- Thrill
- Single second heart sound

Chest radiograph

- Normal sized heart
- 'Boot'-shaped appearance of heart as a result of RVH and concavity on the left heart border because the main pulmonary artery is small
- Oligaemic lung fields

Chest radiograph

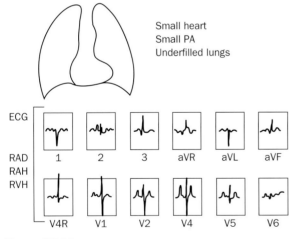

Small heart
Small PA
Underfilled lungs

ECG

RAD   1   2   3   aVR   aVL   aVF
RAH
RVH

V4R   V1   V2   V4   V5   V6

Figure 20.16

ECG

- Right axis deviation (RAD)
- RVH

Management

- Corrective surgery after 4–6 months of age
- Hypercyanotic spells are usually self-limiting, but if prolonged need prompt treatment: sedation and pain relief (morphine), β-adrenergic blocker to relieve infundibular spasm, correction of acidosis

Transposition of the great arteries (TGA)

Two parallel circulations result from the aorta arising from the right ventricle and the pulmonary artery arising from the left ventricle.

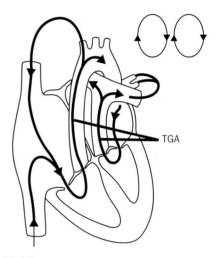

TGA

Figure 20.17

Usually associated with VSD, ASD, PDA which provides mixing between the two circulations.

Symptoms

- Progressive cyanosis within first few hours or days of life, worsens when duct closes
- Breathlessness and heart failure may develop

Signs

- Cyanosis
- Usually no murmurs

Chest radiograph

- Enlarged heart
- Narrow upper mediastinum

Chest radiograph

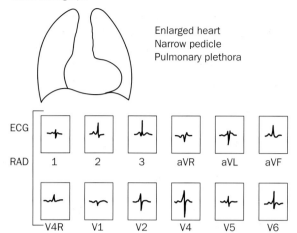

Enlarged heart
Narrow pedicle
Pulmonary plethora

Figure 20.18

- 'Egg on side' appearance of heart
- Pulmonary plethora

ECG

- Rarely helpful in establishing a diagnosis

Management

- Emergency (to improve mixing of saturated and desaturated blood)
- Maintain patency of ductus arteriosus with prostaglandin infusion
- Balloon atrial septostomy

Surgery

- Arterial switch procedure in first few weeks of life to give anatomical correction

A lump found in the groin

Age: 5 months

STEVEN RYAN

Presentation

A paediatric surgeon received the following referral from a general practitioner:

'Please would you see this 5-month-old boy who has a non-painful swollen right testicle and groin. It does not appear to be causing him any discomfort.'

Self-test 1: What are the potential causes of such a swelling? Which are common and which are rare?

Answers: Common: inguinal hernia and hydrocele; rare: tumour.

Initial considerations and action

Lumps, bumps and swellings of various parts of the body are commonly referred to paediatricians and paediatric surgeons. The first thoughts are:

- Is it an acute or urgent problem that requires immediate attention?
- If left is there an ongoing possibility of complications?
- Is it painful?
- Is there a cosmetic effect?

Here the most likely diagnoses are an inguinal hernia (Figure 21.1) and a hydrocele. Inguinal hernia is seen in about 2 per cent of boys. It is less common in girls (0.2 per cent). In young children a hydrocele is unlikely to

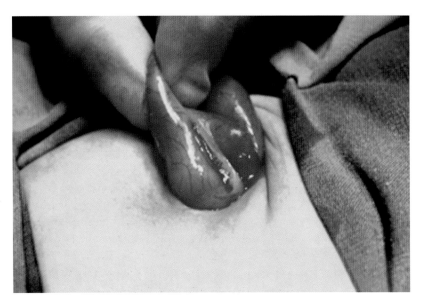

Figure 21.1   An inguinal hernia.

have a serious cause and is unlikely to require urgent attention or develop complications. The condition is not painful and the cosmetic effect is minimal. An inguinal hernia similarly has no cosmetic effect and here it would not be painful, although such hernias can become strangulated and irreducible, in which case ischaemia and necrosis of the bowel may occur. This process is usually very painful and associated with increasing signs of local swelling and evidence of intestinal obstruction.

Self-test 2: When an inguinal hernia is seen in a girl, what condition should be considered?

Answer: Testicular feminization syndrome (tissue insensitivity to androgen) which is seen in about 1 in 100 girls with inguinal hernias.

The surgeon notes the lack of pain and the routine nature of the referral from the GP and arranges for the patient to be seen in the outpatient clinic the following afternoon.

History

Tommy is seen with his mother. He is an only child. He has otherwise been in good health and is the result of an uncomplicated pregnancy and delivery. He was born at full term and weighed 3.86 kg. He has been drinking and feeding well, and has thrived. He vomits small amounts of milk shortly after feeding and has done so for several months. He has his bowels open twice every day and passes solid but soft stools.

Then, specific information about the swelling is noted:

- Right sided
- Appeared about 4 weeks ago with a soft swelling in the right groin
- Simply pressing on it made it go away
- It increased in size and firmness when Tommy was crying
- It has grown bigger since then and the swelling now reaches into the right scrotum
- The parents have not since attempted to reduce it
- It does not appear tender and has not been red or firm

Interpretation of the history

This history is more in keeping with the development of an inguinal hernia although a hydrocele cannot be excluded. Both are abnormalities of the processus vaginalis (see below under 'Background information'), which follows a route from the abdomen through the inguinal canal and into the scrotum. Other inguino-scrotal swellings can occur at various ages through childhood, as seen in Table 21.1.

Examination

When Tommy was examined the following findings were noted:

- Swelling extended from right groin to scrotum
- The swelling was soft and 'squidgy'
- It was not possible to define an upper limit to the swelling on the skin surface, i.e. you could not 'get above it'
- The swelling could be reduced gently up from the scrotum and returned to the abdomen through the inguinal area
- It reappeared in the inguinal canal shortly afterwards when the surgeon's finger was removed
- It was not tender, there was no redness and no overlying tissue swelling
- The abdomen was soft, non-distended, with normal bowel sounds
- After reduction both testes were easily identified in the scrotum – they were of normal size and consistency
- There was no light transmission on transillumination

Interpretation of the examination

These findings are most consistent with a reducible, right-sided, inguinal hernia rather than a hydrocele. A hydrocele would be firmer and it would usually be possible to define the upper limit of the abnormality. The key diagnostic feature of a hydrocele is the brilliant transillumination seen (Figure 21.2).

Table 21.2 is a summary of the findings on examination for inguinoscrotal swellings.

Table 21.1 Inguinoscrotal swellings in childhood

Diagnosis	Age range	Features
Inguinal hernia	Any but especially infancy	Swelling starts in inguinal region May develop to reach scrotum Usually reducible Common in pre-term babies Much less common in girls Not usually present at birth
Hydrocele	Infancy	In line of processus vaginalis Usually irreducible Does not vary much in size Usually first seen in scrotum Usually painless Typically presents at birth Usually resolves by toddler-hood
	Older children	Much rarer May be associated with inflammatory or neoplastic conditions
Testicular torsion	Neonate (rare) Adolescent	Associated with severe pain, redness and systemic upset
Epididymo-orchitis	Adolescent	Acute pain and tenderness – usually less severe than torsion
Lymph glands	Any age	In inguinal area – usually multiple Often bilateral, firm

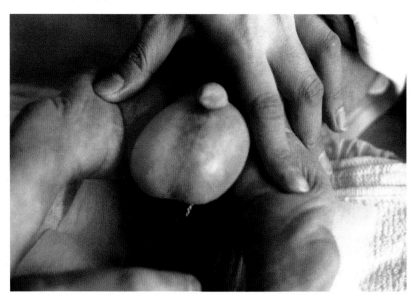

Figure 21.2 Transillumination of the scrotum.

Table 21.2 Findings on examination in scrotal swelling

Diagnosis	Features
Inguinal hernia	
Reducible	Cannot 'get above it'
	Swelling arises from inguinal ring
	Can be pushed back through inguinal canal and ring
	Soft
Irreducible	Immobile
	Tender
	Redness and subcutaneous swelling develop if strangulated
Hydrocele	Smooth
	Transilluminates
	Can 'get above it'
Testicular torsion	Redness and swelling of scrotum
	Hard, exquisitely tender testes and lower cord
	Systemically unwell if diagnosis delayed
Epididymo-orchitis	Very variable swelling and tenderness of testis and scrotum
	May be difficult to differentiate from testicular torsion
Lymph glands	Firm lumps in line of inguinal ligament
	Size, shape and consistency depend on underlying cause

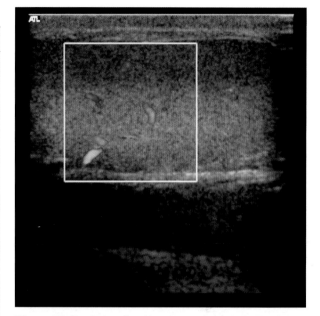

Figure 21.3 Colour flow Doppler study of testis. The bright colours indicate good blood flow and rule-out infarction.

In this situation no investigations were needed.

Self-test 3: Mumps orchitis:

A Is rarer in prepubescent boys than older boys and adults

B Can occur without swollen parotid glands

C Affects both testes in 67 per cent of boys

D Causes testicular atrophy in 33 per cent of cases

E Is commonly associated with a hydrocele

Answers: True: A, B, D; false: C (33 per cent), E (rarely).

Investigations

For most of the above situations, investigations are not usually required to confirm the diagnosis. The area where they are most likely to be required is in the differentiation of testicular torsion from other causes of acute scrotal pain and swelling. Here ultrasonography comes into its own, and in particular Doppler ultrasonography (Figure 21.3). In testicular torsion there is reduced blood flow in the testis, whereas it is usually normal or increased in other inflammatory conditions.

Management and prognosis

Tommy was admitted for corrective surgery 3 weeks later. Tommy made an uneventful recovery and, at follow-up 1 month later, his wound was healing well. He was discharged from further follow-up.

Diagnosis

Right inguinal (indirect) hernia repaired by surgery.

How to undertake an inguinal hernia repair

- Transverse incision through inguinal crease
- External oblique fascia opened
- Blunt dissection of cremaster muscle and tissue
- Hernial sac identified, and spermatic vessels and cord gently dissected free
- Sac contents reduced, and then the sac is cut
- Sac twisted clockwise and neck of sac transfixed
- Wound repaired

Background information

Descent of the testis

Testicular differentiation begins by 6 weeks' gestation in the presence of a Y chromosome and, shortly afterwards, testosterone production occurs from the Leydig cells, which are stimulated by chorionic gonadotrophin. The testis forms at 3 weeks of development, and the germ cells migrate from the yolk sac to the germinal ridge of the mesoderm. Over the next 4 weeks the germ cells coalesce to form the primordial testis. This is located on the posterior wall of the abdomen, just medial to the kidney. The epididymis and vas deferens differentiate from the mesonephric (wolffian) duct under the influence of testosterone and join up with the kidney, which then enlarges and migrates caudally as shown in Table 21.3.

At 13 weeks the processus vaginalis, an outpouching of the parietal peritoneum, forms a developing tunnel that moves medially and caudally between the internal and external abdominal oblique muscles and into the scrotum. At around 30 weeks, the testis enters the processus vaginalis and then descends into the

Table 21.3 The descent of the testis in fetal life

Month of fetal life	Position
3	Iliac fossa
7	Inguinal canal
8	External inguinal ring
9	Scrotum

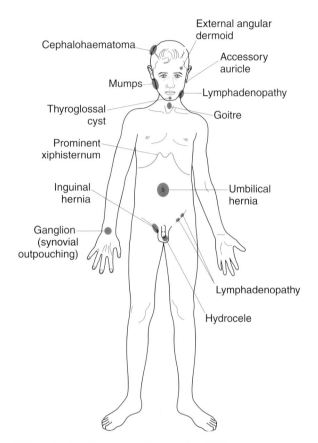

Figure 21.4   Lumps and bumps in childhood.

scrotum and becomes fused with the posterior layers of the scrotum, providing an anchor that prevents the testis from rotating. At 37–40 weeks (full term), the processus vaginalis usually closes, eliminating any communication between the peritoneum and the inguinal canal or scrotum. Failure of closure may present with an indirect inguinal hernia or a hydrocele.

Abnormalities of testicular descent

Two patterns of abnormal testicular descent are recognized:

1 Ectopic
2 Arrested normal descent

In the former, which is seen in two-thirds of cases, the testis becomes located in the superficial inguinal pouch.

Table 21.4 Lumps, bumps and swelling in childhood

Site	Cause	Age group	Details
Scalp	Cephalohaematoma	Neonate	Subperiosteal blood Under one or both parietal bones Never, ever aspirate with needle May increase likelihood of jaundice Settles over a few weeks
	Caput succedaneum	Neonate	Moulding of skull Diffuse scalp oedema Prolonged delivery Settles in hours and over a few days
Face	External angular dermoid	Any age toddler and older	Remove as infection risk Smooth lump at outer margin of 'eyebrow' Sequestration of epidermal cells at skin fusion line
Neck	Thyroglossal cyst	Any age, more likely in younger children	Midline swelling over hyoid bone Remove as infection risk Moves with swallowing
	Goitre	Any age	More common in adolescent girls Swelling in lower anterior neck Moves with swallowing Determine cause and treat
	Lymph nodes	Any age	Commonly caused by viral infections: Usually small, smooth and mobile, and not tender May be large and painful if: – 'adenitis' – bacterial superinfection – catch scratch fever – Epstein–Barr virus infection May be large if: – atypical mycobacterial infection – lymphoma Be concerned if: large, fixed, tender, not smooth systemic symptoms
	Parotid gland	Older children	Swelling which spreads from cheek to neck Obliterates angle of jaw Less common since mumps immunization
Abdomen	Umbilical hernia		Midline Beneath umbilicus Easily reducible Nearly always resolves spontaneously
Groin	Direct inguinal hernia Hydrocele		See above See above

The testis is of normal size and, if it can be relocated in the scrotum by 3 years of age, spermatozoa production is preserved. If normal descent is arrested, the testis is hypoplastic and immobile, and usually infertile. It is conventional to operate to place the testis in the scrotum at about 2–3 years of age. This is partly to reduce the long-term risk of malignancy in a testis that is undescended.

Epidemiology of inguinal hernias

Inguinal hernias present:

- 90 per cent in boys
- 60 per cent on the right
- 25 per cent the left
- 15 per cent bilaterally

There is also increased familial incidence.

Other lumps and bumps in childhood

Figure 21.4 and Table 21.4 show the other common lumps and bumps seen in children.

Further sources of information

Books

Jones PG, Woodward AA (eds). *Clinical Paediatric Surgery: Diagnosis and management*. Melbourne: Blackwell Scientific, 1986

McLachlan J. *Medical Embryology*. Wokingham: Addison-Wesley, 1994

Nixon H, O'Donnell B. *Essentials of Paediatric Surgery*, 4th edn. Oxford: Butterworth-Heinemann, 1993

Article

Kass EJ, Lundak B. The acute scrotum. *Pediatric Clinics of North America* 1997; **44**: 1251–66

Websites

http://yalesurgery.med.yale.edu/surgery/sections/ped_surg/hernia.htm

www.pedisurg.com/PtEduc/Hydrocele.htm

Self-test 4: Eight-year-old Harry was referred by his general practitioner with a midline swelling in the front of his neck that moved up and down as he swallowed. It was smooth and painless. Harry was otherwise well.

A What is the most likely cause for this swelling?
B What should be done about it?
C What tissue might be found within it?
D How could this be shown preoperatively?
E What is the risk of not undertaking surgery?

Answers:
A A thyroglossal cyst
B It should be surgically removed
C Thyroid tissue
D A radionuclide thyroid scan
E Infection

Acute presentation

Sudden collapse

Age: 8 years

STEVEN RYAN

C H A P T E R

22

Presentation

Eight-year-old Samantha is brought to the emergency department by ambulance following a 999 call from her parents. They told the ambulance service that they had found Samantha unconscious and shaking on the floor of the bathroom at 9.30pm. The ambulance arrived within 6 minutes, by which time Samantha had stopped shaking but she remained barely rousable. On arrival at the emergency department she is placed in the recovery position and given high-flow oxygen by facemask. Her heart rate is 120/minute and her blood pressure 118/78 mmHg. She has a capillary refill time of 1 second. She has a finger-prick test that shows her blood glucose concentration is 5.4 mmol/L. Although she has responded to the pain of the lancet, she is not responding to spoken commands other than by groaning. Her pupils are equal and reactive. Her temperature is 36.8°C. At this point her parents arrive by her side.

Self-test 1: List the possible causes for such a sudden collapse in a previously well child.

Answers:

Cardiac: syncope, arrhythmia

Primary neurological: epilepsy, stroke (haemorrhagic or infarctive), migraine

Drugs: deliberate self-harm (e.g. with tricyclic drugs), alcohol

Metabolic: hypoglycaemia

Trauma: may also be a secondary and accompanying event

Respiratory: airway blocked

Initial considerations and action

Life support

The initial approach to caring for Samantha is not the classic pathway of history, examination and investigations. The first priority is to stabilize her condition using a life support pathway. This will have started even before the ambulance arrived and ambulance control would have given telephone advice on:

- What to do (recovery position)
- What not to do (stick anything in her mouth)

The receiving staff:

- 'SHOUT' for help to make sure appropriate medical and nursing staff are available
- 'APPROACH', making sure they do not harm themselves

For example, Samantha could be dripping wet having got out of the bath, and the hospital floor might be slippery

- 'FREE' the patient from any constricting clothing or impediments to her resuscitation

Then:

- AIRWAY
- BREATHING
- CIRCULATION are assessed and dealt with

Here, Samantha's airway is adequate in the recovery position and oxygen is given to complement her breathing. Her circulation is adequate. It is important to check the blood glucose level in children who have had a fit or who are unconscious, because this is a common problem and it is easily and quickly dealt with. Samantha's blood glucose level is normal. Her conscious level is assessed rapidly using the 'AVPU' scale.

The AVPU scale

A alert
V responds to voice only
P responds to pain
U unconscious

She is somewhere between V and P. A patient clearly in category 'P' is at high risk of compromising his or her airway and many such patients need tracheal intubation. Samantha avoids this.

Making the diagnosis

Once the patient has been stabilized, it is possible to think what might be the probable causes of her problem (Figure 22.1). The two most likely systems that could be responsible for sudden episodes such as this are the cardiovascular system and the central nervous system (CNS). Her airway does not appear to be obstructed and her blood sugar is normal, making respiratory or metabolic problems unlikely. Trauma remains a possibility and this could have occurred as a secondary event after, say, a faint. A sudden reduction in cerebral blood flow can cause brain malfunction and result in a collapse. This process is called syncope. This can result from either a classic faint or a primary cardiac arrhythmia. The CNS may have a primary malfunction – a seizure – or it may be disturbed by other events. Head trauma, metabolic disturbance, drug ingestion or infection might be responsible. Features in the history which might suggest these alternatives are:

- **Syncope:**
  Fainting: history of previous faints; occurs on standing up, getting out of the bath, during school assembly, when unwell, after missed meals (especially breakfast)
  Arrhythmia: family history of sudden collapses or death, collapse during exercise, collapse when startled
  Obstructive cardiomyopathy

- **Neurological disorder:**
  Brain haemorrhage
  Stroke
  High blood pressure: hypertensive encephalopathy
- **Seizure:**
  Primary: history of previous seizures with complete recovery, previous investigations ruling out other causes.
  Secondary: other known abnormality of brain function or structure, e.g. cerebral palsy
- **Trauma:**
  Signs of trauma on patient or visible damage or blood on furniture
- **Drug effect:**
  Drugs in the house with compatible effects to overdose (e.g. tricyclic antidepressants)
  History of previous ingestion episodes
- **Infection:**
  Prodromal symptoms including fever and history of rash
- **Metabolic disturbance:**
  History of diabetes, family history of metabolic disorder, previous unexplained episodes of coma

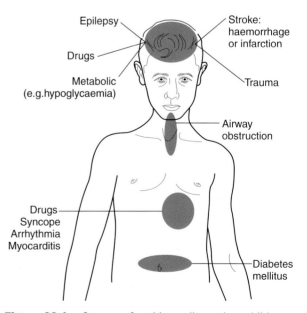

Figure 22.1 Causes of sudden collapse in a child.

A Seizures and hypertension

B Hyperventilation and hypoglycaemia

C Coma and hypoglycaemia

D Seizures and cardiac arrhythmia

E Fixed left pupil and diminished conscious level

Answers:

A False – hypertensive encephalopathy

B False – aspirin poisoning

C False – insulin overdose

D True

E False – trauma or haemorrhage or other focal brain lesion

History

Samantha's parents gave further details. She had gone up to have a bath about 20 minutes previously. The bath had been run but she had not got into it. They heard a strange cry from Samantha and then a thud. They ran upstairs and found Samantha on the bathroom floor. She was lying on her back with her legs and arms extended, and jerking all her limbs vigorously. There was a large amount of frothy saliva around her mouth. She was unresponsive. She appeared to have passed urine during the attack. Within 2–3 minutes the shaking had stopped and Samantha was deeply asleep and snoring. The ambulance arrived shortly afterwards.

Samantha's previous medical history was unremarkable. She had been born at full term following an unremarkable pregnancy and her birth weight was 3.8 kg. She had made normal developmental progress and was progressing well at school. She was up to date with her immunizations. Her mother and father were both well, although her mother suffered from asthma. She had a brother Peter aged 14 who also was currently well. At the age of 12 he had fainted during a school assembly. He recovered quickly and had no further episodes.

On direct questioning there were no medications in the household other than paracetamol, Samantha had been completely well before this episode and had had no previous episodes of collapse or coma.

What Samantha's parents have observed is a generalized (meaning that consciousness was lost), clonic (shaking) seizure. The clonic phase of a generalized seizure may be preceded by a tonic phase in which the whole body goes stiff. The onset of the tonic phase may be accompanied by a loud noise as air is expelled from the compressed lungs. Urinary incontinence and frothing of saliva are also strong supportive features in the history.

Syncope is now much less likely because, although a few brief clonic movements are occasionally seen after a syncopal episode, sustained clonic movements are unusual. Other than the thud, there was no history compatible with trauma and nothing to suggest drug ingestion.

At this point it appears that Samantha has had a generalized seizure. Further examination and investigations will be required to determine its nature and significance.

Examination

While the patient is semiconscious, a general examination can be undertaken together with a partial examination of the nervous system. In this state, neurological condition will be regularly assessed and the nurses caring for her will be asked to perform regular neurological observations. Figure 22.2 shows these regular observations recorded on a chart. It is set out in such a way that it is very easy to spot any deterioration and take appropriate action. The chart incorporates elements of the Glasgow Coma score (Table 22.1), which is a more detailed and formal scale than 'AVPU', the latter being reserved for emergency initial assessment. Here we can see Samantha's conscious level is improving.

General examination of Samantha showed:

- No signs of trauma
- No rash was observed
- Breathing rate 20/minute
- Blood oxygen saturation between 98 and 100 per cent
- Heart rate was 106/minute
- Pulse was regular
- Blood pressure was 114/68 mmHg
- Pupils were bilaterally dilated but equal and reacting to light

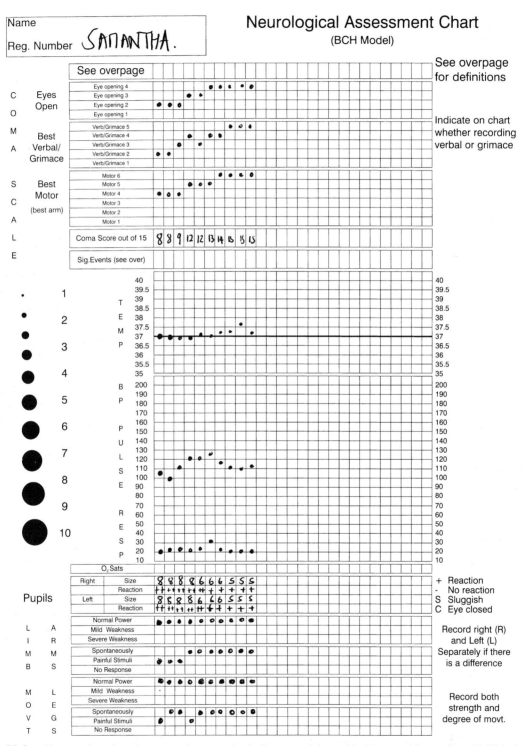

Neurological Assessment Chart
(BCH Model)

Name

Reg. Number SAMANTHA.

Figure 22.2 Observation chart incorporating neurological status. Adapted by Tatmon, Waren, Powell, Whitehouse and Noons, 1997, Birmingham Children's Hospital NHS Trust.

Table 22.1 The Glasgow Coma score for use in children aged 4–15 years

Response	Score
Eye opening:	
Spontaneous	4
To voice	3
To pain	2
No response to pain	1
Best movement response:	
Obeys spoken command	6
Localizes to pain	5
Withdraws from pain	4
Abnormal flexion to pain (also called decorticate)	3
Abnormal extension to pain (also called decerebrate)	2
No response to pain	1
Best verbal response:	
Orientated and converses	5
Disorientated and converses	4
Inappropriate words	3
Incomprehensible sounds	2
No response to pain	1

- Optic fundoscopy revealed no abnormality
- Posture was normal
- All of limb her reflexes were brisk and her plantar reflexes were up-going

Particularly important aspects of the examination are:

- External inspection for signs of head and neck trauma. Look for obvious bruising or swelling. Other important points are to examine the ear canals for bleeding and the nose for bleeding or clear fluid loss, all of which could point to base-of-skull fracture. Look for features of infection such as a non-blanching rash consistent with meningococcal septicaemia

- Continuing monitoring of airway, breathing and blood oxygen saturation by pulse oximeter
- Examination of cardiovascular system for arrhythmias or hypotension, which could indicate a primary cardiovascular problem, a drug-induced problem (such as tricyclic antidepressants which can independently compromise the CNS and the heart) or raised intracranial pressure (with high blood pressure and slow heart rate)
- At this early stage, examination of the nervous system is limited. In addition to conscious level, posture is noted as well as trunk and limb tone and limb reflexes, together with plantar responses. The main purpose is to detect severe brain pathology (decorticate or decerebrate posture) and whether there is a focal abnormality. This could indicate a focal lesion within the brain (such as a tumour or unilateral haemorrhage) or a 'Todd's paresis' which is a transient focal lack of function following a seizure
- It is also important to look at the pupils, which may especially let you know that there is a focal lesion. Inspection of the optic fundi and discs is important to exclude the changes of papilloedema. This would suggest raised intracranial pressure and may be very difficult in an uncooperative child or one with pinpoint pupils

See Figure 25.1, p. 272.

At this stage Samantha begins to regain consciousness, recognizes her parents and asks where she is. She has no recollection of the seizure or subsequent events. At this point Samantha appears to have had an uncomplicated seizure and there are no features to suggest any other significant underlying pathology. The doctors caring for her decide that neuroimaging is not required. The diagnosis at this point is one of primary generalized seizure.

Investigations

In Samantha, when blood was taken for glucose estimation at the bedside, it was also sent for further biochemical analysis (Table 22.2).

Table 22.2 Blood results from Samantha

Parameter	Test value	Expected range
Sodium (mmol/L)	135	138–145
Potassium (mmol/L)	5.2	3.5–6.0
Calcium (mmol/L)	2.3	2.2–2.7
Phosphate (mmol/L)	1.8	0.95–1.75
Magnesium (mmol/L)	0.91	0.6–0.95
Chloride (mmol/L)	98	96–104
Creatinine (μmol/L)	48	44–88
Glucose (mmol/L)	4.8	3.3–5.5
pH	7.42	7.36–7.44
Base excess (mmol/L)	−2	−4–+2
P_{CO_2} (kPa)	4.1	4.3–4.6
P_{O_2} (kPa)	10 (capillary)	11–14.4 (arterial)

Clearly Samantha's biochemistry results are normal. It is important to confirm in the laboratory the results of the bedside glucose test, because the latter is more accurate. It has also been possible to rule out electrolyte and acid–base disturbances in Samantha, which is helpful in making inborn errors of metabolism less likely. Prolonged fits can cause some degree of metabolic acidosis as a result of a build-of lactic acid, but that was not likely here because the fit was short.

Samantha's parents asked whether she would be having a brain scan. The doctors caring for Samantha do not feel that there is any indication for this at present. They explain that they would undertake a scan in this situation only if she did not recover from the convulsion or if the convulsion were focal in nature. However, an electroencephalogram (EEG) is ordered for some weeks later and Samantha is seen in the outpatient clinic with her parents. Since her previous seizure a further 2-minute clonic convulsion has occurred. The EEG result is shown in Figure 22.3.

Self-test 3: Which of these EEG reports is most likely in Samantha?

A   **Centrotemporal spikes on left**

B   **Generalized spike and wave**

C   **Chaotic pattern (hypsarrhythmia)**

D   **Three per second spike and wave**

E   **Localized slow wave activity in right temporal lobe**

Answers:

A   False: benign rolandic epilepsy

B   True

C   False: infantile myoclonic epilepsy

D   False: typical absence epilepsy

E   False: temporal lobe epilepsy

Diagnosis

Primary generalized epilepsy with clonic seizures.

Management

At this consultation the clinician would discuss the following topics.

Explanation of epilepsy and its natural history – what it is and is not

It is important to establish the family's current understanding and also any misconceptions.

Any modifications of lifestyle (remember driving)

Samantha's EEG did not show any evidence of photosensitivity and, as none of her fits have been provoked by a flickering light, no special precautions need to be taken about computer use or watching television. Samantha was a keen swimmer and asked if she could continue. The doctor said she could – as long as she was well supervised. It was also safe for her to cycle, providing that she avoided busy roads and wore a helmet. If Samantha had been of driving age she would have been unable to drive legally for a period of 1 year. She would be allowed to drive again when next seizure free for 1 year. Some careers are blocked by regulations, even after a single fit, and these include airline pilot, train driver and taxi driver, the navy and the fire brigade. In other situations remission of epilepsy in childhood is not a bar and this includes the army.

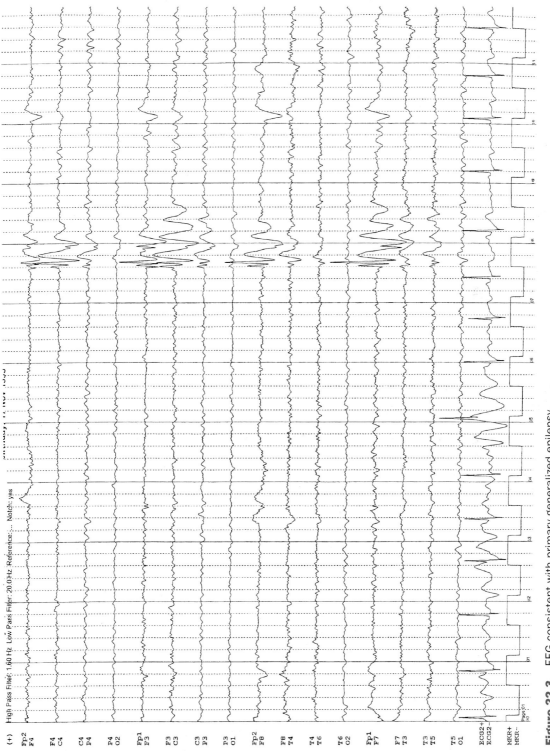

High Pass Filter: 1.60 Hz Low Pass Filter: 20.0 Hz Reference:... Notch: yes

(+)

Fp2
F4

F4
C4

C4
P4

P4
O2

Fp1
F3

F3
C3

C3
P3

P3
O1

Fp2
F8

F8
T4

T4
T6

T6
O2

Fp1
F7

F7
T3

T3
T5

T5
O1

ECG2+
ECG2−

MKR+
MKR−

Figure 22.3 EEG consistent with primary generalized epilepsy.

Drug treatment – benefits and risks – duration of treatment

Samantha is advised to commence regular twice-daily treatment with sodium valproate. She and her parents are warned about the potential common side effects (weight gain, increased appetite and possible temporary hair loss) and uncommon serious side effects (hepatitis). An initial 2-year course is recommended and, if no seizures occur, the drug will be discontinued at that point. The possible side effect of drugs on behaviour and cognition is also important for school-age children. It was pointed out that, although sodium valproate rarely causes cognitive impairment, it could occasionally cause behavioural problems.

How to recognize seizures, and when and how to give first aid in established epilepsy

- Keep calm
- Remove sources of danger
- Recovery position if possible
- Let the seizure run its course
- A period of rest
- Do not force anything into the child's mouth
- Shout for help if seizure prolonged

Frequently nowadays the clinician is a nurse specialist. Good practice is to give written material to summarize the information that has been given. It is also important to decide who else needs to be told and what information they receive. Teachers, for example, should be told about the nature of the condition, first aid measures and the educationally relevant side effects, together with any restrictions on activity. Problems of psychological adjustment are commonly seen in teenagers and it is helpful to families to know that these can occur.

Background information

Definition

An epileptic seizure is the clinical manifestation of cortical neuronal discharge. This manifestation can result in disturbed consciousness, behaviour, emotion, motor function, perception or sensation. The types of episode tend to be similar (stereotyped) and usually recur spontaneously. Two main types of epilepsy are recognized – generalized and partial (focal) (Table 22.3).

Table 22.3 Types of seizure seen in school-aged children

Generalized		
Tonic–clonic	Cry, loss of consciousness, falls, stiff then twitching	Can be just tonic or clonic, can be brief Urinary incontinence, tongue biting
Typical absence	Stops, stares, maybe eye flickering and chewing	Stops in adolescence
Myoclonic	Sudden major muscle contraction, may fall to ground, momentary loss of consciousness	Significant risk of injury – may need head protector, often occurs when waking
Atonic	Sudden loss of major muscle tone, momentary loss of consciousness	Very significant risk of injury, head protector may be needed
Partial		
Simple partial	Normal activity of part of brain interrupted	Localized twitching, turning head and neck, tingling, visual disturbance, altered perception, including déjà vu
Complex partial	Altered or impaired consciousness	Fidgeting, fumbling, lip smacking with ongoing unusual behaviour

Diagnostic tests

The EEG is not used to diagnose epilepsy but confirms its nature and is an aid to determining treatment. An EEG is an amplified tracing of the electrical activity over the brain surface measured from electrodes placed on to the scalp. Normal brain activity (waves) consists of four types of wave.

How to read an EEG

The first aspect to consider is the underlying rhythms of the EEG (Table 22.4).

The second aspect is significant abnormalities and whether they are localized, generalized or typical:

- Localized, e.g. over a temporal lobe in temporal lobe epilepsy
- Generalized, e.g. over both hemispheres – consistent with primary generalized epilepsy
- Typical:
  3/second spike and wave: typical absence epilepsy (Figure 22.4)
  centrotemporal spikes: benign rolandic epilepsy

Drug management

Commonly used drugs and their indications and side effects are shown in Table 22.5. The mechanism of action of anticonvulsant drugs is to interfere with polarization changes of neuronal membranes, most typically by interacting with receptors on neuronal membranes and at synaptic junctions. γ-Aminobutyric acid (GABA) is released from presynaptic neurons and inhibits depolarization by down-activating adjacent chloride channels. Drugs that work through the GABA mechanism include the benzodiazepines, phenobarbital/phenobarbitone, sodium valproate and vigabatrin. Phenobarbital and carbamazepine work through their effect on sodium channels on the neuronal membranes.

Prognosis

Children with generalized epilepsy and those without an anatomical abnormality are more likely to stop having seizures, and this is especially true of those with typical absences. Those who develop seizures before 2 years of age and those with multiple seizure types are less likely to grow out of their seizures. Around three-quarters of children with seizures will stop having them.

Samantha continued her treatment for 2 years and remained seizure free. The treatment was then stopped by reducing the dose over 2 months. She has had no further seizures for 2 years.

Further sources of information

Book

Appleton R, Baker G, Chadwick D, Smith D. *Textbook of Epilepsy*, 3rd edn. London: Martin Dunitz, 1994

Websites

www.epilepsy.org.uk

www.efa.org

Self-test 4: Eleanor is a tall thin teenager who is seen after her fifth 'collapse' in 2 years. Two have occurred in the shower and two during the morning at school. On each occasion she has felt peculiar and her eyesight has become dark, and she has

Table 22.4 First considerations when reading an electroencephalogram (EEG)

Wave	Frequency (Hz)	Feature
Alpha	8–12	Main type in healthy individuals, tend to reduce during mental activity and on opening eyes
Beta	6–10	Normal but also some anticonvulsants and stress can increase them
Theta	4–7	More likely if drowsy
Delta	<4	Deep sleep but also brain disorders

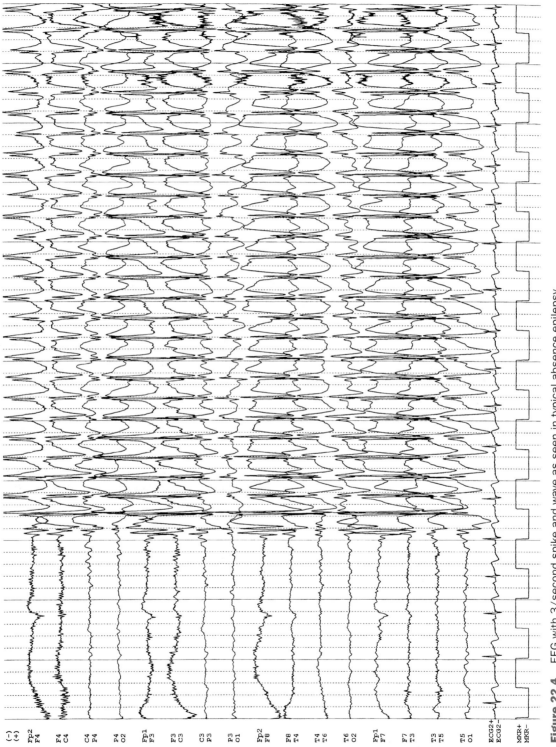

(−)
(+)

Fp2
F4

F4
C4

C4
P4

P4
O2

Fp1
F3

F3
C3

C3
P3

P3
O1

Fp2
F8

F8
T4

T4
T6

T6
O2

Fp1
F7

F7
T3

T3
T5

T5
O1

ECG2+
ECG2−

MKR+
MKR−

Figure 22.4   EEG with 3/second spike and wave as seen in typical absence epilepsy.

Table 22.5 Commonly used anticonvulsant drugs

Drug	Seizure types	Common side effects	Rare side effects
Carbamazepine	Local	Dizziness, drowsiness	Erythema multiforme Marrow suppression
Lamotrigine	Local, generalized	Erythema multiforme (avoided by gradual introduction)	
Phenytoin (Second/third line)	Local, generalized	Gum swelling, hirsutism Acne	Ataxia (in overdose)
Valproate	Generalized	Weight gain, hair loss Behaviour changes	Teratogenicity, liver failure

fallen down and taken a few minutes to come round. She was then pale and shaking and was observed to have a fast heart rate that slowly settled down. There are no shaking movements, tongue biting or urinary incontinence. She has had an ECG test, which was normal. She is now well; the last attack was 4 weeks previously.

A What system is responsible for the episodes?
B What change in heart rate, if any, would there be during the episode?
C What factor might be predisposing to the morning episodes?
D What other factors may initiate such episodes?
E What is the cause of the fast heart rate and pallor?

Answers:
A Cardiovascular
B These are syncopal episodes (also known as vasovagal) and bradycardia occurs at the time of collapse

C Missing breakfast
D Standing up; hot environments; intercurrent illness; emotional shock; pain
E An adrenaline (epinephrine) surge by which bradycardia is overcome

Self-test 5: Ian, an 11-year-old boy with diabetes, faints and becomes unconscious. He was well until a few minutes before the episode.
A What is the likely cause of his problem?
B How should it be dealt with?

Answers:
A Hypoglycaemia
B Give sugar or use subcutaneous glucagon. Remember that the airway may be compromised by low conscious level. Glucose jellies are available for smearing on to the buccal mucosa

A rash that fails the glass test

Age: 3 years

LEENA PATEL

Presentation

Sarah is 3 years old. This morning she woke up with a few red and purple spots on her face. Having found that the spots did not fade with the 'glass test', her mother became extremely worried and rushed her to the local hospital. Sarah has had flu-like symptoms and a fever for a day. She also vomited twice yesterday evening.

Self-test 1: What is a 'glass test' and what is its significance?

Answer: A glass pressed against the skin distinguishes whether a rash is blanching or non-blanching. A non-blanching rash does not fade under pressure because of leakage of blood into the skin and subcutaneous tissue rather than congestion in capillaries (when skin blanches on pressure). The most common cause is a viral infection but meningococcal septicaemia should be considered in any febrile child presenting with a non-blanching rash, because it is a life-threatening condition and the most common cause of death outside the neonatal period. Laypeople and paramedics are taught to recognize it and to seek medical advice promptly.

Initial considerations and action

Sarah's story of an acute illness and petechial rash raises a number of questions:

- Does she have the more serious meningococcal septicaemia or a relatively innocuous viral illness?

- Is it more likely to be the latter because viral infections are common in early childhood and she has had flu-like symptoms?
- Could the two coexist or has one (a viral infection) predisposed to the other (meningococcal septicaemia)?
- Vomiting is a common non-specific symptom in ill children, but may be a sign of meningitis and raised intracranial pressure. Is there any association between the vomiting yesterday evening and waking this morning with the purplish spots?
- Are there other conditions that need to be considered?

The history and examination should provide some answers.

History

Sarah has not had any rash other than the spots on her face. She has been unusually quiet and clingy this morning. She has not been crying or irritable and her mother does not think that she has a headache.

The previous day she was hot and whingey, and had a runny nose, and did not go to playgroup. Her mother felt that Sarah had picked up the same bug that Sarah's two older siblings had had – they had had colds and been hot for a few days. Sarah did not eat much and mother put it down to a sore throat. She managed to keep drinks down till the evening when she was sick twice. The vomiting was quite forceful but she only brought back milk – no bile or blood.

Sarah's mother was asked about other symptoms that might explain the fever and vomiting, but Sarah has not had any respiratory, gastrointestinal or urinary symptoms.

Sarah's birth and previous medical history are unremarkable except for chickenpox when she was 2 years old. She has had all the immunizations that she has been sent appointments for.

Self-test 2: Do you think Sarah has a headache and what might be the relevance?

Answer: No. Although she may not be able to complain of headache at her age, she might be expected to cry inconsolably because of the pain or be irritable. Parents can usually tell whether their child is in pain. A headache is a symptom of meningitis.

Interpretation of the history

The history of the acute febrile illness, runny nose and similar symptoms in the siblings suggests a viral infection rather than focal infections such as a urinary tract infection.

This possibility does not rule out septicaemia because this is commonly preceded by a viral upper respiratory tract infection.

As the vomiting has not been persistent and does not appear to be associated with a headache, it is less likely to result from meningitis and raised intracranial pressure.

Self-test 3: Is Sarah likely to get septicaemia, considering that she has had all the routine immunizations?

Answer: Yes – they would protect Sarah against meningococcal C infection but not serotypes A and B or other bacteria such as pneumococci.

Examination

Observation shows that Sarah:

- Is quiet and clings to her mother
- Does not appear drowsy or lethargic
- Has pale skin but her mucous membrane is pink
- Has non-blanching spots on her face

When Sarah is undressed, the following are noted:

- A petechial rash on the face and also all over her body, which her mother says is new
- The spots are <2 mm in diameter and are not confluent
- Ear temperature 39.5°C
- Respiratory rate 30/min, no difficulty in breathing, no intercostal recessions, arterial oxygen saturation (Sao_2) 97 per cent in air
- Hands and feet warm, capillary refill time <2 seconds, pulse 110/min, normal volume and regular, blood pressure (BP) 94/56 mm Hg
- Does not resent bright light or the noise in A&E, no neck stiffness
- Clear nasal discharge, red pharynx, a few petechiae on the palate
- No swelling on hands and feet
- No generalized lymphadenopathy or hepatosplenomegaly

Interpretation of the examination

Important features from the examination

The purpose of the examination in a child presenting acutely with a febrile illness and a petechial rash is:

- To assess whether the child is seriously ill and has septicaemia
- To obtain additional clues to the diagnosis

Features of serious illness and septicaemia

- Appear seriously ill
- Lethargic, irritable, altered level of consciousness
- Signs of circulatory collapse or inadequate systemic perfusion

An assessment of the airway, breathing and circulation and appropriate resuscitation must be performed without delay.

Sarah does not have any of these features.

Children with Henoch–Schoenlein purpura and idiopathic thrombocytopenic purpura are relatively well and the principal feature is a non-blanching rash.

Self-test 4: Define lethargy.

Answer: Lethargy is a level of consciousness characterized by poor or absent eye contact or failure to recognize carers or to interact with people or objects in the environment.

Self-test 5: What are the signs of circulatory failure and inadequate systemic perfusion?

Answer:

- Poor peripheral perfusion
  - capillary refill time prolonged (>5 seconds)
  - cold extremities (peripheral core temperature gradient > 2°C)
  - thready pulse
- Tachycardia out of proportion to the fever or bradycardia
- Hypotension
- Irritability, lethargy and decreasing conscious state
- Poor urine output (<0.5 ml/kg per hour)
- Low oxygen saturation

Features of meningeal irritation

Sarah does not have any signs of meningeal irritation or meningitis (see Chapter 14).

The timing of the eruption of the rash in relation to the fever and progress

- A petechial rash during an acute febrile illness favours a viral infection
- Rapid development of purpuric lesions is an ominous sign and would suggest septicaemia
- Idiopathic thrombocytopenic purpura presents some weeks after a viral infection

Size and distribution of the non-blanching rash

Sarah's rash is generalized when she is examined and petechial.

The non-blanching rash of septicaemia is usually generalized in distribution and purpuric or petechial, and may be necrotic in the centre (Figure 23.1).

Petechiae on the face, neck, upper arms and upper chest above the nipple line (distribution of drainage of the superior vena cava) are observed after bouts of severe coughing, forceful vomiting, crying or a generalized convulsion caused by rupture of capillaries from intrinsic mechanical forces generated by increased intrathoracic pressure.

The lesions of Henoch–Schoenlein purpura are symmetrically distributed over the extensor surfaces of the lower limbs, buttocks and lower back. They vary in appearance and can be petechial, maculopapular, urticarial or haemorrhagic bullae (Figure 23.2, p. 244).

Bruises are seen in:

- Mobile children from everyday activities – usually on extensor surfaces of the limbs and the forehead
- Non-accidental injury – suspect if the bruises are:
  - unexplained (i.e. no history of injury)
  - on the neck, trunk or genital area (see Chapter 16)
- Idiopathic thrombocytopenic purpura (Figure 23.3, p. 244)
- Coagulation factor deficiency (e.g. haemophilia):
  - on any part of the body
  - may occur after trivial injury
  - may be raised and palpable rather than flat (palpable purpura)
- Self-inflicted injury from sucking:
  - well-defined, round, deep purple in the centre
  - on areas accessible to the child's mouth, usually the upper limbs, and not seen on the back

Associated features

Associated features helpful in diagnosing a petechial rash are shown below:

- **Microcirculatory bleeding:** nose bleeds, oozing from gums, haematuria, melaena (uncommon with thrombocytopenia)
- **Serious internal bleeding:** gastrointestinal or intracranial bleeding (uncommon with thrombocytopenia)
- **Systemic features:**
  - fever (septicaemia, Henoch–Schoenlein purpura, leukaemia)
  - swelling of hands and feet, rarely the forehead and scalp (Henoch–Schoenlein purpura)
  - abdominal pain (Henoch–Schoenlein purpura, haemolytic–uraemic syndrome)

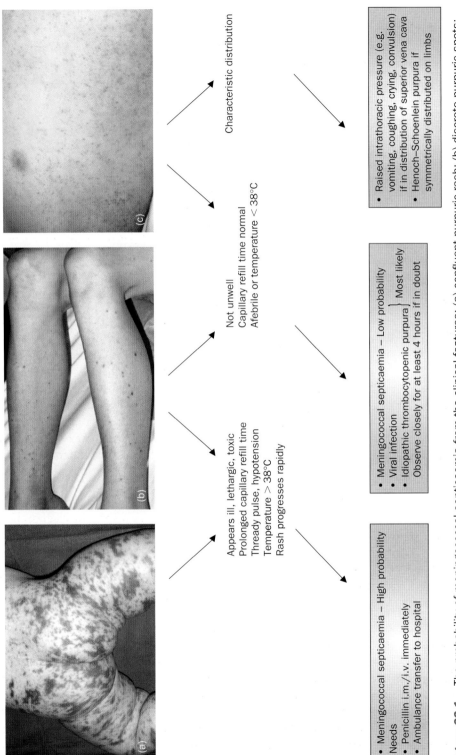

Appears ill, lethargic, toxic
Prolonged capillary refill time
Thready pulse, hypotension
Temperature > 38°C
Rash progresses rapidly

Not unwell
Capillary refill time normal
Afebrile or temperature < 38°C

Characteristic distribution

- Meningococcal septicaemia – High probability
Needs
- Penicillin i.m./i.v. immediately
- Ambulance transfer to hospital

- Meningococcal septicaemia – Low probability
- Viral infection   } Most likely
- Idiopathic thrombocytopenic purpura
Observe closely for at least 4 hours if in doubt

- Raised intrathoracic pressure (e.g. vomiting, coughing, crying, convulsion) if in distribution of superior vena cava
- Henoch–Schoenlein purpura if symmetrically distributed on limbs

Figure 23.1   The probability of meningococcal septicaemia from the clinical features: (a) confluent purpuric rash; (b) discrete purpuric spots; and (c) fine petechial rash.

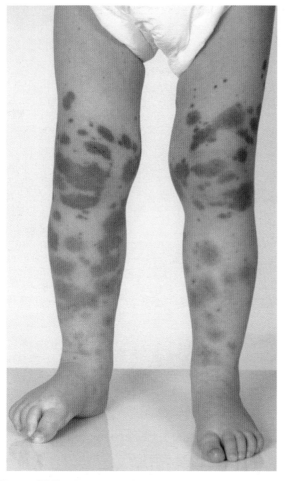

Figure 23.2 Symmetrical distribution of lesions in Henoch–Schoenlein purpura.

- bloody diarrhoea, vomiting, oliguria (haemolytic–uraemic syndrome)
- hypertension (haemolytic–uraemic syndrome)
- arthritis (Henoch–Schoenlein purpura)
- haematuria (Henoch–Schoenlein purpura)
- anaemia (haemolytic–uraemic syndrome, leukaemia)
- lymphadenopathy, hepatosplenomegaly (leukaemia)
- jaundice (liver disease)
- steatorrhoea (vitamin K deficiency)
- **Immunization:** measles/mumps/rubella (MMR) vaccine (self-limiting thrombocytopenia with rubella component)
- **Medication history:**
  - aspirin
  - anticonvulsants, antibiotics
- **Contact history at home or school:**
  - meningococcal infection
  - flu-like illness (viral infection)

As Sarah does not appear to be seriously ill and her rash is petechial, the most likely diagnosis might be a viral upper respiratory tract infection. However, she has a temperature >38°C and the rash has rapidly progressed. Therefore, septicaemia cannot be confidently excluded: children with it may not appear severely ill initially, but can deteriorate rapidly after admission to hospital. Sarah is therefore admitted for close monitoring and is managed as though she has septicaemia.

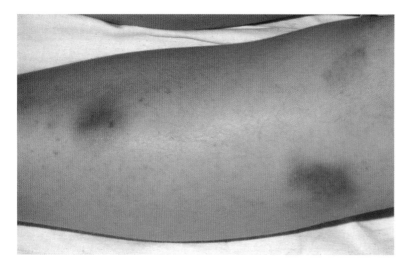

Figure 23.3 Bruises in a girl with idiopathic thrombocytopenic purpura. She presented with a 3-day history of spontaneous bruising. Her platelet count was 5×10^9/L.

Investigations and results

Investigations are helpful in diagnosis and to monitor progress and predict outcome, as in meningococcal septicaemia. Investigations to consider:

- **Bacterial culture:**
  - blood
  - throat swab
  - skin lesion aspirate
  - (cerebrospinal fluid [CSF] if meningitis suspected)
- **Polymerase chain reaction:** blood (or CSF) to detect meningococci and pneumococci: helpful in patients who have already had antibiotics and in whom blood culture will be negative
- **Full blood count (FBC):**
  - low or raised neutrophil count (systemic bacterial infection)
  - low platelet count (thrombocytopenia, disseminated intravascular coagulation [DIC])
  - pancytopenia (leukaemia, bone marrow suppression)
- **Coagulation screen:**
  - prolonged international normalized ratio (INR) (DIC)
  - prolonged activated partial prothrombin time (APTT) (DIC)
  - prolonged prothrombin time (PT) (vitamin K deficiency)
- **Blood film:**
  - large platelets (i.e. young platelets, suggests active production and increased turnover as in idiopathic thrombocytopenic purpura)
  - fragmented red blood cells (RBCs) (haemolytic–uraemic syndrome)

The principal reason for investigating Sarah is to exclude or confirm septicaemia. The FBC, clotting screen and plasma electrolytes are available soon after she is admitted (Table 23.1). They are normal but that does not exclude the possibility of septicaemia. The crucial results are the blood culture and bacterial polymerase chain reaction (PCR), but these will be available only after 48 hours. A lumbar puncture is not done because Sarah does not have signs of meningitis.

Table 23.1 Sarah's investigation results

Investigation	Time when result available	Result
FBC	Within 1 h	
Hb		10.5 g/dL
WBC		8.3×10^9/L
Neutrophils		56%
Lymphocytes		35%
Platelet count		278×10^9/L
Clotting screen	Within 1 h	
PT		14 s (control 14 s)
APTT		34 s (control 35 s)
INR		1.0
Plasma U&Es	Within 1 h	
Sodium		138 mmol/L
Potassium		3.9 mmol/L
Bicarbonate		22 mmol/L
Urea		3.1 mmol/L
Creatinine		45 μmol/L
Plasma glucose	Within 1 h	4.5 mmol/L
Urine microscopy	Within 1 h	No WBCs, no RBCs
Urine culture	After 24 h	No organisms
Throat swab	After 48 h	Upper respiratory flora only
Blood culture	After 48 h	No organisms
Blood for meningococcal and pneumococcal PCR	After 1 week	Negative

APTT, activated partial thromboplastin time; FBC, full blood count; INR, international normalized ratio; PCR, polymerase chain reaction; PT, prothrombin time; RBC, red blood cell count; U&Es, urea and electrolytes; WBC, white blood cell count.

Diagnosis

Sarah is a 3 year old, fully immunized, with an acute febrile illness, high temperature (39.5°C) and rapidly progressing petechial rash. She has no signs of circulatory collapse, no alteration in her level of consciousness, no signs of meningeal irritation and does not appear seriously ill. The most likely diagnosis is a viral infection but septicaemia cannot be excluded clinically.

Management and follow-up

The two possible diagnoses are explained to Sarah's mother. She is reassured that Sarah does not appear seriously ill at present but that she requires:

- Admission to hospital for observation (see below) and treatment for a minimum of 48 hours, but longer if observation and investigations reveal that she has septicaemia
- Investigations for septicaemia, although all the results will not be available immediately
- Treatment with a broad-spectrum antibiotic intravenously and doses recommended for serious infections (e.g. cefotaxime 50 mg/kg per dose 6-hourly) without further delay and continued for at least 48 hours, when the result of the blood culture and meningococcal PCR will be available

Observations in a child suspected of having septicaemia

- Any deterioration in the previous hour
- Level of consciousness
- Oxygen saturation
- Respiratory rate
- Core temperature, skin temperature and the difference
- Capillary refill time
- Pulse rate and volume
- Blood pressure
- Urine output
- Progress and extent of the rash
- Signs of meningeal irritation

Sarah's progress in hospital

Sarah does not deteriorate while in hospital. On the ward round the following day, she is bright and playful. She has not had any vomiting and is regaining her appetite. She is now afebrile and the rash is beginning to fade. The blood culture result 48 hours after admission reveals no growth. As Sarah is also well, intravenous antibiotic treatment is stopped, she is discharged and no follow-up is arranged. The final diagnosis is a viral infection.

Background information

Terms used to describe various rashes

- **Non-blanching or purpuric lesions:**
  - Petechiae: flat, red or reddish-purple, pinpoint to <2mm in diameter
  - Purpura: larger than petechiae and usually >5mm in diameter, purple or blue in early stages
  - Bruise: large areas of haemorrhage into the superficial layers of the skin
- **Other skin lesions:**
  - Macule: discrete, flat (i.e. not raised) discoloration of the skin that is <5mm in diameter and blanches on pressure
  - Papule: lesion raised above the skin surface and usually >5mm diameter
  - Plaque: elevated lesion with diameter greater than the height above the skin surface
  - Vesicle: fluid-filled lesion <5mm in diameter
  - Bulla: fluid-filled lesion >5mm in diameter
  - Pustule: lesion filled with pus, an opaque fluid
  - Weals: raised flat-topped lesions of variable size

Pathophysiology of purpura

Purpura occurs when haemostasis is deranged and blood leaks from blood vessels into the skin, mucous membrane or other tissues. Colour changes from red/purple/blue to brownish and then yellow when extravasated haemoglobin is converted to haemosiderin.

Normal haemostasis requires:

- Intact vascular endothelium
- Normal number and function of circulating platelets
- Adequate amounts of coagulation factors (Figure 23.4)

It is helpful to think of these when categorizing the conditions that lead to purpura.

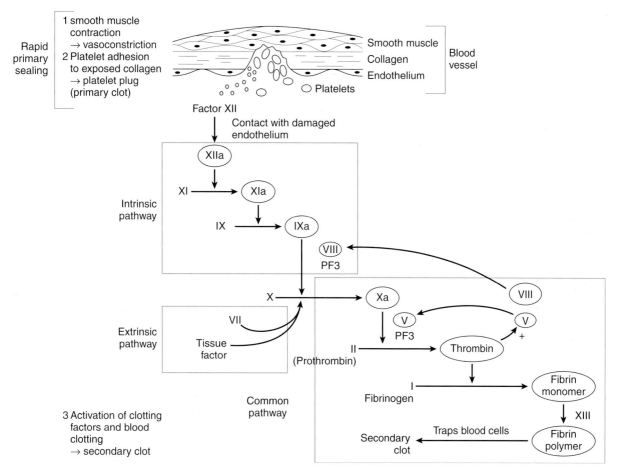

Figure 23.4 Normal haemostasis.

Differential diagnosis of purpura in children

- **Injury to blood vessel:**
  Extrinsic injury:
  - accidental
  - non-accidental
  - self-inflicted

  Intrinsic mechanical forces: forceful vomiting, coughing, generalized tonic–clonic convulsion

  Vasculitis: Henoch–Schoenlein purpura
- **Abnormal number and function of circulating platelets:**
  Thrombocytopenia

  Reduced platelet production:
  - bone marrow suppression, e.g. viral infection, live virus vaccines especially MMR, drugs
  - bone marrow infiltration, e.g. leukaemia, lymphoma
  - congenital aplastic anaemia, e.g. Fanconi's anaemia

  Increased platelet destruction:
  - consumptive coagulopathy
  - idiopathic thrombocytopenic purpura
  - immune mediated, e.g. systemic lupus erythematosus

  Increased destruction and reduced production:
  - intrauterine infections (TORCH)
  - Wiskott–Aldrich syndrome

  Abnormal platelet distribution:
  - hypersplenism (splenic pooling)
  - giant haemangioma

Microangiopathic: haemolytic–uraemic syndrome:
- abnormal platelet function:
- von Willebrand's disease
- drugs, e.g. aspirin
- **Inadequate amounts of coagulation factors:**
Congenital/inherited deficiency:
- intrinsic factors: XI (haemophilia C), IX (haemophilia B or Christmas disease) and VIII (haemophilia A or classic haemophilia)
- extrinsic factors: VII
- common pathway factors: V, X, II (prothrombin), I (fibrinogen)
Acquired deficiency:
- liver disease: reduced synthesis of vitamin K-dependent (II, VII, IX, X) and non-vitamin K-dependent (V, XI, XII) factors
- vitamin K deficiency secondary to steatorrhoea
- **Consumptive coagulopathy, disseminated intravascular coagulation:**
Septicaemia: *Neisseria meningitides, Streptococcus pneumoniae*
Viraemia: echovirus
Cyanotic congenital heart disease

Meningococcal septicaemia

Incidence

- 1–3 per 100 000 population per year
- Most common in children <5 years age; a second peak occurs between 15 and 24 years of age (rare in infants <3 months age)
- Highest in late winter and early spring
- Case fatality rate is approximately 10–20 per cent

Meningococcal infection is the most common infectious cause of death in the UK. It can be a fulminant, rapidly progressive disease resulting in circulatory collapse, disseminated intravascular coagulation (DIC) and death within hours of presentation if untreated. Identifying the characteristic purpuric rash, prompt diagnosis, early pre-emptive treatment with a bactericidal antibiotic and emergency lifesaving treatment are crucial in reducing mortality.

Table 23.2 Epidemiology of meningococci serotypes

Serogroup	Epidemiology
A	Epidemics in Africa and Asia
B	Most common in the UK
C	Significantly reduced since routine immunization was implemented in 1999
	Main cause of small outbreaks in teenagers and young adults
Y and W135	Uncommon in the UK
	W135 serogroup outbreaks among pilgrims to Mecca and Medina

Meningococcal serotypes that cause invasive disease

Encapsulated strains are virulent (Table 23.2).

Pathology

- *Neisseria meningitidis* is a Gram-negative diplococcus
- Asymptomatic nasopharyngeal carriage of the organism is common (5–10 per cent of the population)
- Mode of transmission is direct contact with respiratory secretions

Meningococcal disease peaks during the winter months and appears to be associated with infection with respiratory viruses. Endotoxin (lipid A) released from the outer membrane of the bacteria mediates the disease process and is associated with release of other mediators – cytokines (e.g. tumour necrosis factor α [TNF-α], interleukin 1 [IL-1], and 6 [IL-6]), chemokines (e.g. IL-8) and nitric oxide. These lead to diffuse vasculitis, disseminated intravascular coagulation and involvement of multiple systems (Figure 23.5). The level of endotoxin is 50- to 100-fold greater in meningococcal septicaemia than in other Gram-negative infections, and correlates with mortality.

Presentation

Meningococcal infection presents as septicaemia, meningitis or both (Table 23.3). Septicaemia is usually more fulminant than meningitis.

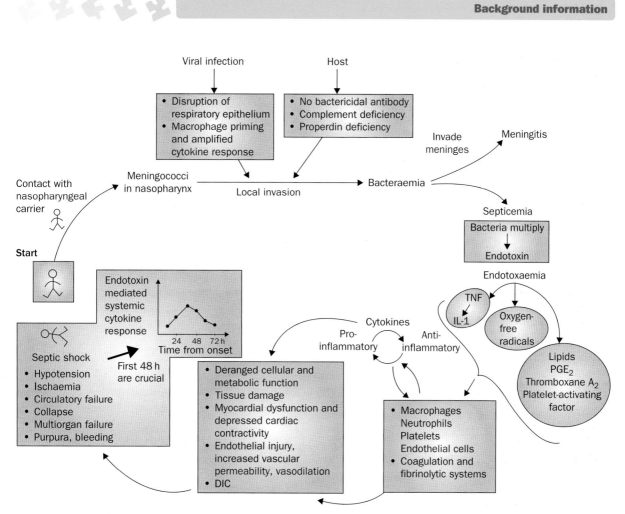

Figure 23.5 The pathogenesis of meningococcal septicaemia. DIC, disseminated intravascular coagulation; IL-1, interleukin 1; PGE$_2$, prostaglandin E$_2$; TNF, tumour necrosis factor.

Table 23.3 Spectrum and modes of presentation in invasive meningococcal disease

Fulminant septicaemia[a]	Mild septicaemia[b]	Meningitis and septicaemia	Meningitis[c]
Shock	Unwell		Headache
Lethargy	Fever		Vomiting
Joint pain	Purpuric rash		Neck stiffness
Muscle pain			Convulsions
↓			↓
Poorer prognosis			Better prognosis

[a]Ten per cent of patients.
[b]Ten to twenty per cent of patients.
[c]About 30 per cent of patients.

A prodrome with fever and upper respiratory symptoms (coryza, sore throat, tonsillitis) is common. The rash can be:

- Purpuric: the cardinal feature of meningococcaemia is a purpuric rash in an ill child (see Figure 23.1). It may progress to become confluent or with extensive purple bruises and necrosis
- Petechial
- Maculopapular – rarely. In a child with a maculopapular blanching rash, meningococcal disease should be suspected if:
  - the child is more unwell than might be expected with a viral illness and
  - the fever has not settled by the time the rash appears

Features associated with a poor prognosis

- Age < 2 years
- Extensive purpura with skin necrosis (purpura fulminans)
- Petechial rash for <12 hours before admission (rapid progression)
- Absence of meningitis
- Hypotension (systolic BP < 70 mmHg) (high level of circulating endotoxin)
- Low core temperature and core skin temperature difference >3°C
- White blood cell (WBC) count < 5000 × 10⁹/L (failure of neutrophils to mount an appropriate response)
- Platelet count < 100 × 10⁹/L
- Erythrocyte sedimentation rate (ESR) < 10 mm/h (represents low levels of fibrinogen and ongoing DIC)
- Deranged clotting
- High plasma lactate
- (High endotoxin load, high cytokine levels especially TNF-α, high nitric oxide levels)

Differential diagnosis

See Figure 23.1, p. 243. Fulminant pneumococcal septicaemia can be indistinguishable from meningococcal septicaemia clinically.

Management

Antibiotics
Meningococci are sensitive to penicillin and early treatment reduces the risk of death. A child seen at home by the GP should be given intramuscular penicillin before ambulance transfer to hospital (about 15 per cent of patients with a petechial–purpuric rash presenting to a GP will have meningococcal disease).

A bactericidal antibiotic such as a third-generation cephalosporin (e.g. cefotaxime) is given in appropriate doses intravenously in hospital.

Resuscitation and supportive treatment
Antibiotics do not treat the endotoxaemia and destruction of bacteria by antibiotics leads to further release of endotoxin. An important aspect of management is supporting the patient until the disease process runs its course. A child in shock requires immediate resuscitation, anticipation and early recognition of complications, and interventions to support all major systems (Table 23.4). It involves a team of A&E staff, paediatricians, intensivists, anaesthetists and specialist nurses.

Course and prognosis

Septicaemia
The course of the disease is influenced by the level of endotoxaemia and endotoxin-mediated cytokine response. The first 48 hours are critical and, even with prompt diagnosis and antibiotic treatment, death can occur as a result of irreversible shock. The mortality rate remains as high as 40–50 per cent.

Gangrene and limb loss may occur as a consequence of vasculitis and DIC, and require psychological support and rehabilitation.

Meningitis
Unlike other causes of bacterial meningitis (especially *Streptococcus pneumoniae*), neurological morbidity after meningococcal meningitis is low (see Chapter 14).

Prophylaxis

Asymptomatic carrier state is common because the organism tends to colonize the nasopharynx. All household members and close contacts should receive antibiotic chemoprophylaxis to prevent secondary cases.

Table 23.4 The management of fulminant meningococcal septicaemia

Assessment of ABC and immediate resuscitation
Assessment with Glasgow Meningococcal Septicaemia Prognostic Score: • Transfer to a paediatric intensive care unit • Elective ventilation • Continuous cardiac, arterial blood pressure and blood gas monitoring, central venous pressure monitoring
Reducing cardiovascular complications: • Aggressive volume replacement to maintain perfusion to vital organs – 20 ml/kg crystalloid or colloid intravenous boluses and repeated until perfusion improves • Inotropes to optimize cardiac output and peripheral perfusion – dopamine, dobutamine, adrenaline (epinephrine), noradrenaline (norepinephrine) • Vasoactive agents to prevent limb loss – sodium nitroprusside, prostacyclin
Reducing haematological complications: treatment of coagulopathy to reduce complications of liver and kidney failure, life-threatening haemorrhage and peripheral limb loss: • Avoid intramuscular injections • Vitamin K • Fresh frozen plasma, platelets, cryoprecipitate
Reducing pulmonary complications: pulmonary oedema from endotoxin-mediated increase in pulmonary capillary permeability, fluid resuscitation and ventricular dysfunction; adult respiratory distress syndrome: • Intubation and mechanical ventilation to optimize oxygen delivery
Reducing renal complications: prerenal renal failure from reduced perfusion, intrarenal failure from acute tubular necrosis or microemboli: • Maintain euvolaemia and normal electrolyte balance • Renal doses of dopamine to improve renal blood flow • Haemodialysis and haemofiltration for acidosis, hyperkalaemia
Reducing neurological complications: cerebral oedema, increased cerebral intracranial pressure, syndrome of inappropriate ADH if coexistent meningitis: • Head of bed elevated 30° • Correcting fluid and electrolyte disturbances • Mannitol
Reducing skin, soft tissue and skeletal complications: extensive necrosis, bone ischaemia, gangrene: • Surface skin lesions are treated like burns and may require excision and grafting • Amputation

ABC, airway, breathing, circulation; ADH, antidiuretic hormone.

Oral rifampicin is the drug of choice:

- <12 months age: 5 mg/kg twice daily for 2 days
- 1–12 years: 10 mg/kg twice daily for 2 days
- >12 years: 600 mg twice daily for 2 days

Viral infections – a snapshot

A rash occurs with many of the common childhood viral infections and may be blanching or non-blanching.

The rash is usually associated with a febrile illness and is self-limiting, and only supportive management is required. An accurate diagnosis is important mainly for epidemiological purposes. Infection with echovirus type 9 may be difficult to differentiate clinically from meningococcal septicaemia. Patients present with a non-specific febrile illness and pharyngitis. Aseptic meningitis may be a feature.

Idiopathic thrombocytopenic purpura – a snapshot

Incidence

The incidence is 4 per 100 000 children per year (similar to acute leukaemia). It affects children between 2 and 10 years of age, and boys more commonly than girls.

Aetiology

Idiopathic thrombocytopenic purpura (ITP) may occur after a viral infection or immunization (e.g. measles/mumps/rubella or MMR vaccine). It results from an altered immune response and formation of anti-platelet antibodies.

Pathophysiology

Circulating anti-platelet antibodies (possibly produced in response to a viral infection or defect in immune regulation) bind to epitopes on the platelet membrane. Antibody-coated platelets are destroyed by the spleen and reticuloendothelial system. More platelets are produced in the bone marrow, but not enough to compensate for the rapid destruction.

Presentation

An otherwise well, apyrexial child presents acutely (after a viral infection) with:

- A generalized, widespread petechial rash – usually – or
- Bruising: this can occur spontaneously when the platelet count is $<30 \times 10^9$/L (Figure 23.3) or with relatively trivial injury when it is $<50 \times 10^9$/L

Bleeding from the mucous membranes, e.g. epistaxis or gum bleeds, may occur. There is no:

- Associated hepatosplenomegaly or lymphadenopathy
- Family history of bleeding disorder

Diagnosis

The diagnosis is clinical and supported by a low platelet count, often $<20 \times 10^9$/L.

Differential diagnosis

Idiopathic thrombocytopenic purpura may need to be differentiated from the more serious causes of thrombocytopenia (such as leukaemia) with bone marrow aspiration, especially if there are any atypical features:

- Lymphadenopathy
- Hepatosplenomegaly
- Anaemia
- Abnormal WBC count

Bone marrow aspirate

This helps to differentiate increased destruction (ITP) from failure of production (leukaemia, bone marrow suppression) of platelets.

Treatment

Idiopathic thrombocytopenic purpura is usually self-limiting, associated with petechiae alone or minor bleeding and remits spontaneously within 8 weeks. Most children do not require active treatment.

- Petechiae, minor bleeding:
  Observe patient at home
  Inform and reassure parents:
  – risks of intracranial haemorrhage low
  – prevent forceful contact injury
  – minor injury to an active preschooler cannot be prevented
  – course: resolves within 6 months of diagnosis in 90 per cent of children
  – treatment does not alter course but shortens period of profound thrombocytopenia
- Life-threatening bleeding in central nervous system (CNS) or gastrointestinal (GI) tract: treat

regardless of platelet count. Treatment is symptomatic because it merely raises the platelet count:

Intravenous immunoglobulin (Ig): Fc receptor blockade by Ig allows antibody-coated platelets to remain in circulation longer and the platelet count rises rapidly

Polyclonal anti-D IgG (WinRho) in rhesus-positive patients

Prednisolone for 10–21 days: leukaemia must be ruled out with bone marrow aspirate before starting treatment with prednisolone

Henoch–Schoenlein purpura (anaphylactoid purpura) – a snapshot

Incidence

- The incidence is 14–18 per 100 000 children per year
- Most common vasculitic disease in children
- More common in preschool children and in boys

Aetiology

Henoch–Schoenlein purpura is an immune-complex mediated systemic vasculitis most commonly involving the skin, joints, GI tract and kidneys. It is associated with IgA abnormalities, including high serum IgA concentrations and IgA deposits in involved tissues.

Henoch–Schoenlein purpura often follows a viral or bacterial upper respiratory tract infection.

Presentation

The presenting feature is usually a petechial, purpuric or urticarial rash (Figure 23.2), which starts over the buttocks and extensor surfaces of the lower limbs but may spread all over the body. Other features are shown in Table 23.5.

Diagnosis

The diagnosis is clinical and the platelet count is normal.

Table 23.5 Other features of Henoch–Schoenlein purpura

Other features	Common	Rare
Vasculitis	Fever	
Skin	Petechial, purpuric or urticarial rash Oedema on hands and feet	Haemorrhagic bullae Oedema on scalp or forehead
Joints	Pain and swelling of ankles, knees, other large joints	
GI tract	Colicky abdominal pain Vomiting Intestinal ischaemia	Intestinal bleeding and melaena Intussusception
Kidneys	Haematuria Mild proteinuria End-stage renal failure	Acute nephritis Nephrotic syndrome
CNS	Headache Motor deficit Unconsciousness	Convulsions

CNS, central nervous system; GI, gastrointestinal.

Treatment and follow-up

Henoch–Schoenlein purpura is usually self-limiting and management is symptomatic. Inform parents about:

- Good prognosis for the majority of children
- Probability of renal disease

All children should be monitored for 3 months after presentation with regular:

- Urine dipstick for blood and protein
- BP measurement to identify significant renal disease

Further sources of information

Book

Anderson MS, Glodé MP, Smith AL. Meningococcal disease. In: Feigin RD, Cherry JD (eds). *Textbook*

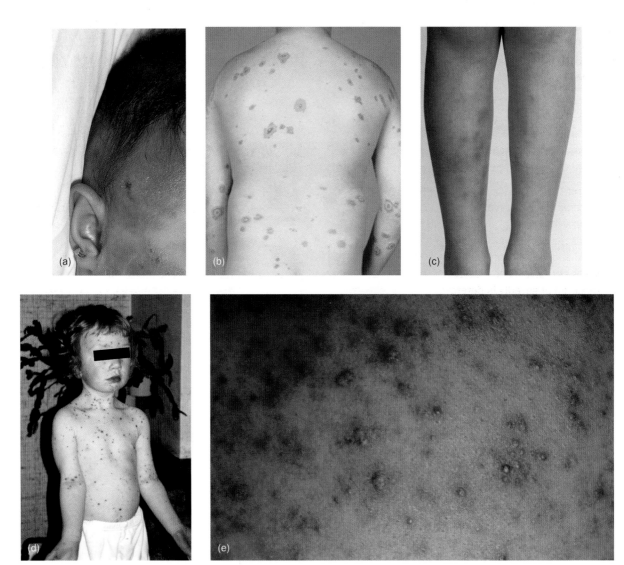

Figure 23.6 Self-test 7.

of Pediatric Infectious Diseases, Vol 1, 4th edn. Philadelphia: WB Saunders, 1998: 1143–56

Articles

Brogan PA, Raffles A. The management of fever and petechiae: making sense of rash decisions. *Archives of Disease in Childhood* 2000; **83**: 506–7

Tizard EJ. Henoch–Schönlein purpura. *Archives of Disease in Childhood* 1999; **80**: 380–3

Wells LC, Smith JC, Weston VC, Collier J, Rutter N. The child with a non-blanching rash: how likely is meningococcal disease? *Archives of Disease in Childhood* 2001; **85**: 218–22

Self-test 6: What are the major pathophysiological differences of bacteraemia, septicaemia and septic shock?

Answers:
- Bacteraemia is the presence of viable bacteria in the blood
- Septicaemia is the proliferation of bacteria in the blood and the release of endotoxin. It is associated with a systemic inflammatory response. The spectrum of severity is determined by the level of endotoxaemia and systemic inflammatory response: it ranges from mild septicaemia with no organ dysfunction to septic shock and multiorgan failure. Toxin damage to endothelium causes leakage of blood into tissues (therefore purpura) and microthrombi (therefore tissue ischaemia and necrosis)
- Septic shock is septicaemia associated with hypotension and the failure of cardiac output to meet the metabolic demands of the body. Damage and activation of endothelium lead to leakage of fluid from blood vessels (therefore hypovolaemia) and production of vasodilator substances (therefore more severe hypotension)

Self-test 7: The children in Figure 23.6 presented acutely with a fever and a rash that was not purpuric: (a) followed ear piercing, (b) had not taken any medicines, (c) had a painful rash localized over the shins and (d) and (e) was a healthy little girl. Identify the rash and the most likely micro-organism.

Answers:
(a) Erysipelas – streptococcal infection associated with ear piercing
(b) Erythema multiforme – herpes simplex
(c) Erythema nodosum – streptococci
(d) and (e) Chickenpox – varicella-zoster

Acute presentation

A child with severe abdominal pain

Age: 8 years

LEENA PATEL

Presentation

On Saturday evening Andy's mother calls the emergency GP service. Andy is 8 years old and the tummy ache that started this morning has just not settled. He felt hot in the afternoon and has stayed in bed since. He has not eaten anything all day and the little he has drunk seems to have come straight back up.

Self-test 1: What is an 'acute abdomen'?

Answer: An 'acute abdomen' (or 'surgical abdomen') implies an emergency surgical condition as the cause of a patient's acute abdominal pain. The clues to this are:
- Acute abdominal pain continuing for more than 4–6 hours and getting progressively worse
- Associated anorexia and nausea
- Vomiting, especially if it contains bile

Initial considerations and action

Acute abdominal pain is a common symptom in childhood. The underlying problem may be medical or surgical (Table 24.1). The most common diagnoses in decreasing order of frequency are:

- Non-specific abdominal pain
- Gastroenteritis
- Acute appendicitis
- Constipation
- Urinary tract infection
- Viral illness and mesenteric adenitis

- Streptococcal pharyngitis
- Lower lobe pneumonia

The on-call GP suspects an 'acute abdomen' from the mother's message and goes to see Andy at home. The priority is to identify a:

- Surgical cause ('acute abdomen') or
- Medical condition that requires urgent attention

History

The on-call GP obtains a history from Andy's mother:

Andy complained of a tummy ache around his belly button soon after getting up in the morning. He felt sick and picked at breakfast. Mother persuaded him to have some milkshake but he vomited soon after. He could not keep paracetamol down either. At first mother put it down to a 'tummy bug' as he had unexpectedly been on the toilet twice that morning for motions. Andy was not hungry even at lunch time. In the afternoon, he was hot and sweaty and lay down. The tummy ache had not eased and it was now hurting on the right side of his belly. Mother became more concerned when he did not want to get up and was not even interested in his new computer game. With direct questioning, the GP learns that Andy has not vomited any bile and passed urine twice in the morning.

The GP asks about any recent illnesses, injuries and problems in the past. Andy has not had a high fever, respiratory symptoms, urinary frequency, dysuria or rash in the last few days. He played football yesterday but there were no untoward injuries. He has not previously had troublesome tummy ache, diarrhoea, constipation or operations.

Table 24.1 Classification of acute abdominal pain in children and adolescents

	Medical	Surgical
Abdominal		
Gastrointestinal	Non-specific abdominal pain	Appendicitis
	Viral gastroenteritis	Intussusception
	Bacterial enterocolitis, e.g. *Campylobacter*, *Salmonella* species	Intestinal obstruction
	Mesenteric adenitis	Peritonitis
	Inflammatory bowel disease	Meckel's diverticulitis
Urinary tract	Pyelonephritis	
Liver and gallbladder	Infectious hepatitis	Laceration after blunt injury
Spleen		Laceration after blunt injury
Non-abdominal		
Respiratory	Tonsillitis, pharyngitis	
	Lower lobe pneumonia with pleuritis	
Other systems	Diabetic ketoacidosis	
	Sickle-cell crisis	
	Henoch–Schoenlein purpura	

Common in children <2 years	Consider in adolescent girls	Uncommon in children and adolescents
Intussusception	Ectopic pregnancy	Peptic ulcer
Strangulated inguinal hernia	Pelvic inflammatory disease	Acute pancreatitis
Malrotation	Torsion of ovary or cyst	Acute cholecystitis, gallbladder stones
		Renal stones
		Herpes zoster

Self-test 2: Why does Andy not want to get up?

Answer: There are a number of possible explanations why Andy wants to stay in bed.

When there is peritoneal irritation, the pain is worse on movement as a result of rebound tenderness. This is noticeable with walking, a jerk to the bed, jolt in the car on the way to hospital and coughing. Pain and tenderness are more intense with perforation and generalized peritonitis, and children tend to lie still.

When adjacent to the psoas muscle, the inflamed appendix causes spasm of the muscle and hip flexion. An attempt to extend the hip, which Andy would have to do if he were to get up from his bed, makes the abdominal pain worse.

Important points in the history and examination of a child with acute abdominal pain

- **History:**
  - abdominal pain: onset, duration and progress, site, character, aggravating factors, alleviating factors, previous similar episodes
  - vomiting: onset before or after abdominal pain, isolated or repeated, containing bile or blood
  - anorexia, nausea

- diarrhoea (volume and nature of stools) or constipation
- urinary symptoms
- non-abdominal symptoms: respiratory symptoms, rash
- recent history of abdominal injury
- pre-existing condition such as urinary tract abnormality, inflammatory bowel disease, type 1 diabetes mellitus, sickle-cell anaemia or cystic fibrosis
- past history of abdominal surgery
- family history: recent gastroenteritis or respiratory symptoms
- ethnic origin: sickle-cell anaemia
- **Examination:**
  - gentle non-threatening approach is essential
  - general appearance, posture, pallor, breathing, pulse, capillary refill time, temperature, fetor oris
    Abdomen:
    - inspection (from end of bed and side of bed): abdominal distension, operative scars, skin colour
    - palpation (forearm and hand should be horizontal and level with the abdomen): tenderness, guarding, rigidity, masses, costovertebral angle
    - percussion: tenderness, fluid
    - auscultation: bowel sounds
    - hernial sites
    - rectal examination is unpleasant for the child and should be undertaken only by an experienced person
    Respiratory system:
    - pharynx, ears, neck for lymph nodes, chest skin for rash of Henoch–Schoenlein purpura

Interpretation of the history

The site and nature of abdominal pain and associated symptoms provide useful clues to the organ involved and the likely pathology (Figure 24.1). Andy's symptoms of pain around the umbilicus that does not ease but shifts to the right lower abdomen, and food refusal as a result of anorexia and vomiting, are typical of acute appendicitis. It contrasts with non-specific abdominal pain that remains periumbilical, does not worsen and

is self-limiting. Vomiting is stimulated by inflammation and distension of the appendix, but it is not a universal symptom in appendicitis. Other symptoms are related to the anatomical position of the appendix, which normally varies between different individuals (Figure 24.2). Diarrhoea results from irritation of the small intestine, caecum or rectum by a neighbouring inflamed appendix and also from irritation of the rectosigmoid by peritoneal fluid in the pelvis after perforation. The stools are likely to contain mucus and slime, and are not large in volume as in gastroenteritis. In gastroenteritis, vomiting is more likely to precede the abdominal pain and the periumbilical pain is colicky because of rapid peristalsis. An inflamed appendix in contact with the bladder may cause frequency of micturition, urgency and dysuria. Urine microscopy and culture are required to exclude a urinary tract infection. A high fever is expected with acute pyelonephritis and respiratory infections, but is unusual with uncomplicated acute appendicitis.

The absence of previous abdominal surgery excludes intestinal obstruction caused by adhesions. Obstipation is rare with acute appendicitis, but is seen in mechanical intestinal obstruction along with abdominal distension and bilious vomiting.

Beyond infancy, intussusception is uncommon (Table 24.2) and associated with conditions such as:

- Cystic fibrosis
- Henoch–Schoenlein purpura
- Meckel's diverticulitis

The symptoms of intussusception differ from acute appendicitis in that:

- Onset is more sudden and dramatic
- Abdominal pain is colicky or paroxysmal
- Vomiting is persistent and often bilious

In addition to differentiating acute appendicitis from other surgical causes of abdominal pain, the history also helps differentiate it from medical non-abdominal conditions, especially when the pain is atypical and intermittent (see Table 24.1). Pain is referred to the abdomen through the tenth and eleventh thoracic nerves in lower lobe pneumonia.

Injury to the spleen, liver, kidneys and/or pancreas should be suspected when a child develops abdominal

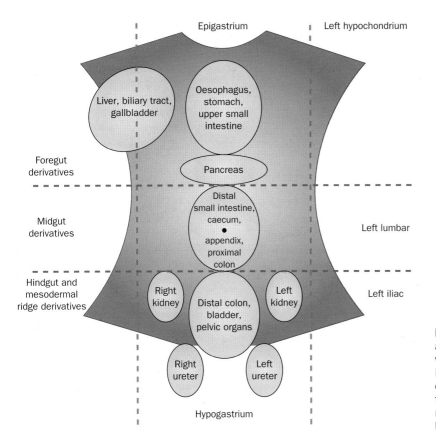

Figure 24.1 labels:
- Epigastrium
- Left hypochondrium
- Liver, biliary tract, gallbladder
- Oesophagus, stomach, upper small intestine
- Foregut derivatives
- Pancreas
- Distal small intestine, caecum, appendix, proximal colon
- Midgut derivatives
- Left lumbar
- Hindgut and mesodermal ridge derivatives
- Right kidney
- Distal colon, bladder, pelvic organs
- Left kidney
- Left iliac
- Right ureter
- Left ureter
- Hypogastrium

Figure 24.1 The regions of the abdomen and surface areas to which visceral pain is referred. This is often far from the involved organ, corresponds to the dermatome from which the affected organ receives innervation and tends to be felt in the midline.

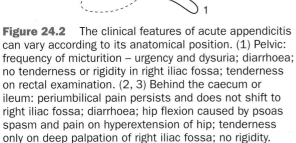

Figure 24.2 The clinical features of acute appendicitis can vary according to its anatomical position. (1) Pelvic: frequency of micturition – urgency and dysuria; diarrhoea; no tenderness or rigidity in right iliac fossa; tenderness on rectal examination. (2, 3) Behind the caecum or ileum: periumbilical pain persists and does not shift to right iliac fossa; diarrhoea; hip flexion caused by psoas spasm and pain on hyperextension of hip; tenderness only on deep palpation of right iliac fossa; no rigidity.

Table 24.2 Annual incidence of common surgical causes of acute abdominal pain

Cause	Annual incidence	Most common age group
Intussusception	1 in 1000 live births	Infants
Appendicitis	4 in 1000 children aged 5–14 years	School-age

pain with or without vomiting after blunt abdominal injury, such as a fall from a bicycle.

Self-test 3: Explain why the typical pain from acute appendicitis is first felt around the umbilicus and then shifts to the area directly overlying the appendix.

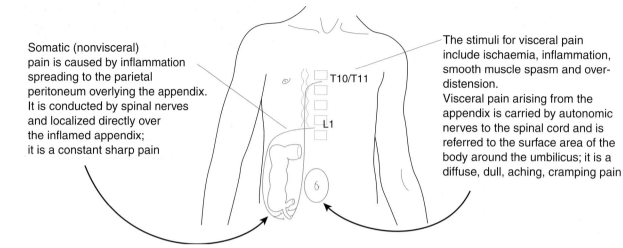

Somatic (nonvisceral) pain is caused by inflammation spreading to the parietal peritoneum overlying the appendix. It is conducted by spinal nerves and localized directly over the inflamed appendix; it is a constant sharp pain

The stimuli for visceral pain include ischaemia, inflammation, smooth muscle spasm and over-distension.
Visceral pain arising from the appendix is carried by autonomic nerves to the spinal cord and is referred to the surface area of the body around the umbilicus; it is a diffuse, dull, aching, cramping pain

T10/T11

L1

6

Figure 24.3 The mechanism of visceral and somatic (non-visceral) pain from an inflamed appendix.

Answer: Pain from an organ such as the appendix can be visceral as well as somatic (or non-visceral) (Figure 24.3):

- Visceral pain: inflammation and distension of the appendix initially gives rise to visceral pain. Signals from the stretch receptors are carried by autonomic nerve fibres to the spinal cord and the tenth thoracic spinal nerve which supplies the dermatome at the level of the umbilicus. The pain is referred around the umbilicus and is diffuse dull aching
- Somatic pain: subsequent spread of inflammation to the anterior parietal peritoneum overlying the appendix gives rise to somatic pain which is more localized and intense than visceral pain. It serves as a counterirritant and suppresses the periumbilical pain. Thus, the periumbilical pain shifts to the point directly above the position of the inflamed appendix. When the inflamed appendix lies behind the caecum, there is no right iliac fossa pain and periumbilical pain persists

Examination

The GP examines Andy with the aim of:

- Eliciting signs of acute appendicitis
- Identifying whether there is generalized peritonitis

- Excluding other possible causes of acute abdominal pain

The GP observes and examines Andy while talking with him and his mother. He notes the following:

General examination

- Alert and apprehensive
- Looks pale and mother mentions that he is not normally so white
- Pulse 112/minute and regular
- Capillary refill time 2 seconds and not delayed
- Does not appear to be in shock
- Temperature 38°C

Abdominal examination

- Points to the area of maximum pain in the right iliac fossa
- No abdominal distension
- No generalized tenderness or rigidity and no mass (the GP began gentle palpation from the left upper quadrant and away from the site of pain)
- Localized tenderness and guarding in the right lower quadrant (when this quadrant was palpated, Andy winced and pushed the GP's hand away)
- Normal bowel sounds

The GP does not persevere with eliciting rebound tenderness or with rectal examination because he does not wish to make the examination more unpleasant for Andy. Bearing in mind the extra-abdominal causes of acute abdominal pain, the GP examines Andy's throat, ears, neck for lymph nodes, chest and the skin for a vasculitic rash, but does not find anything abnormal.

Interpretation of the examination

Andy has the typical features of acute appendicitis seen in under 50 per cent of school-age children:

- An acute history of abdominal pain and persisting for more than 4–6 hours
- Pain starting in the umbilical region and shifting to the right lower quadrant within 24 hours
- Pain worse on movement, walking or coughing as a result of peritoneal irritation
- Anorexia
- Nausea and vomiting
- Signs of peritoneal irritation (tenderness and guarding) localized to the right lower quadrant

The clinical features of acute appendicitis can be atypical especially in younger preschool children, who cannot localize pain so well and who usually point to the umbilicus irrespective of the site of pain. Tenderness may be diffuse or only noted on rectal examination (which is not routinely done in children). There is also a considerable overlap between the various clinical features of acute appendicitis and the common medical causes of acute abdominal pain (especially non-specific abdominal pain and acute gastroenteritis). Thus the diagnosis may not be as obvious as it is with Andy.

Andy does not have any features suggestive of generalized peritonitis. Perforation and generalized peritonitis can occur if acute appendicitis is left untreated for 24–36 hours or longer. When this occurs, the child becomes progressively more unwell, appears pale, and has tachycardia and a high fever. Signs of shock may develop. Inflammatory fluid and intestinal contents leak into the peritoneal cavity. The abdominal pain is severe and generalized. As it is worse with movement and breathing, the child appears anxious, usually lies still, breathes with the mouth open and takes shallow breaths, and the end of each inspiration is stopped short. The child will not cough or take deep breaths if requested. The abdomen is extremely tender and rigid (guarding is voluntary spasm and rigidity is involuntary spasm of the abdominal muscles). Bowel sounds are initially reduced and subsequently the abdomen will be silent as paralytic ileus develops. This is associated with more frequent vomiting, which may be faeculent. Bowel sounds are normal or reduced in uncomplicated acute appendicitis. Increased high-pitched sounds or borborygmi suggest mechanical intestinal obstruction.

Self-test 4: Which of the following fluids can cause abdominal pain if present in the peritoneal cavity?

A Stomach contents

B Bile

C Pancreatic enzymes

D Intestinal contents

E Urine

F Ascites fluid

G Chyle

H Blood

I Inflammatory fluid or pus

J Dialysis fluid

Answer: Hydrochloric acid (A), bile (B), pancreatic enzymes (C), faecal material (D), urine (E), blood (H), inflammatory fluid and pus (I) can cause abdominal pain.

Self-test 5: What is paralytic ileus and does it always require surgery?

Answer: Absence of peristalsis results in paralytic ileus. Fluid and gas pool in the intestine. The clinical features are:

- Abdominal distension ('drum-like')
- Effortless vomiting containing bile
- Absent or minimal bowel sounds
- Failure to pass flatus

Paralytic ileus is common after abdominal surgery and other causes are peritonitis, renal failure and hypokalaemia (e.g. during fluid management of diabetic ketoacidosis). Surgery is required when paralytic ileus is associated with peritonitis.

Differential diagnosis of acute abdominal pain

Onset with acute central abdominal pain, nausea and vomiting is common to both non-specific abdominal pain and acute appendicitis. Features that help differentiate the two are shown in Table 24.3.

Table 24.3 Features most likely to help in differentiating non-specific abdominal pain and acute appendicitis

	Non-specific abdominal pain	Acute appendicitis
Appetite	May be reduced	Anorexia
Abdominal pain	Colicky	Constant, worse with movement
Progress	Self-limiting	Progressive
Appearance	Normal	Anxious
Pulse	<100/min	>100/min
Palpation	No localized tenderness	Right iliac fossa tenderness, guarding

In gastroenteritis, the diarrhoea tends to be profuse, watery and more troublesome than abdominal pain. Vomiting usually precedes abdominal pain. The abdominal pain is periumbilical and colicky. There may be mild abdominal tenderness and bowel sounds are active and of normal pitch. There may be other family members with similar symptoms.

Inflammatory bowel disease involving the terminal ileum may mimic acute appendicitis. A right iliac fossa mass may be palpable but is unusual in uncomplicated acute appendicitis.

Mesenteric adenitis is associated with colicky periumbilical abdominal pain and prodromal upper respiratory tract symptoms. Mild abdominal tenderness may be present. Urinary tract infection and an extra-abdominal cause, particularly a lower lobe pneumonia (Figure 24.4), should be sought when pain is out of proportion to the abdominal examination findings. High fever with chills is usual. Abdominal tenderness, if present, is not likely to be localized to the right iliac fossa.

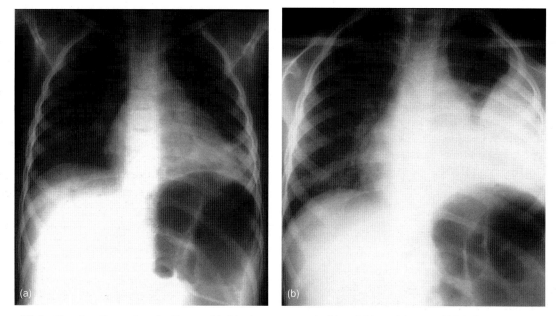

(a) (b)

Figure 24.4 Chest radiographs of a 6-year-old girl who presented with a 24-hour history of high fever, progressively severe pain in the left side of the abdomen and anorexia, but no cough. The pain was worse on deep breathing. Air entry was reduced at the left base on auscultation. (a) Her initial chest radiograph showed a left lower lobe pneumonia and small pleural effusion; (b) 4 days later, her fever had not settled despite intravenous broad-spectrum antibiotics. Her trachea was deviated to the right and the left lower chest was dull on percussion. She had developed an empyema and required thoracotomy and decortication.

Investigations and results

The diagnosis of acute abdominal pain is principally based on the history and examination.

Ultrasonography of the abdomen may be helpful when the clinical features are not clear cut. However, a negative result does not preclude acute appendicitis or other surgical cause such as intussusception.

Plain abdominal radiograph may show a faecolith in appendicitis, soft tissue mass in intussusception, air–fluid levels in intestinal obstruction, free intra-abdominal air with a perforated viscus, faecal loading in colon with constipation or radio-opaque renal stones.

Abdominal computed tomography (CT) exposes the child to radiation, is expensive, of limited value in decision-making and therefore undertaken only in exceptional cases.

The white blood cell (WBC) count will reveal mild neutrophil leucocytosis (WBC $10–20 \times 10^9$/L) in uncomplicated appendicitis. Significant leucocytosis (WBC $>20 \times 10^9$/L) suggests perforation and abscess or a bacterial infection (lower lobe pneumonia, streptococcal tonsillitis, pyelonephritis).

Other appropriate investigations, such as urine microscopy and culture and chest radiograph, are arranged according to the clinical suspicion.

Diagnosis

Andy has acute appendicitis but does not have features suggestive of perforation and generalized peritonitis.

Self-test 6: Why are perforation and peritonitis more likely in infants and toddlers with acute appendicitis?

Answer: Acute appendicitis is the most common surgical cause of acute abdominal pain in children, but is not common under 2 years of age. The symptoms of acute appendicitis in infants and preschool children tend to be non-specific and are more likely to be mistaken for more common medical conditions such as gastroenteritis, and so admission to hospital may be delayed. In addition, the greater omentum is relatively small in infants and young children and may be of little help in localizing the inflammation and preventing widespread peritonitis.

Management and follow-up

The GP is certain about the diagnosis and refers Andy urgently to the on-call surgical team at the local hospital. He has an appendicectomy that night.

When there is uncertainty about the diagnosis, an early surgical opinion and a period of active observation are crucial because the danger of missing appendicitis is perforation. Reassessment in 2–3 hours and at frequent intervals if necessary, preferably by the same person, will reveal whether there is steady improvement or deterioration. Intravenous broad-spectrum antibiotics are given if perforation is suspected.

Complications of acute appendicitis

- **Perforated appendix:** generalized peritonitis, intra-abdominal abscess, septicaemia
- **Postoperative:** wound infection, postoperative paralytic ileus, late intestinal obstruction from adhesions, abscess
- **Appendix mass or abscess:** the greater omentum and intestine can wall off an inflamed appendix and prevent diffuse peritonitis. The abdominal pain may ease and a right iliac fossa mass may be felt a few days later. This is treated with intravenous broad-spectrum antibiotics and an elective appendicectomy is done after 4–6 weeks. A high swinging fever with a mass suggests an appendix abscess. Ultrasonography and CT may be helpful

Background information

Intussusception

Intussusception occurs when a segment of the intestine telescopes into the lumen of another segment adjacent to it (Figure 24.5). It is the most common cause of

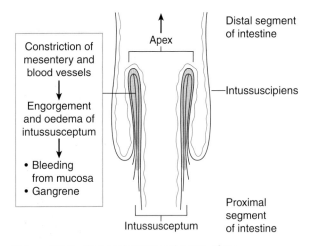

Distal segment of intestine

Apex

Intussuscipiens

Constriction of mesentery and blood vessels

↓

Engorgement and oedema of intussusceptum

↓

• Bleeding from mucosa
• Gangrene

Proximal segment of intestine

Intussusceptum

Figure 24.5 The pathology and parts of an intussusception.

intestinal obstruction between 3 months and 3 years of age. The peak incidence is between 4 and 10 months of age and it is more common in boys. Most cases are idiopathic, but an association with the following is recognized:

- Weaning and change in diet
- Gastroenteritis
- Viral upper respiratory tract infections and peak seasonal incidence in spring and autumn

It is possible that an inflamed Peyer's patch protrudes into the intestinal lumen and forms the apex of an intussusception.

In a few cases, and especially in older children, the advancing apex of the intussusception is a:

- Meckel's diverticulum
- Haematoma in the wall of the intestine in Henoch–Schoenlein purpura
- Polyp

Clinical features

The typical features are:

- Sudden onset
- Paroxysms of inconsolable crying or screaming and drawing up of the legs as a result of colicky abdominal pain with the child quiet, lethargic

and weak in between these paroxysms (abdominal pain lasts several seconds and recurs every 5–15 minutes)
- Pallor
- Vomiting
- Abdomen not distended, emptiness in the right iliac fossa on palpation and sausage-shaped lump felt in the mid or upper abdomen

Stools may be normal or contain mucus and fresh blood ('redcurrant jelly' stools). Intussusception should be suspected in a child with gastroenteritis if there is acute deterioration and a change in the pattern of the illness.

Investigation and management

Fluid resuscitation should be commenced promptly and while awaiting investigations. Hypovolaemia and shock can result from engorgement of the intussusceptum.

An abdominal radiograph is not always informative but may show:

- Small intestinal obstruction
- Free intraperitoneal gas from perforation
- A sausage-shaped soft tissue mass formed by the head of the intussusception and an absence of gas in the right iliac fossa (Figure 24.6a)

Ultrasonography and an air-contrast enema are most useful in confirming the diagnosis. An intussusception may reduce spontaneously or during an air enema. A surgeon needs to be on stand-by because emergency surgical reduction is required if the air enema fails or is complicated by perforation (Figure 24.6b).

What to look at when interpreting a plain radiograph of the abdomen

- Patient's name and date of examination
- Marker for right and left sides
- Position of liver and stomach bubble
- Diaphragm and peritoneum:
  - free air under diaphragm
  - peritoneal calcification (meconium peritonitis secondary to meconium ileus)

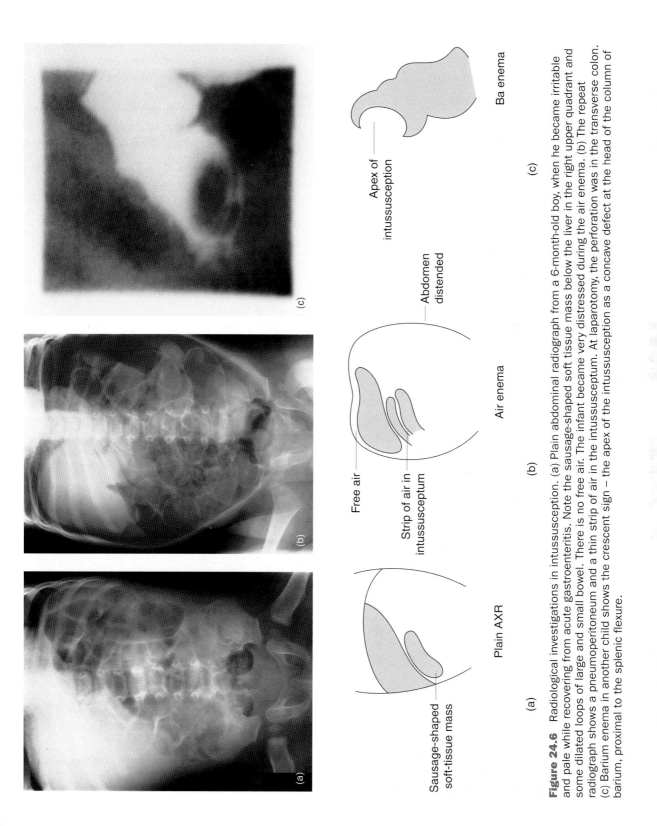

Figure 24.6 Radiological investigations in intussusception. (a) Plain abdominal radiograph from a 6-month-old boy, when he became irritable and pale while recovering from acute gastroenteritis. Note the sausage-shaped soft tissue mass below the liver in the right upper quadrant and some dilated loops of large and small bowel. There is no free air. The infant became very distressed during the air enema. (b) The repeat radiograph shows a pneumoperitoneum and a thin strip of air in the intussusceptum. At laparotomy, the perforation was in the transverse colon. (c) Barium enema in another child shows the crescent sign – the apex of the intussusception as a concave defect at the head of the column of barium, proximal to the splenic flexure.

- Lower part of chest above the diaphragm:
  - pleural effusion
  - collapse/consolidation of the lung
- Shape of the abdomen
- Bowel distension with air, air–fluid levels or frothy material:
  - gastroenteritis (air in rectum excludes intestinal obstruction)
  - paralytic ileus
  - pyloric stenosis (stomach distended and very little air distally)
  - duodenal atresia ('double bubble' sign from air–fluid levels in the stomach and duodenum)
  - small intestinal obstruction
  - large intestinal obstruction (Hirschsprung's disease)
- Masses: sausage-shaped mass of intussusception
- Air in bowel wall and portal venous system (necrotizing enterocolitis)
- Calcified opacities:
  - faecolith
  - ureter or renal stone
- Foreign bodies, artefacts, tubes and drains

Sickle-cell disease

Sickle-cell disease is an autosomal recessive condition in which synthesis of haemoglobin is abnormal. It occurs mainly in people of African, Indian, middle Eastern and Mediterranean descent. The incidence varies from 1 in 400 (African descent) to 1 in 60 000 (whites) live births. It is characterized by the following:

- Chronic haemolytic anaemia
- Vaso-occlusion leading to ischaemia and infarction, and manifesting as:
  - acute pain crises
  - chronic pain from aseptic necrosis or bony infarction
  - acute gross ischaemia involving the lungs (acute chest syndrome) and brain (cerebrovascular occlusion)
  - organ dysfunction from repeated episodes of ischaemia and infarction in the kidneys

(glomerular and tubular dysfunction leading to hyposthenuria) and spleen (autosplenectomy)
- Increased susceptibility to invasive infection with encapsulated bacteria such as *Streptococcus pneumoniae*, *Haemophilus influenzae* b, meningococci and *Salmonella* species associated with functional hyposplenism (decreased phagocytosis and opsonization)

Acute worsening of the anaemia can occur with:

- Aplastic crises, usually resulting from infection with parvovirus B19
- Splenic sequestration crisis from pooling of blood in the spleen, which results in gross enlargement of the spleen and hypovolaemia
- Hyperhaemolytic crisis secondary to infection

Acute pain crises

Sickled cells can occlude any small blood vessel in the body and cause ischaemic injury. Hand–foot syndrome (dactylitis) with acute painful swelling of the hands and feet, caused by infarction in the small bones, is often the initial presentation in children under 2 years of age. Pain in the bones of the lower back and limbs is common in older children. Abdominal pain can occur as a result of vaso-occlusion in the mesenteric circulation. The pain is usually severe and can resemble a surgical emergency, especially when associated with vomiting, fever, abdominal distension and guarding.

Self-test 7: Why are clinical features of sickle-cell disease unusual before the age of 4–6 months?

Answer: HbF (fetal haemoglobin) is the major normal Hb at birth and it does not sickle. It binds more oxygen than adult haemoglobins and is essential for increased oxygen release in the fetus. Normally, more and more HbA (containing β-globin chains) is synthesized after birth and the proportion of HbF falls to 10–15 per cent by 4 months of age (Table 24.4). In sickle-cell disease, HbS-containing abnormal β-globin chains are produced. When deoxygenated, HbS polymerizes into rigid crystal-like rods (sickling) (Figure 24.7). The relatively higher proportion of HbF during the first few months of life prevents polymerization of HbS and sickling.

Table 24.4   Normal and abnormal haemoglobins[a]

Type of haemoglobin	Globin chains	Proportion of total Hb concentration
Normal Hb		
HbF	$\alpha_2\ \gamma_2$	50–85% at birth, 10–15% at 4-month age, <2% after 3 years
HbA	$\alpha_2\ \beta_2$	15–40% at birth, 95–98% after 3 years
HbA$_2$	$\alpha_2\ \delta_2$	Virtually absent at birth, 1–3% after 6 months
Abnormal Hb		
HbS	α_2 abnormal β_2 (amino acid valine substituted for glutamic acid at position 6)	Relatively low compared with HbF for age 4–6 months

[a]Haemoglobin is made up of four haem molecules (protoporphyrin IX combined with iron) and four globin chains. Globin chains differ according to the type of haemoglobin.

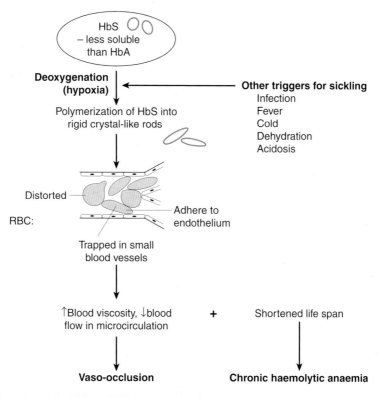

Figure 24.7   Pathophysiology of sickling. RBC, red blood cells.

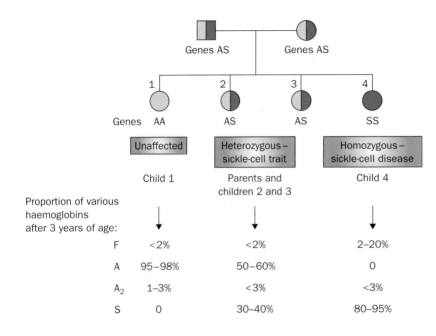

Child 1 — Unaffected
Parents and children 2 and 3 — Heterozygous – sickle-cell trait
Child 4 — Homozygous – sickle-cell disease

Proportion of various haemoglobins after 3 years of age:

	Child 1	Parents and children 2 and 3	Child 4
F	<2%	<2%	2–20%
A	95–98%	50–60%	0
A$_2$	1–3%	<3%	<3%
S	0	30–40%	80–95%

Figure 24.8 Autosomal recessive inheritance in sickle-cell disease.

Self-test 8: What specific pathological conditions will you consider in a child with sickle-cell disease presenting with acute abdominal pain?

Answer:

- Vaso-occlusive crisis involving structures in the abdomen
- Pigmented gallstones, cholecystitis
- Lower respiratory infection with *Streptococcus pneumoniae* or *Haemophilus influenzae* b

Self-test 9: The following are true of sickle-cell disease:

A The anaemia is microcytic/hypochromic
B The reticulocyte count is usually low
C Splenic sequestration crisis is rare in adults
D HbS completely replaces HbA
E A sickle solubility test (e.g. Sickledex) is a reliable screening test in infants

Answers:

A False: it is normochromic/normocytic in sickle-cell disease and microcytic/hypochromic in thalassaemia major and trait

B False: as with other chronic haemolytic anaemias, the reticulocyte count is usually high; it is low during aplastic crises

C True: as a result of autosplenectomy from repeated episodes of splenic infarction

D True: homozygotes with the disease have no HbA; heterozygote carriers of the sickle-cell trait have some HbA (Figure 24.8)

E False: high levels of HbF interfere with the test and can give a false-negative result in infants with sickle-cell disease. A positive test does not differentiate sickle-cell disease from sickle-cell trait. Haemoglobin electophoresis is more reliable and also identifies other abnormal haemoglobins

Further sources of information

Articles

Davenport M. ABC of general surgery in children: acute abdominal pain in children. *British Medical Journal* 1996; **312**: 498–501

Davies SC, Oni L. Management of patients with sickle cell disease. *British Medical Journal* 1997; **315**: 656–60

Harrington L, Connolly B, Hu X et al. Ultrasonographic and clinical predictors of intussusception. *Journal of Pediatrics* 1998; **132**: 836–9

Jack DB. Diagnosis of appendicitis: getting it right every time? *The Lancet* 1997; **349**: 1076

Steinberg MH. Management of sickle cell disease. *New England Journal of Medicine* 1999; **340**: 1021–30

Self-test 10: The salient clinical features of a number of school-age children presenting with acute abdominal pain are given below. Match each with the most likely diagnosis from Table 24.1.

Clinical features

A Colicky periumbilical pain, bilious vomiting, abdominal distension and visible peristalsis

B Colicky periumbilical pain, persistent vomiting of clear fluid, profuse watery diarrhoea and mild abdominal distension

C Colicky periumbilical pain, pain and swelling of the left elbow, and non-blanching rash on the legs

D Persistent dull periumbilical pain, vomited once and diarrhoea with small stools containing mucus

E Right-sided abdominal pain, high fever with rigors, tachypnoea, shallow breathing and reduced air entry on auscultation of the right side of the chest

F Pain on right side of the abdomen, high fever with rigors, vomiting, passing urine frequently

Answers:

A Mechanical intestinal obstruction

B Gastroenteritis

C Henoch–Schoenlein purpura

D Acute appendicitis

E Right lower lobe pneumonia

F Right pyelonephritis

Self-test 11: How might a child with a Meckel's diverticulum present?

Answer: A Meckel's diverticulum is a remnant of the vitelline duct and is present in a small number of people. It may contain heterotopic gastric epithelium or pancreatic tissue and the following problems occasionally arise:

- Bleeding from ulcerated gastric mucosa presenting as bloody stools
- Inflamed epithelium at the base of the diverticulum serves as the apex of an intussusception
- Obstruction and inflammation with clinical features similar to acute appendicitis

Self-test 12: If a mother and father have the sickle-cell trait, what is their risk of having a child with sickle-cell disease?

Answer: The risk is 1 in 4 (or 25 per cent) with each pregnancy.

Acute presentation

A girl who is unsteady and vomiting

Age: 9 years

STEVEN RYAN

Presentation

Jane, aged 9, was taken to the accident and emergency department (A&E) of her local hospital. She had been referred there by her general practitioner who had sought an urgent opinion. In his brief referral letter he had stated:

Dear Doctor

Please could you see and assess this patient. She has been unwell for about 1 week with dizziness and vomiting. She is not eating much and drinking little and I am concerned she may become dehydrated. Until this episode she has been in good health. She has mild asthma, which is well controlled with a low-dose steroid inhaler.

Initial considerations and action

A brief and to-the-point referral from the GP. Note that the GP has not reported her examination findings, so this part of the assessment will be especially important.

Self-test 1: What are the causes of both vomiting and dizziness?

Answer: Inner-ear disease, brain disorders, systemic infection, anxiety, drugs and poisons (Tables 25.1 and 25.2).

Table 25.1 Causes of vomiting

- Any infection, e.g. urine infection
- Gastrointestinal infection
- Inner-ear disease, e.g. labyrinthitis
- Brain disease, e.g. raised intracranial pressure
- Gastrointestinal obstruction
- Gastrointestinal dysfunction, e.g. gastrointestinal reflux
- Psychological, e.g. anxiety, bulimia
- Metabolic – ketosis
- Drug related
- Poisoning, e.g. ethanol

Table 25.2 Causes of dizziness

- A common unexplained symptom
- Psychological – anxiety
- Hyperventilation
- Inner ear, e.g. labyrinthitis
- Brain related, e.g. migraine, postviral cerebellar dysfunction
- General infection
- Syncopal, e.g. vasovagal episodes
- Drug side effects
- Poisoning
- Motion sickness
- Metabolic, e.g. hypoglycaemia

Initial thoughts will be:

- To determine the cause of the problem
- To determine the effect of the symptoms, e.g. is there evidence of dehydration?

History

Jane's mother gives the following history.

Presenting complaint

Jane has actually been unwell for about 3 weeks, although she not been her usual self for about 3 months really. Over the last 3 weeks:

- Her vomiting has become steadily worse
- She tends to be worse in the morning and better later in they day
- The vomit on occasions has had bile in it
- She complains of dizziness – she feels that the room is spinning round much of the time
- The dizziness is not worse on movement
- She is taking regular sips of fluid
- She has also complained of an intermittent frontal headache
- She is also unsteady on her feet, though her mother feels that this is because she is weak through lack of nourishment
- She looks thinner and has lost a little weight through this illness

Other relevant history

- There is no family history of migraine
- Her asthma is indeed well controlled
- She was taking no other medication and no medicines were missing at home
- Jane denied having taken any medicines, recreational drugs or alcohol
- There has been no change in bowel habit and no abdominal pain

Self-test 2: What is the potential meaning of these specific items in the history?
A Worse in the morning
B Not worse on head movement
C Unsteadiness

Answer: Symptoms related to raised intracranial pressure are worse first thing in the morning and get better during the day. Lack of exacerbation on head movement makes inner-ear problems less likely. The unsteadiness could represent underlying brain dysfunction. The history is therefore suggestive of a brain problem and hence neurological examination will be important.

Interpretation of the history

The history seems to be more prolonged than at first appeared and the spells appear to be progressive which is worrying. Dizziness is a frequently reported symptom at all ages and it is important to determine whether it involves perception of movement (vertigo) or a feeling of light-headedness. Other symptoms are individually non-specific, such as headache and unsteadiness, but is a jigsaw building up with an underlying picture emerging?

Examination

General inspection

- Height and weight: 125 cm and 20.2 kg – some evidence of recent weight loss
- Dry mouth and lips but eyes not sunken and normal skin turgor
- Capillary refill time <2 seconds and peripheries warm
- Minor cervical lymphadenopathy only

Cardiovascular system

- Pulse 82/minute, good volume and regular
- Blood pressure 98/66 mmHg

Respiratory system, ear, nose and throat, abdomen

- No abnormality found

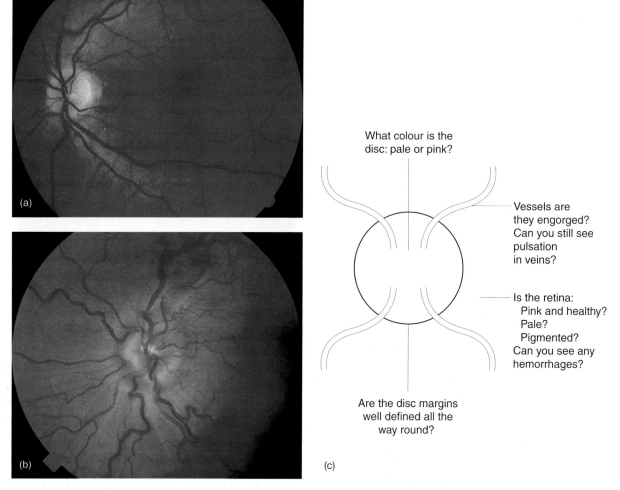

Figure 25.1 (a, b) Normal optic fundus and one showing papilloedema; (c) how to report the findings on fundoscopy.

Nervous system

- Nystagmus when looking to left, otherwise full range of eye movements
- Pupils equal, reacting to light and accommodation
- Consensual light reflex present bilaterally
- Visual fields unimpaired
- Optic fundal examination (Figure 25.1) – both disc margins are blurred and veins are engorged
- No facial weakness
- General body tone diminished
- Deep tendon reflexes diminished – especially on left
- Plantar reflexes down-going bilaterally

Assessment of coordination

- Past-pointing and very unsteady on finger–nose test
- Dysdiadochokinesis on hand-pat test
- Worse on left side
- Tends to stagger to left when walking – heel–toe walking impossible

Urine bedside testing

- **Ketones:** + + +
- **Glucose:** −
- **Protein:** trace
- **Blood:** nil

- **Leucocytes:** nil
- **Specific gravity:** nil

Self-test 3: What do each of the following features indicate?
A Dry lips and mucous membranes
B Ketones in urine
C Nystagmus to left and staggering to left
D Blurred disc margins and venous engorgement
E Reduced tone and reduced reflexes

Answers:
A Mild dehydration
B Starvation – oxidation of fat
C Left-sided cerebellar lesion
D Papilloedema – raised intracranial pressure
E Cerebellar lesion

There is mild dehydration but skin turgor and cardio-vascular status are normal. This would put the dehydration at less than 5 per cent.

There is ketosis, indicating that carbohydrate stores are depleted and fat oxidation has been increased. Dehydration and starvation are a potent cause of this. Unfortunately, excessive ketone production is a metabolic derangement that can worsen nausea, vomiting and anorexia

There are clear signs of a significant abnormality within the central nervous system (CNS). The nystagmus, incoordination, low tone and diminished reflexes point to a cerebellar problem.

The lateralization of the findings to the left indicates that the lesion is in the left cerebellum. This would tend to rule out a general cause of cerebellar dysfunction.

The findings on optic fundal examination are consistent with papilloedema and this is in keeping with raised intracranial pressure.

In summary, the findings are consistent with a lesion in the left cerebellum associated with raised pressure in the skull vault.

Investigations

Blood count, urea, electrolytes and acid–base status are assessed (Table 25.3) and an urgent computed tomography (CT) brain scan is requested (Figure 25.2).

Table 25.3 Results

Test	Result
Full blood count	Normal
Sodium	128 mmol/L (low)
Potassium	3.8 mmol/L (low)
Chloride	88 mmol/L (low)
Urea	10.4 mmol/L (high)
pH	7.36 (normal)
Base deficit	6 mmol/L (high)
Anion gap	28 mmol/L (high)
Carbon dioxide	3.6 mmol/L (low)

Self-test 4: Summarize and interpret these results.

Answer: Salt depleted and with compensated metabolic acidosis (caused by ketones).

There is evidence of salt loss of both potassium and sodium, probably related to vomiting. There is also dehydration (high urea) as well as excess metabolic acid with compensatory hyperventilation, which has lowered the carbon dioxide levels. The ketones, previously identified, are the likely culprit.

The brain scan shows a mass within the left cerebellar hemisphere. This is causing obstruction to the flow of cerebrospinal fluid (CSF), which has resulted in hydrocephalus.

Diagnosis

Left cerebellar tumour with secondary hydrocephalus.

Progress

Jane's parents are asked to see the consultant without Jane. Her primary nurse stays with her. A junior doctor is present and the senior nurse from the ward (for details about breaking bad news, see Chapter 5). The parents are plainly told the diagnosis and given time to express their grief and ask what happens next. Jane is referred to a

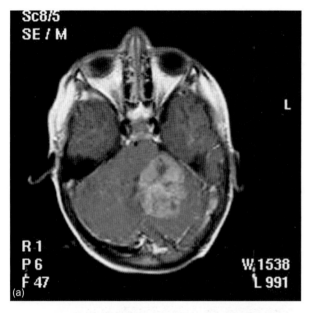

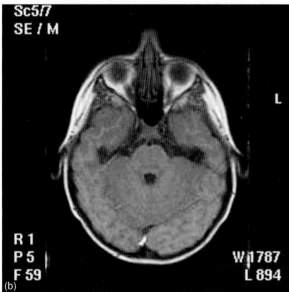

Figure 25.2 Brain scan showing left-sided cerebellar tumour with secondary hydrocephalus. (a) Cerebellar tumour; (b) hydrocephalus.

specialist children's hospital with an oncology unit supported by a neurosurgical department. She is to be sent there the following day by ambulance. The oncology consultant asks that Jane be prescribed the corticosteroid dexamethasone because this reduces the tissue swelling related to brain tumours and can temporarily reduce raised pressure.

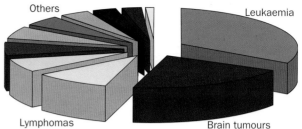

Figure 25.3 The relative incidence of childhood cancers in the UK.

Background knowledge

Paediatric malignancy

The epithelial cancers of adulthood – lung, gastrointestinal tract, breast and skin – are very uncommon in children. The three main groups of malignant conditions are:

1 Leukaemia and lymphomas
2 Brain tumours
3 Other solid tumours

They are rare because only one child in 600 will develop a malignancy throughout childhood. In the UK around 1200 malignancies are diagnosed annually. Figure 25.3 shows the relative incidences of various childhood malignancies.

Brain tumours

Therapy may involve a CSF shunt to relieve intracranial pressure, resection of the tumour if possible and radiation in a number of types. Chemotherapy is generally much less useful. Survival rates vary widely between 25 per cent and 100 per cent, dependent on tumour type and position.

Leukaemia

- Peak age 3–5 years
- Mostly acute lymphoblastic leukaemia
- Treatment comprises:
  – induction – typically 4 weeks
  – intensification
  – CNS treatment
  – maintenance for 2–3 years

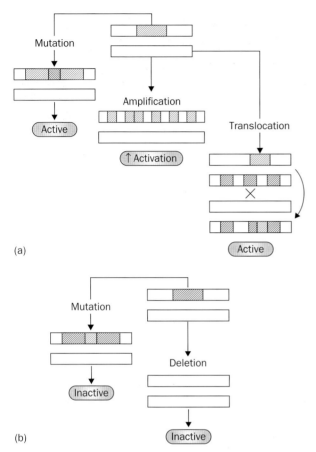

(a)

(b)

Figure 25.4 Gene mechanisms in malignancy.
(a) Activation of oncogenes; (b) deactivation of tumour suppressor genes.

- Five-year survival rate increased from 40 per cent in 1962 to 92 per cent in 1991

Cancer genes

Increasingly the role of abnormal genes in cancer development is being recognized. Figure 25.4 demonstrates the role of two contrasting types of gene: oncogenes that promote cancer when activated and tumour-suppressor genes that allow it to develop when deactivated.

Care

As well as definitive and hopefully curative treatment, care of such patients also involves:

- Psychological support
- Family and social support
- Nutritional support
- Symptom relief and palliation – pain control, antiemetics
- Treatment of side effects of therapy – unlike other areas of medicine these are universal; an example would be infection as a result of immunosuppression being combated by antibiotics and colony-stimulating factors
- Immunization against possible infections acquired during immunosuppression

Websites

www.spade39.ncl.ac.uk/ccw/guide2.htm

www.cancerbacup.org.uk/info/index.htm

Self-test 5: Peter is 14 and went out with his friends and was found late at night semi-conscious. He was placed in the recovery position and an ambulance was summoned. On arrival in hospital he was vaguely responding to voice and definitely to pain. By this time his parents had arrived and gave the history that he had been in good health until he had gone out. He had slurred speech and nystagmus when he moved his head. He improved his conscious level but was very unsteady with diminished reflexes.

A What are the key conditions to consider?

B What is the most likely cause?

C What investigations might be considered – especially if Peter did not show signs of recovery?

Answers:

A Poisoning with alcohol or other recreational drugs; traumatic head injury; a combination of these two; an acute vascular problem (ischaemia or haemorrhage)

B Alcohol poisoning

C Blood alcohol level; CT of brain; blood sugar level (hypoglycaemia is a common complication of alcohol poisoning in children)

Self-test 6: Elaine is 4. Over a period of 2 days she becomes very unsteady on her feet and seems like she is drunk. There is no vomiting. Examination reveals that there is no localization but she has diminished reflexes, low general tone, past-pointing and nystagmus laterally in both directions. She is well nourished and is known to have constipation occasionally. She had chickenpox 2 weeks previously along with her twin sister. Both girls made a good recovery from the chickenpox and did not require any specific medical treatment. Elaine's mother suffers from migraine. Elaine is due to start her new school the following week.

A What is the most likely cause for the findings?
B What is the prognosis?
C What investigation would be best for showing the abnormality?

Answers:
A Postinfectious cerebellar demyelination
B Usually excellent – complete recovery is the norm
C Magnetic resonance imaging – much better for showing demyelination than CT

A boy with recurrent wheezing and breathlessness

Age: 5 years

LEENA PATEL

Presentation

Terence is 5 years old and is taken to see the general practitioner. Yet again he has been wheezy and unable to catch his breath. His class teacher has also noticed it and the school nurse asked his mother whether Terence had asthma.

Self-test 1: What do you understand by wheeze? Think of what else you might wish to know to decide whether Terence has asthma.

Answer: Check your response with Tables 26.1 and 26.2.

Initial considerations and action

Wheeze is a high-pitched, musical, whistling or squeaky noise from the airway. It is a common respiratory symptom (see Chapter 9). Knowing that Terence has recurrent, as opposed to acute, wheeze helps in the diagnosis, although there is some overlap in that a condition that usually presents as acute wheeze may rarely give rise to recurrent or chronic wheeze, and vice versa (see Chapter 9, Table 9.1). Asthma is the first diagnosis that most professionals think of in a school-age child with recurrent wheeze and breathlessness. However, it is important to clarify what the mother calls wheeze and what she means by 'unable to catch his breath'. Parents may mislabel noises from mucus in the upper airway, snoring or stridor as wheeze. In addition, all children who wheeze do not necessarily have asthma, and other conditions must not be overlooked.

Table 26.1 Features of asthma from a history

Presenting features
Recurrent wheeze
Dry cough
Difficulty breathing
Chest tightness
Symptoms triggered or made worse
With colds and viral infections
At night
With physical activity, overexcitement, laughing or crying
On contact with furry or feathery animals
In a dusty environment
In a smoky atmosphere
By chemical irritants, e.g. paint, aerosols
When the pollen count is high
With changes in environmental temperature
Symptoms respond to inhaled bronchodilator
History of eczema, runny nose without colds (hayfever)
Family history of asthma, eczema or hayfever

Table 26.2 'Non-asthma' features

Persistent/chronic productive or wet cough

Green purulent sputum

Recurrent ear infections

Clubbing

Localized wheeze

Crackles

Focal and/or persistent chest radiograph abnormality

Poor response to asthma treatment

Recurrent skin infections

Poor weight gain

Frequent offensive stools

Recurrent vomiting

For all these need to consider:

- Diagnoses other than asthma, e.g.
  - Cystic fibrosis
  - Ciliary dyskinesia
  - Primary immunodeficiency
  - Congenital bronchial wall defect
  - Gastro-oesophageal reflux
- A specialist opinion
- Investigations
  - Chest radiograph
  - Sputum or cough swab for bacterial culture
  - Sweat test
  - Full blood count, lymphocyte subsets
  - Immunoglobulins, IgG subclasses, functional antibodies and response to test immunization

History

From the practice records the GP notes that Terence has been seen at the practice a number of times with wheezing, including 6 weeks ago when the impression was 'viral infection'. His first wheezy episode was at 16 months of age when he was prescribed amoxicillin and salbutamol syrup for 5 days. The GP then obtains a history from mother.

Although Terence was first wheezy when he was 16 months old, it has only been bad since he started school last year. Mother is asked to describe what she calls wheeze and in what way it has been bad. She explains that Terence's wheeze is the whistling sound he makes when he breathes out. Since starting school Terence has been wheezy most days. It is worse when he has a cold and he has had about three colds in the past 6 months. Colds 'go straight to his chest' and he coughs and wheezes almost continuously for a few days. The cough is dry. Terence coughs and wheezes more when he runs around a lot and is up two or three nights every week. He appears breathless when the wheeze is especially loud. Terence often has to sit and watch other children play. He has missed 4 days from school this term.

Mother is not sure whether the medicines that Terence had at 16 months helped in any way. He has not had any other treatment since, but his father thinks that he may need inhalers. Terence had chickenpox when he was 2 years old. He has not had eczema, runny nose without colds, ear discharge or infections, persistent diarrhoea, vomiting or poor weight gain.

Terence's mother smoked when she was pregnant with him and still smokes but only outdoors. His birth was uneventful. He has had all his vaccines. His mother has no concerns about his development. She is healthy but his father and an 8-year-old half-sister from his father's previous partner have asthma. There are no chest illnesses other than asthma in the family. His mother got the dog before Terence was born. Terence loves playing with him and it does not seem to make the wheeze or cough worse.

Interpretation of the history

The history helps identify the following:

- The range, frequency and severity of symptoms
- The precipitating/exacerbating factors
- The response to treatment
- Any features that might refute the diagnosis of asthma

Terence does have many features of asthma (Table 26.1).

Chest tightness is commonly reported by older children as a tightness, pain or tickle over the sternum but 5 year olds like Terence may not be able to describe it.

Antibiotics (amoxicillin) and orally administered β_2 agonists (salbutamol syrup) would not be expected to relieve the symptoms of asthma. β_2 Agonists administered orally are ineffective as bronchodilators.

The impact of symptoms on sleep, activity and schooling helps assess their severity. Although Terence has not missed many days off school, his symptoms would be considered to be sufficiently troublesome to warrant treatment because he has:

- Had more frequent exacerbations associated with colds in the past 6 months
- Interval symptoms almost daily
- Symptoms that regularly disturb sleep
- Symptoms that restrict activities

As Terence has had symptoms for a long time, it is reassuring to know that the cough is dry and not productive. If a child with asthma produces any mucus (phlegm) it is white and not purulent, yellow, green, brown or foul in nature. A persistent productive cough with purulent mucus would raise the possibility of other pathology, such as cystic fibrosis or a primary immunodeficiency (Table 26.2).

Recurrent wheeze and cough may be the presenting features of repeated aspiration associated with gastro-oesophageal reflux. This is uncommon in school-age children. In addition, Terence has no history of vomiting.

Self-test 2: What is 'viral wheeze' and how might you differentiate it from asthma?

Answer: Many infants and young children wheeze when they have a cold or viral respiratory infection – 'viral wheeze' (Figure 26.1). Some of these will have transient wheeze and others will turn out to have asthma. Distinguishing whether a child has transient virus-induced wheeze or asthma might be possible only by watching the child's progress over time or by hindsight.

Self-test 3: What is the relevance of a history of passive smoking and pets?

Answer: Maternal smoking during pregnancy affects the developing lungs of the fetus and the airway is likely to be hyperreactive after birth. Passive smoking, irrespective of whether the smoker is indoors or out, is associated with

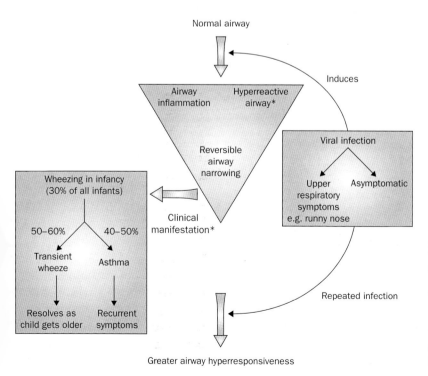

Figure 26.1 Sequence of events following a virus infection in infants and young children, and outcome in infants and young children who wheeze with viral respiratory infections.
*Airway hyperresponsiveness induced by viral infection lasts several weeks. It does not always lead to symptoms.

increased frequency and severity of asthma symptoms in children. Allergens from pets (with fur or feathers) enhance airway hyperreactivity in atopic children.

Examination

In a child suspected of having asthma, the main purpose of the examination is:

- To check for features that suggest a diagnosis other than asthma (Table 26.2), such as underweight, clubbing, purulent nasal discharge, moist cough, localized wheeze or reduced air entry, and crackles
- To assess the severity of asthma from the shape of the chest and any deformities, and peak expiratory flow measurement if the child is old enough to understand and cooperate

Terence is happy and chatty during the consultation and did not appear short of breath at any stage. He appears well nourished and his weight and height are 20 kg (75th centile) and 109 cm (50th centile). He does not have pallor or clubbing. His eardrums appear normal and are not dull or retracted. Examination of the nose reveals no discharge and no inflamed mucous membrane. He does not have nasal flaring, intercostal recessions or tachypnoea. His chest is not barrel shaped but he has Harrison's sulci. Auscultation reveals good air entry over both lungs. A high-pitched expiratory wheeze is heard bilaterally but expiration is not prolonged. There are no crackles. Peak flow measurement is not attempted.

Meaning of the examination

- A barrel-shaped chest is seen with an increase in the anteroposterior diameter, a prominent sternum and relatively horizontal ribs. It indicates persistent overinflation of the lungs from chronic obstruction
- Harrison's sulci are symmetrical horizontal grooves along the attachment of the diaphragm extending laterally from the lower end of the sternum and above the anterior costal margins, which are everted. These sulci are a sign of a chronic respiratory condition (such as troublesome asthma, cystic fibrosis, chronic lung disease)

in early childhood when the chest wall is more compliant. They occur as a result of overuse of the diaphragm and contraction of abdominal muscles during respiration
- Bilateral wheeze indicates generalized airway obstruction (as opposed to a localized wheeze heard when there is a focal abnormality)
- Prolonged expiration suggests airway obstruction and is especially heard during acute exacerbations of asthma (see Chapter 35)
- Peak flow readings can be obtained in children older than 6–7 years but even then children need to have had clear explanations from an asthma nurse or physiotherapist and some practice before the measurements can be considered reliable

Interpretation of the examination

Terence's examination findings support the history of asthma

- His symptoms are worse with colds, physical activity and at night
- The recurrent troublesome symptoms and presence of Harrison's sulci indicate that airway obstruction has been persistent for some time and there is a need for treatment
- The history and examination do not point to respiratory conditions other than asthma

Investigations and results

The diagnosis of asthma is based on the history and examination findings and no investigations are required routinely.

A symptom diary completed by the parents is helpful when there is uncertainty about the frequency, timing and duration of symptoms.

Parents often ask about allergy tests but they are not recommended because they are not diagnostic and have a number of limitations, including poor reliability.

Spirometry is helpful in monitoring progress but can be done only in children aged over 6–7 years. Features of 'non-asthma' from the history and examination warrant further investigations (see Table 26.2, p. 278).

Diagnosis

Terence is a 5-year-old boy with recurrent wheeze, dry cough and breathlessness since 16 months of age. He has had frequent exacerbations associated with colds in the past 6 months and symptoms that regularly disturb sleep and are worse with activity. There is a family history of asthma, his mother smokes and they have a dog. He does not have any 'non-asthma' features (see Table 26.2) and is diagnosed to have troublesome asthma.

As many as one in five children have asthma at some time. The airway obstruction in asthma is reversible (as opposed to fixed) and improves with inhaled bronchodilator treatment. This needs to be confirmed for Terence.

Management and follow-up

The aims of management are to:

- Provide information to the family about asthma and its management
- Avoid known triggers such as furry or feathered animals and cigarette smoke
- Control daytime and night-time symptoms, normalize routine activity and encourage physical activity
- Prevent acute exacerbations
- Minimize need for reliever, short-acting, inhaled bronchodilator
- Maintain control with lowest possible dose of inhaled corticosteroid

Drugs for the management of chronic asthma (Table 26.3)

Inhaled bronchodilators (short acting and long acting) and corticosteroids are the drugs of choice. The success of treatment depends on:

- Tailoring the treatment for the child
- Selecting the most appropriate delivery device according to the age and ability of the child (Table 26.4 and Figure 26.2)
- Providing information and support for children and parents with the help of asthma nurse specialists

Table 26.3 Drugs used in chronic asthma

Drug	Mechanism of action	Mode of delivery
Inhaled short-acting β_2 agonist Salbutamol Terbutaline	Bronchodilator	Aerosol with spacer or breath-actuated device Dry powder inhalers (e.g. Accuhaler or Turbohaler) Nebulizer solution
Inhaled anticholinergic Ipratropium bromide	Bronchodilator	Aerosol with spacer Nebulizer solution
Inhaled corticosteroid Beclomethasone Budesonide Fluticasone	Anti-inflammatory	Aerosol with spacer Dry powder inhalers
Inhaled long-acting β_2 agonist Salmeterol Formoterol	Bronchodilator Synergistic with inhaled corticosteroid	Aerosol with spacer Dry powder inhalers
Anti-leukotriene Montelukast	Leukotriene receptor antagonist	Oral
Sodium cromoglycate	Controversial but may prevent mediator release	Aerosol with spacer Dry powder

Table 26.4 Choice of delivery device for inhaled medication according to age (Figure 26.2)

Age group	Most appropriate delivery device
Infants and toddlers	MDI aerosol with spacer and mask
2–7 years	MDI aerosol with spacer
Older children	Dry powder inhaler for mild–moderate asthma but MDI aerosol with spacer for moderate–severe asthma

Note:

The child should be able to use the device correctly.

The inhaler technique should be checked regularly to identify and correct difficulties.

A pressurized MDI alone without a spacer requires precise coordination of actuation and inspiration and is not suitable for children.

MDI, metered dose inhaler.

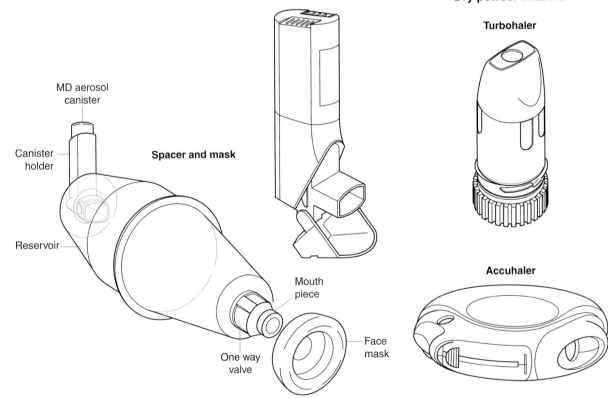

Figure 26.2 Delivery devices in Table 26.4. MDI, metered dose inhaler.

A stepwise approach to management is recommended with:

- Inhaled short-acting β_2 agonist as a 'reliever', to be taken as required
- Inhaled corticosteroid as a long-term preventive in patients with frequent and persistent symptoms
- Inhaled long-acting β_2 agonist in combination with inhaled corticosteroid

The step-up approach is safer than the step-down approach (starting with a higher dose of inhaled corticosteroid to gain control, and then titrating to the lowest effective dose to minimize systemic effects). Children should be reviewed at least every 3 months to:

Step-down if symptoms are controlled	Step-up if symptoms are not controlled
↓	↓
Reduce inhaled corticosteroid to lowest effective dose	Check inhaler technique and adherence Reinforce avoidance of potential allergens Step-up treatment

Initial treatment with a bronchodilator for Terence (Table 26.5)

Table 26.5 How to use a large-volume spacer

1 Shake aerosol canister and fit into end of spacer

2 Ask child to put mouthpiece in mouth, seal with lips and continue to take normal breaths; spacer should be kept horizontal or tilted slightly up

3 Press canister

4 Hold spacer in place until child has taken five normal breaths; valve should click with each breath

Repeat steps 1–4 for each puff required

Care of the spacer

Wash once a week in warm soapy water, rinse and leave to dry naturally

Replace every 6 months

The GP:

- Recommends a short-acting β_2 agonist inhaler with a large-volume spacer (salbutamol 100 μg/puff or terbutaline 250 μg/puff aerosol, two puffs with a volumatic or Nebuhaler) as a 'reliever' when Terence has symptoms, before any physical activity and before bedtime
- Asks mother to keep a diary of the symptoms, doses of the treatment given and whether treatment relieves Terence's symptoms
- Arranges to review Terence after 1 week
- Introduces Terence and his mother to the asthma nurse

Self-test 4: Why did the GP recommend administering the bronchodilator with a spacer rather than a nebulizer?

Answer: A nebulizer is more effective than other ways of administering inhaled bronchodilators simply because a much larger dose is given. This is illustrated in Table 26.6. Children with acute symptoms severe enough to warrant the doses of bronchodilator delivered by a nebulizer require medical supervision. For all others who do not need high doses, a large-volume spacer is just as effective as a nebulizer. Therefore nebulizers are not routinely recommended for home use and are reserved for use in general practices, ambulances and hospitals.

Information for the family

The asthma nurse

- Spends time with the mother and Terence explaining asthma and the treatment (see Self-test 5)
- Teaches the mother and Terence how to take the 'reliever' with the spacer device
- Gives Terence's mother leaflets about asthma and its management

Table 26.6 Potential systemic effects of prolonged high-dose inhaled corticosteroid treatment

	Nebulized dose	Dose per puff (metered inhalation) with a spacer	No. of puffs with spacer equivalent to nebulized dose
Terbutaline	2.5–5 mg	250 µg	10–20
Salbutamol	2.5–5 mg	100 µg	25–50
Ipratropium	125–250 µg	18 µg	7–14

Self-test 5: What might you expect the asthma nurse to explain to Terence and his mother?

Answer: The asthma nurse might explain the following:
- Asthma symptoms and that they occur as a result of airway inflammation, spasm and narrowing
- The common triggers that children with asthma are sensitive to and avoidance measures
- Inhaled bronchodilators (quick 'relievers') relieve symptoms by allowing the narrow airway to relax
- Inhaled corticosteroids (long-term 'preventers') control and prevent symptoms and exacerbations by reducing the airway inflammation
- The rationale for the delivery device recommended (Table 26.7) and the correct technique
- The warning signs of an asthma attack (increase in symptoms)
- What to do during an attack:
  - give the reliever (five puffs) and repeat the treatment after 5–10 minutes if it does not have an effect
  - consult the GP or nurse because Terence may need additional treatment such as a short course of an oral steroid (prednisolone)
- The danger signs during an attack that indicate the need to seek medical help urgently:
  - the effect of the reliever treatment lasts less than 3 hours so repeated doses are required more often than every 3 hours
  - Terence becomes very distressed with wheeze or breathlessness
  - Terence becomes too breathless to talk or eat
  - Terence becomes pale and his lips go blue

Table 26.7 Reasons for delivery of aerosol medication with rather than without a large-volume spacer

Easier to use – inhalation does not have to be synchronized with inspiration

Greater proportion of drug delivered to the airway

Less drug deposited in the oropharynx, so reduced local side effects, reduced absorption through the gut and reduced risk of systemic effects

Work just as well as nebulizers in mild-to-moderately severe acute attacks of asthma

Self-test 6: What are the common indoor allergens and irritants that trigger asthma and what relatively simple or easy avoidance measures will you advise?

Answer:

Trigger	Avoidance measure
House-dust mite (fond of bedding, carpets and soft furnishings, loves warm humid environments and detests the sun)	Wash bed linen, curtains and cuddly toys at 60°C regularly Minimize clutter and number of cuddly toys Vacuum frequently Damp-dust surfaces regularly Avoid woollen blankets and carpets, and upholstered furniture Open windows and avoid overheating the house

Cigarette smoke	Avoid smoky places
	Parents (and patients) who smoke will need support to stop smoking
Pets with fur or feathers (allergens in dander)	Avoid acquiring them
	Keep out of bedroom
	Bathe cats and dogs regularly

Terence's progress after 1 week and treatment with inhaled corticosteroid

When Terence is reviewed after 1 week, the mother reports that he has had the inhaler before bedtime and once or twice every day. She thinks that it has helped because the wheeze and cough have eased considerably.

This improvement in symptoms with inhaled bronchodilator provides further support for the diagnosis of asthma. The GP now recommends regular treatment with an inhaled corticosteroid. Arrangements are made to review Terence's progress after 4 weeks because an improvement is expected within this period.

Review and monitoring

As a result of the potential risk of growth suppression with prolonged inhaled corticosteroid treatment, Terence's height and weight are carefully measured and his mother is told that his growth will be monitored every 3 months. Any fears that his mother might have about steroid treatment are addressed. Figure 26.3 shows the pharmacokinetics of inhaled corticosteroids.

Self-test 7: Terence's mother asks whether he will grow out of the asthma. What should she be told?

Answer: She should be told:
- Asthma is a condition in which the airways have a tendency to narrow and this brings about the symptoms
- The tendency for the airways to narrow is inherited and also influenced by various things in the environment, such as house-dust mite, animal dander, pollen, cigarette smoke and pollutants

- People with asthma cannot grow out of this tendency
- However, as Terence gets older, his asthma is likely to become less troublesome and it will also become easier to control with treatment. Many children with asthma will have no symptoms when they are teenagers and adults

Background information

Atopy

Atopy is defined as the predisposition to produce immunoglobulin E (IgE) antibodies to common environmental allergens such as house-dust mite, pollens and moulds. It runs in families but the mode of inheritance does not follow any recognized pattern. The expression of disease in the form of asthma, atopic dermatitis and allergic rhinoconjunctivitis is complex and possibly determined by:

- Several genes that predispose to atopy (polygenic)
- Modifying environmental factors (multifactorial)
- Other genetic and environmental triggers that influence specific end-organ (airways, skin, conjunctiva and nose) sensitivity

Whether breast-feeding protects against atopic diseases is controversial.

Pathophysiology of asthma

Asthma is a chronic inflammation of the airways in which many cells (including T-helper 2 lymphocytes, mast cells and eosinophils) play a role. This is associated with reversible narrowing and increased responsiveness of the airways to various triggers (Figures 26.4 and 26.5, p. 287).

Mechanism of action of drugs used in asthma

Figure 26.6 (p. 288) shows mast cell (1) activation, (2) degranulation and (3) release of secondary mediators and the mechanism of action of different drugs used in asthma.

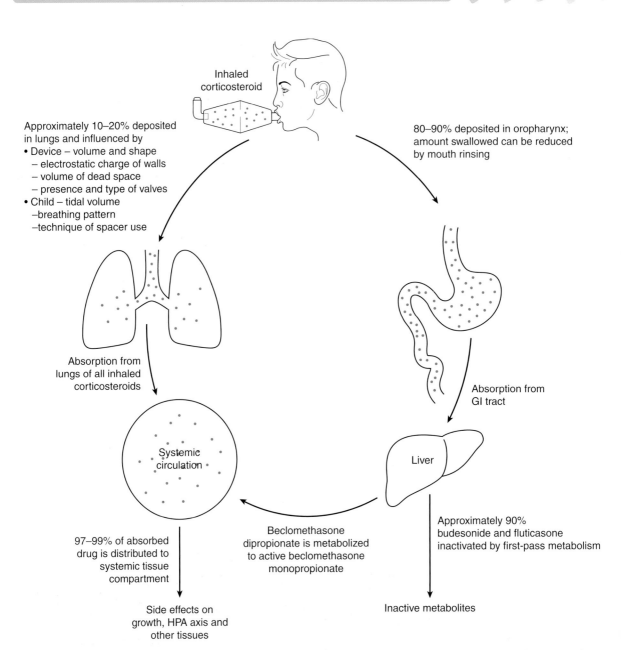

Inhaled
corticosteroid

Approximately 10–20% deposited
in lungs and influenced by
• Device – volume and shape
  – electrostatic charge of walls
  – volume of dead space
  – presence and type of valves
• Child – tidal volume
  –breathing pattern
  –technique of spacer use

80–90% deposited in oropharynx;
amount swallowed can be reduced
by mouth rinsing

Absorption from
lungs of all inhaled
corticosteroids

Absorption from
GI tract

Systemic
circulation

Liver

97–99% of absorbed
drug is distributed to
systemic tissue
compartment

Beclomethasone
dipropionate is metabolized
to active beclomethasone
monopropionate

Approximately 90%
budesonide and fluticasone
inactivated by first-pass metabolism

Side effects on
growth, HPA axis and
other tissues

Inactive metabolites

Figure 26.3   The pharmacokinetics of inhaled corticosteroids. GI, gastrointestinal.

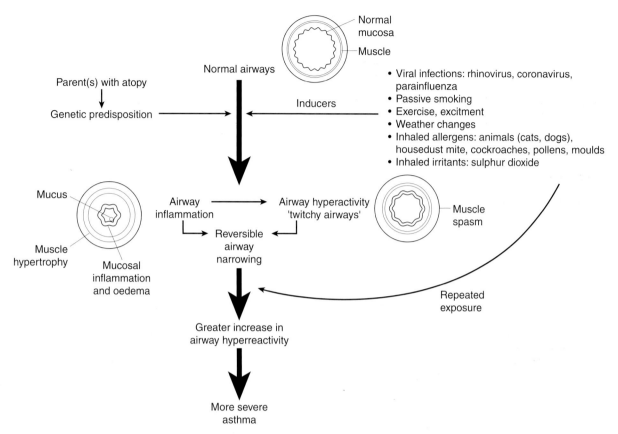

Figure 26.4   The pathogenesis of asthma.

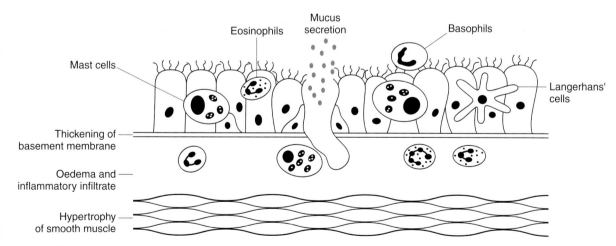

Figure 26.5   Pathological changes in the airway in asthma.

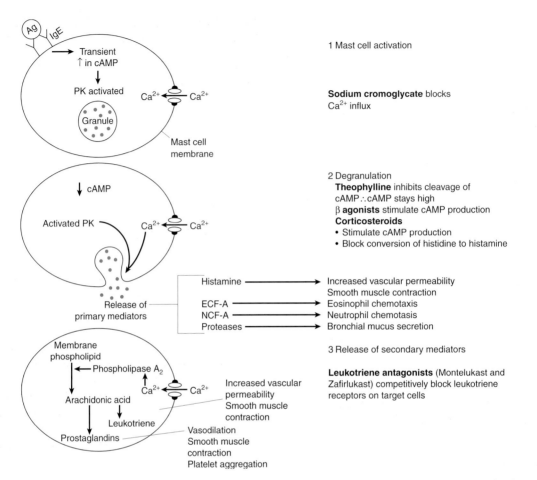

1 Mast cell activation

Sodium cromoglycate blocks Ca^{2+} influx

2 Degranulation
Theophylline inhibits cleavage of cAMP ∴ cAMP stays high
β **agonists** stimulate cAMP production
Corticosteroids
• Stimulate cAMP production
• Block conversion of histidine to histamine

3 Release of secondary mediators

Leukotriene antagonists (Montelukast and Zafirlukast) competitively block leukotriene receptors on target cells

Figure 26.6   Mast cell (1) activation, (2) degranulation and (3) release of secondary mediators and the mechanism of action of different drugs used in asthma. From Janis Kuby *Immunology*, 3rd edn. © 1992, 1994, 1997 by W.H. Freeman and Company. Used with permission.

Table 26.8   Passive smoking and maternal smoking and their effects

Passive smoking increases the risk of	Effects of maternal smoking in pregnancy
Sudden infant death	Increased risk of miscarriages and premature labour
Respiratory infections	Increased perinatal mortality
Wheeze and cough	Increased risk of sudden infant death syndrome
Bronchial hyperreactivity	Intrauterine growth retardation and low birthweight
Asthma symptom severity, frequency, need for treatment	Poor postnatal growth
Persistent middle-ear effusion	Interferes with normal development of the fetal lungs and airways, and postnatally leads to irreversible airway disease
Chronic obstructive airway disease in adulthood	

The risks of passive smoking – a snapshot

The components of the cigarette smoke of a smoker that are inhaled passively are:

- **Mainstream smoke:** the exhaled aerosol after the smoker has inhaled and filtered in his or her lungs
- **Sidestream smoke:** the smoke that comes directly from the burning tip, which therefore contains higher concentrations of toxins
- The toxins in tobacco smoke include carbon monoxide, nicotine, ammonia, hydrogen cyanide and numerous carcinogens

Mechanisms by which passive smoking affects the lungs

- Changes in antibody and cell-mediated immune responses
- Enhanced sensitization in atopic children
- Damage to cilia and impaired mucociliary transport
- Hyperplasia of goblet cells and increased mucus secretion
- Altered number and function of alveolar macrophages and polymorphs

Table 26.8 shows the effects of passive smoking and maternal smoking.

Further sources of information

Book

Brand PLP. Practical interpretation of lung function tests in asthma. In: David TJ (ed.), *Recent Advances in Paediatrics* 18. Edinburgh: Churchill Livingstone, 2000: 77–109

Articles

British Thoracic Society, Scottish Intercollegiate Guidelines Network. British guidelines on the management of asthma. *Thorax* 2003; **58**(suppl 1): i1–94 (also available on BTS website)

Cates C. Chronic asthma. Extracts from 'Clinical Evidence'. *British Medical Journal* 2001; **323**: 976–9

Lipworth BJ. Modern drug treatment of chronic asthma. *British Medical Journal* 1999; **318**: 380–4

Websites

www.brit-thoracic.org.uk

British Thoracic Society's website.

wwww.asthma.org.uk

National Asthma Campaign website.

www.sign.ac.uk/guidelines/published/

Scottish Intercollegiate Guidelines Network (SIGN) Clinical Guidelines website.

Self-test 8: An 8-year-old boy with asthma has been on beclomethasone 200 μg twice daily with a volumatic for the past year and his mother is pleased that his asthma is 'controlled'. He coughs and wheezes when he plays football and requires a couple of doses of salbutamol 200 μg with a volumatic on most days. Will you make any changes to his management?

Answer: Yes, as he has exercise-induced symptoms and the use of salbutamol needs to be minimized:
1 Add in inhaled salmeterol to improve control and
2 Supply a salbutamol dry powder inhaler because it is easier to carry than a volumatic

Self-test 9: A 4-year-old girl has had recurrent wheeze and a bad chest since 1 year of age. Her symptoms have been more troublesome in the past year. An inhaled short-acting bronchodilator did not work and she was subsequently given high-dose, inhaled corticosteroid treatment as well as salmeterol. Her mother gives her the inhalers regularly and the asthma nurse has checked her spacer technique at each review visit. She continues to have troublesome symptoms.
A Does she have 'difficult asthma'?
B What course of action will you take?

Answer:

A: No. 'Difficult asthma' may be described as asthma symptoms on 3 or more days a week, despite treatment with inhaled corticosteroids in doses high enough to increase the risk of systemic side effects. Persistent asthma symptoms and lack of response to treatment can result from:

1 Poor inhaler technique, treatment supervision and adherence (most common reason)
2 Adverse home environment – smoking by a household member, pets, dampness
3 An alternative diagnosis – organic as well as non-organic conditions
4 Genuine unresponsive asthma (rare and needs referral to a respiratory paediatrician)

B: Review history and examination for non-asthma features because conditions other than asthma need to be considered (see Table 26.2).

Self-test 10: What are the local side effects of inhaled corticosteroids and how might they be prevented?

Answer: Oropharyngeal candidiasis: prevented by rinsing the mouth after each dose. Hoarseness, possibly related to myopathy of vocal cords – improves on reducing dose or stopping.

Self-test 11: What are the potential systemic effects of prolonged high-dose inhaled corticosteroid treatment and how might you recognize them?

Answer: The systemic effects are given below. The doses that are more likely to be associated with systemic side effects are given in Table 26.9.

Table 26.9 Doses of inhaled corticosteroids more likely to be associated with an increased risk of systemic side effects

Preparation	Daily dose
Beclomethasone dipropionate	>400 µg
Budesonide	>800 µg
Fluticasone propionate	>400 µg

Systemic effect	Clinical manifestation
Impaired growth	Fall in height from personal centile (i.e. decline in height velocity)
Hypothalamic–pituitary–adrenal suppression with Cushing's syndrome	Cushingoid face ('moonface')
	Weight gain, central obesity
	Hirsutism
	Acne
	Striae
	Weakness, tiredness
Hypothalamic–pituitary–adrenal suppression without Cushing's syndrome	Weight loss
	Weakness, tiredness
	Poor appetite
	Vomiting
	Hypoglycaemia
Reduced bone mineralization	None

Starting school with a disability (cerebral palsy)

Age: 3 years

JACKIE GREGG

Presentation

George is a 3-year-old boy who has cerebral palsy (CP) and is due to start the nursery class of a mainstream school in 6 months' time. He has a review appointment at the child development centre (CDC) with the community paediatrician, physiotherapist, speech and language therapist and occupational therapist. Formal assessment of his educational needs has already started. In view of George's motor difficulties, the paediatrician invites the educational psychologist and preschool advisory teacher to the review.

Initial considerations and action

Professionals should start to think about and plan for starting school and nursery as soon as it is apparent that a child has difficulties that may affect their ability to learn or access the curriculum. George has been attending the CDC and should already have been referred to the local education authority (LEA).

History

George attends the appointment with his mother and grandmother.

George is the only child of Susan and Frank. They are unmarried and their relationship finished shortly after George was diagnosed as having cerebral palsy. George's father has had no involvement with him since then. Susan is worried about how George will cope in nursery and whether others will be able to understand him because his speech is indistinct.

Self-test 1: How does cerebral palsy present?

Answer: Delayed motor milestones with abnormal tone and posturing.

Self-test 2: Which risk factors in the child are associated with cerebral palsy?

Answer: The risk of CP increases with declining birthweight and gestation. Although the two are related they have independent effects. Other risk factors are intrauterine growth retardation, severe birth asphyxia and multiple births (i.e. twins, etc.).

George was born at 29 weeks' gestation weighing 1.1 kg and was admitted to the special care baby unit. He was ventilated for 4 weeks and discharged at 9 weeks of age. Ultrasonography of the head showed bilateral intraventricular haemorrhage and germinal matrix haemorrhage around the lateral ventricles. Serial scans showed the development of periventricular leucomalacia (PVL) with cystic changes. (Leucomalacia literally means softening of the brain's white matter.) Close follow-up was arranged and George's parents were advised that he was at increased risk of developing motor difficulties. By 8 months of age George hadn't acquired sitting balance, he couldn't roll over and he had developed a right-hand preference. Tone was increased in his legs and left arm and the reflexes were brisk. George was lively and sociable.

George was referred to the CDC by the neonatologist. He had a detailed assessment by the child development team (see Chapter 7) and paediatric neurologist, and a diagnosis of spastic diplegia was made. Magnetic resonance imaging (MRI) of the brain showed bilateral PVL. The family were given information on cerebral palsy and referred to Scope – a charity providing information and support to families of individuals with CP.

Following the diagnosis, George's physiotherapist was identified as the key worker and a family service plan was written identifying the services that George would receive. The therapists planned programmes of therapy and arranged regular joint reviews to coordinate the therapy programmes. (Table 27.1 outlines the roles of the therapists.) The developmental paediatrician arranged vision and hearing assessment and continued to see George regularly to monitor his health, review his progress and update the service plan. George is also regularly reviewed by an orthopaedic surgeon with an interest in CP.

A key worker is both a source of support for the families of disabled children and a link by which other services are accessed and used effectively. They have responsibility for working together with the family and with professionals from their own and other services, and for ensuring delivery of the service plan.

Table 27.1   Role of therapists

Physiotherapist

- To assess and advise on motor development
- To advise on positioning and handling to encourage normal development and improve abnormal tone
- To prevent abnormal use of muscles
- Key role in planning of orthopaedic surgery and postoperative rehabilitation

Occupational therapist

- To advise on equipment such as seating, wheelchairs, bath aids
- To assess independence and self-care skills
- To advise on play materials and activities
- To assess hand function, coordination and perceptual skills

Speech and language therapist

To promote:
- Listening
- Play
- Understanding and using language
- Non-verbal communication
- Chewing and swallowing (after feeding assessment)

How to prepare a family service plan

This is an agreed account by the family and professionals of the needs of the child and his or her family and should include:

- A description of the nature of the child's disability and the impact on the family
- List of the key professionals who will be involved including:
  - what sort of work they will be doing and what they are hoping to achieve
  - the goals they are working towards (must be achievable and regularly reviewed and updated)
  - methods to be used and the rationale for the choice of a particular approach
  - how often the child will be seen/the home will be visited
  - how professionals will link with each other
  - agreed role of parents
- List of equipment required and who will provide it
- An agreement on who will be the key worker
- An agreement on how and when the plan will be reviewed (times of transition are very important such as starting school, changing school and moving on to adult services)

George was referred to the Portage service shortly after the diagnosis of cerebral palsy was made (Table 27.2). In George's area, the Portage service is part of the LEA's early years' department, so George was automatically allocated

Table 27.2   Portage

Portage is a home-based teaching service for preschool children, providing:
- Regular visits to the home from a Portage worker
- Assessment of the child's strengths and weaknesses
- Advice on activities to try at home to advance the child's skills

an educational psychologist. If a referral to the Portage service had not triggered a referral to the LEA, the paediatrician would have had a statutory responsibility to refer George at the age of 2 years.

George has a typical diplegic stance (Figure 27.1). He has increased tone in his legs and left arm with brisk reflexes. Although there is marked increased tone around his ankle joints, he has a full range of movements in his joints. He wears ankle–foot orthoses and walks with a walking aid, but can manage short distances at home unaided. George's right-hand function is good, but the left is poor. He therefore struggles to get dressed without help and needs assistance with toileting. George is in good health, eats well and doesn't have any swallowing difficulties.

George is an outgoing child who easily makes friends and he enjoys toddler group. He is chatty, but his mum is worried that he can be difficult to understand and he tends to dribble.

Interpretation of the history

Cerebral palsy is defined as a disorder of movement and posture resulting from a non-progressive lesion of

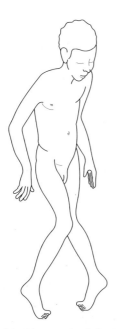

Figure 27.1   Child with spastic diplegia – note that the hips are flexed and internally rotated, and there is flexion at the knees and equinus at the ankles. (From Hall DMB, Hill PD. *The Child with a Disability*, 2nd edn. Oxford: Blackwell Science, 1996.)

the motor pathways in the developing brain. Although the lesion is non-progressive, the clinical manifestations evolve with cerebral maturation. The cerebral palsies are a group of conditions and not a single pathological entity, and are classified by the predominant type of motor disturbance.

Self-test 3: What other problems are associated with cerebral palsy?

Answer: Epilepsy, impaired swallowing, learning disability, vision impairment.

Spastic or spasticity

This refers to increased muscle tone (hypertonia).

Spastic hemiplegia
One half of the body is affected, usually with the arm worse than the leg. Most have normal/near normal intellectual ability. Seizures are the most commonly associated problem. Walking is usually only slightly delayed.

Aetiology Cerebrovascular event in third trimester of pregnancy, infarction of middle cerebral artery, cerebral malformation.

Spastic diplegia
All four limbs are affected, but the arms less so than the legs; it may be asymmetrical. A third have learning disability. Most will achieve walking, but frequently require walking aids.

Aetiology There is hypoperfusion of periventricular area or haemorrhage, leading to PVL and loss of white matter (Figure 27.2).

Spastic tetraplegia/quadriplegia
There is severe involvement of all four limbs, and often poor truncal tone and bulbar involvement. Most individuals need assistance with mobility and have severe learning disability.

Aetiology Pre-term: perinatal cerebrovascular disease; term: prenatal cerebrovascular disease, hypoxic ischaemic encephalopathy caused by birth asphyxia and congenital infection.

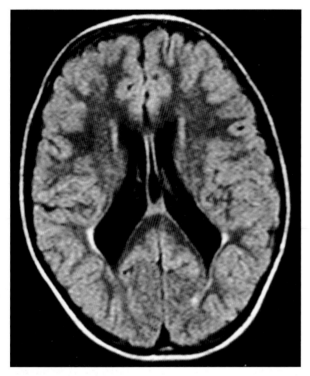

Figure 27.2   Magnetic resonance image of a child with spastic diplegia, showing bilateral ventricular dilatation with loss of periventricular white matter posteriorly. (With thanks to Dr L Abernethy for providing the MRI.)

Ataxic or ataxia

This refers to disordered movements characterized by short and jerky movements. Classic or pure ataxia is present where muscle tone is normal or decreased.

Ataxic
The findings are usually symmetrical, with incoordinate movements and intention tremor.

Ataxic diplegia
The findings are tremor and ataxia with spasticity of the legs.

Aetiology Cerebellar hypoplasia. In those born at term, half are the result of genetic conditions.

Dyskinetic or dyskinesia

This refers to disordered movement comprising slow and writhing movements where muscle tone fluctuates between increased and decreased tone. Most individuals are unable to walk because of incoordination and unwanted movements. Involvement of orofacial muscles leads to problems with articulation and feeding.

Athetosis
There is poor postural control, generalized incoordination and hyperkinetic movements. There is often normal intelligence.

Aetiology Asphyxia in the term infant leading to damage to the basal ganglia.

Choreoathetoid
There is slow writhing movement with reduced voluntary control.

Aetiology Kernicterus, now rare.

Dystonia
There is changing tone, usually affecting all four limbs and associated with severe disability.

Cerebral palsy is a disorder that can result in considerable impairment leading to disability and handicap.

Definitions

- **Disorder:** a medically definable condition or disease entity
- **Impairment:** any loss or abnormality of psychological, physiological or anatomical structure or function
- **Disability:** any restriction or lack (resulting from an impairment) of ability to perform an activity in the manner or within the range considered normal for a human being
- **Handicap:** the impact of the impairment or disability on the person's pursuit or achievement of the goals which are desired by him or her or expected of him or her by society

Diagnosis of cerebral palsy

The diagnosis is based on a careful history, examination and consideration of the development and cause of the motor disorder. Magnetic resonance imaging (MRI) can show evidence of hypoxic or vascular damage to the brain. Where the finding doesn't quite fit or there is a suggestion of regression, a neurology opinion should be sought to consider other conditions that may be mistaken for CP:

- Tumours around the skull base
- Spinal cord lesions
- Hereditary spastic paraplegia
- Metachromatic leucodystrophy
- Dopa-responsive dystonias
- Organic acidaemias
- Hereditary ataxias

Management of cerebral palsy

A multidisciplinary approach is required. As well as therapy input, there needs to be input from the orthotist and an orthopaedic surgeon with an interest in CP. Management of spasticity is becoming increasingly complex with the development of gait analysis and new therapies such as botulinum toxin. Increasingly, specialist spasticity services are being set up, which bring together neurologists, orthopaedic surgeons and physiotherapists who have developed expertise in this area.

Children with cerebral palsy often have other problems, reflecting more widespread damage to the brain:

- Learning difficulties
- Visual impairment
- Squint
- Hearing loss
- Speech and language disorders
- Swallowing difficulties leading to lung disease and growth failure
- Epilepsy
- Behaviour disorders

These too will need to be addressed and may mean the child attending several specialist clinics. It is important that the paediatrician overseeing the child's care pulls together all the different strands of the various interventions.

Table 27.3   Presenting features of cerebral palsy

- Abnormal tone and posturing in infancy
- Delayed motor milestones
- Abnormal gait once walking is achieved
- Feeding difficulties
- Cognitive developmental delay

Meaning of the history in George

Many children who develop CP are identified as being at risk in the neonatal period because of hypoxic–ischaemic encephalopathy, abnormality on cranial ultrasonography or prematurity. Presenting features of cerebral palsy are shown in Table 27.3. The early history and subsequent delay in motor development with abnormality of tone and increased reflexes indicated that CP was the likely diagnosis. The findings on the head scan fit with the clinical picture of spastic diplegia.

Spastic diplegia has a lower risk of associated medical problems, such as feeding difficulties. George is healthy and hasn't developed chronic lung disease. His hearing and vision have been normal on previous testing.

George's main problems relate to his motor impairment. Careful assessment will be required to determine the help he will need to access the school curriculum educationally and socially. He has good social skills and appears to benefit from mixing with his peers. It is not uncommon for parents to be anxious about finding the right school placement. They face difficult choices, particularly in choosing between special and mainstream schools.

Educational assessment

Formal assessment of a child's needs is a comprehensive look at their health, educational and social needs.

Self-test 4: Who of the following may be asked to contribute to formal educational assessment?
A Parents
B Social worker
C Teacher

D Physiotherapist
E Paediatrician
F Psychiatrist

Answer: All of them.

All the professionals involved with George are asked for a contribution and George's parents will be asked to state their views of his needs and their preferred school.

The following issues need to be considered when a child with a disability such as cerebral palsy is due to start school and the paediatrician should cover all these points in his report:

- Medical needs
- Motor skills
- Communication
- Sensory
- Cognitive
- Self-help skills
- Social

Medical needs

The medical problems and how they should be managed must be clearly stated.

Children with severe disability often have additional problems, e.g. spastic tetraplegia is usually associated with feeding difficulties. Incoordination of swallowing caused by bulbar involvement may lead to aspiration and chronic lung problems. Children often require calorie supplementation and, for some, a feeding gastrostomy is the only way that they can be safely fed and receive adequate nutrition.

Epilepsy, too, is common and may be difficult to control fully. Carers need to be aware of the first-aid management of epilepsy and be able to administer treatment for prolonged seizures.

Motor skills

The LEA need to know the extent of the child's motor impairment and what this means in practical terms. The occupational therapist's and physiotherapist's reports will expand on this and advise on management of the motor difficulties and use of mobility aids, equipment

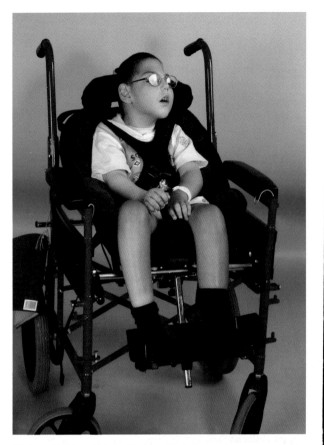

Figure 27.3 Child with spastic tetraplegia in moulded seat to provide optimal positioning and support. (Reproduced with permission of the patient's mother.)

and seating (Figure 27.3). Fine motor difficulties may cause problems with writing and drawing, and other means of recording may need to be developed.

Communication

Communication may be difficult for children who have bulbar involvement and particularly those with athetoid cerebral palsy. Alternative means of communication may be necessary, such as use of symbols or electronic devices.

Sensory

Sensory impairment is common. A significant proportion of children with spastic tetraplegia have cortical vision impairment with very limited vision. Children with a hemiplegia may have an associated visual field defect.

Cognitive

Children with spastic tetraplegia often have severe cognitive impairment whereas children born pre-term who have a diplegia may have good intellectual ability. Some children may have specific difficulties with reading, writing, or attention and perceptual problems.

Self-help skills

The ability to carry out these skills will depend on the child's cognitive ability and motor skills. The child's ability to manage toileting, feeding and dressing needs to be considered.

Social

All children need the opportunity to be with other children to develop their social skills and play. There may be few preschool opportunities for a child with a disability, who consequently may be shy and not sure how to mix and make friends. The school needs to be aware of this and have the ability to develop the child's social skills as well as meeting the educational needs.

Interpretation of the assessment

It is apparent that George's major problem is his limited mobility and the need for assistance with self-help skills. George enjoys being with his peers and should cope socially in a busy nursery class of 30 children. His development is age appropriate. The professionals are confident that he will manage in a mainstream nursery class, with the right physical support. The school will need to have an appropriate physical environment, so that George can easily get around.

Investigations

Careful planning should mean that no further investigations are needed at this stage. However, in view of Susan's concerns about his phonology, the speech and language therapist arranges to assess George further.

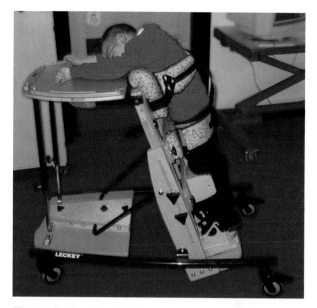

Figure 27.4　Standing frame.

Health needs

The physiotherapist has advised that George's progress be monitored by a physiotherapist who will put in place a programme of therapy depending on the goals and objectives from regular assessments. In the short term, George needs input to improve his mobility and to work towards independent walking. Some time in a standing frame each day is advised (Figure 27.4).

The occupational therapist (OT) has recommended a special chair to improve George's stability when sitting, which will facilitate fine motor skills. The OT will need to monitor his progress and devise therapy programmes according to need.

The speech and language therapist does not consider that speech and language therapy is required. She has found that George's articulation is immature but is developing along normal lines, and should continue to improve with time. His parents and the classroom assistant can be given some pointers on how to help him with this.

George will require a support assistant to ensure his physical safety, to help with his mobility, to carry out programmes of intervention devised by the therapists and to assist him accessing all aspects of school life. The assistant will also help with any toileting or dressing needs.

Management and follow-up plan

The paediatrician, therapists and advisory teacher discuss George's progress and his educational needs with his mother. The advisory teacher answers some specific questions about the educational assessment process and ensures that Susan has the contact number for the educational officer administering the process, and the Parent Partnership officer who is available to support parents through the assessment. This can be a very anxious time for parents:

- Starting school can be a distressing time for the family of a child with a disability. Visiting schools, especially a special school, may result in parents becoming much more aware of the reality of their child's problems
- Starting school is an important time for any child and many parents feel anxious about how their child will cope. George's mother may be concerned that he won't have the support he needs
- Choosing the right school is never easy. Professionals can provide information, but the final decision is that of the parents

The therapists and paediatrician will continue to review George regularly in clinic. The health team must liaise with the school and provide reports for school reviews. Attendance at such reviews may be helpful, particularly if problems occur. School needs to keep a careful watch on George's progress. He may have some specific learning difficulties and perceptual problems, which become apparent as the academic work becomes more challenging. Poor attention and concentration are a relatively common feature in children born prematurely.

Careful review will be required for transfer to senior school, for leaving school and at transfer to adult services.

Background information

Cerebral palsy

Epidemiology

Prevalence figures in developed countries are 2–2.5 per 1000 live births and have remained unchanged over

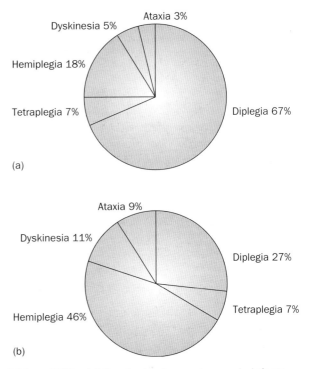

(a)

(b)

Figure 27.5 (a) Cerebral palsy syndromes in infants born pre-term; (b) cerebral palsy syndromes in infants born at term. (Taken from: Parkes J, Donnelly M, Hill N. *Focusing on Cerebral Palsy*. London: Scope, 2001.)

recent years. Between 25 and 40 per cent of cases are found in the 6–7 per cent of children who weighed under 2500 g at birth. The distribution of subtypes differs between pre-term infants (dominated by spastic diplegia) and term infants with CP (dominated by spastic hemiplegia). Spastic subtypes account for more than 90 per cent of CP overall (Figure 27.5).

Aetiology

Approximately 80 per cent have a prenatal aetiology – genetic, cerebral dysgenesis, intrauterine infection, maternal placental disease in term infants, and intra- or periventricular haemorrhage and periventricular leucomalacia in pre-term babies. Intrapartum and postnatal events each account for 10 per cent of cases. Causes include perinatal hypoxic–ischaemic encephalopathy, meningitis, cardiorespiratory arrest and trauma often resulting from non-accidental injury.

Neurophysiology

Spastic CP results from damage to the pyramidal system (motor cortex and internal capsule), which is responsible for voluntary movements that result in:

- Impaired voluntary control
- Abnormal muscle tone and muscle weakness
- Dependence on primitive patterns of mobility
- Agonist/antagonist muscle imbalance around joints leading to fixed joint positions and contractures
- Preserved primitive reflexes

Dyskinetic CP and ataxic CP result from damage to the extrapyramidal system (basal ganglia and cerebellum, respectively).

Legal framework

Meeting the needs of children with special needs is a statutory matter as determined by the 1981, 1993 and 1996 Education Acts and the Special Educational Needs and Disability Act 2001.

The 1981 Education Act

The Act made considerable changes to the way children with a disability should be educated:

- The concept of handicap should be replaced by that of special educational needs
- Parents should have more say in the education of their children
- Children should be integrated into mainstream school if this meets their needs and that of their classmates

The Act recognized that up to 20 per cent of children experience difficulties, needing special help at some stage of their schooling. The Act defined a child with special needs as one who has 'significantly greater difficulty in learning than the majority of children of his age or has a disability which prevents or hinders him making use of the educational facilities generally provided for children of his age'. The LEA must make special educational provision available for such children.

Most children with severe disabilities are known to the paediatrician long before they are of school age.

The health authority must notify the LEA that a child may have special educational needs when the child reaches the age of 2 years.

Such children, particularly if they have complex needs, require a more detailed multidisciplinary assessment. Professional's written advice is submitted to the LEA who decide whether the child's difficulties are sufficiently severe to require a 'Statement of Special Educational Need'.

Later Acts have updated this legislation, included a Code of Practice (recently revised) on identification and assessment of special educational needs, and strengthened the presumption of mainstream schooling for children with special needs.

Further sources of information

Article

Rosenbloom L. Diagnosis and management of cerebral palsy. *Archives of Disease in Childhood* 1995; **72**: 350–4

Report

Parkes J, Donnelly M, Hill N. *Focusing on Cerebral Palsy*. London: Scope, 2001

Website

www.scope.org.uk

Self-test 5: Seven-year-old Brian has sustained a severe head injury. He is an inpatient being managed by the head injury rehabilitation team. It is apparent that he will have long-term motor impairment and learning difficulties. The team are preparing Brian for discharge.

A **What should the team arrange to facilitate discharge?**

B **Which professionals need to be involved?**

C **What needs to be done to ensure that Brian's educational needs will be met?**

Answers:

A A discharge planning meeting involving the hospital team and the community team who will be taking over Brian's care once discharged

B The community paediatrician would usually coordinate the child's care, involving therapists, social worker and educational psychologist, according to the child's needs

C As soon as it was apparent that Brian would have additional educational needs, a formal referral should have been sent to the education authority. A representative from the LEA could also be asked to the discharge planning meeting

Wetting the bed

Age: 8 years

JACKIE GREGG

Presentation

Referral letter from GP:
Please see this 8-year-old girl with bed-wetting. Jayne wets the bed most nights but is otherwise healthy. Her mother wet the bed up until the age of 10 years. I've sent a urine specimen for culture.

Initial considerations and action

Nocturnal enuresis, or wetting during sleep, may be defined as the reflex action of micturition occurring in an individual who has failed to gain bladder control at the normal age without organic pathology.

It is not a single entity and a number of factors may be involved in any one child, so individual assessment is necessary. Primary enuresis occurs in a child who has always been wet at night and secondary enuresis occurs after a period of established bladder control – it is likely to be associated with a precipitating event such as starting school or a urinary tract infection.

Enuresis is very common and a medical or anatomical cause is extremely rare. An appointment is made for the enuresis clinic run by the clinical nurse specialist, who has access to the paediatrician, should further medical assessment be required.

Self-test 1: Which factors in the history would suggest a medical or anatomical cause for the enuresis?

Answer: Daytime wetting, poor stream, recurrent urinary tract infections (UTIs), poor bowel control.

History

Jayne attends the clinic with her mother and a detailed history is taken. The list below outlines the key areas to be covered. The family had been asked to keep a record of wetting for the 2 weeks before the clinic visit.

- **Wetting:**
  - how many times per night/week/month – is there a pattern?
  - at what time of night?
  - fluid intake
  - daytime wetting: time of day, severity
  - urgency, frequency, urinary stream
  - size of wet patch
- Bowel control
- **Bedroom:**
  - sharing room, sharing bed
  - heating
  - access to toilet/potty
- **Family reaction:**
  - are nappies worn?
  - what happens when child wets?
  - what gain does the child/parent obtain?
  - previous management used: rewards, punishment, lifting, fluid restriction
  - previous treatment failures
- **Sleep routine:**
  - bedtime, sleep time, getting up time
  - spontaneous waking, getting up to urinate
- Family history of enuresis
- **Education:**
  - academic progress, developmental milestones
  - bullying at school
  - friends who are also enuretic

- **Medical conditions:** urinary tact infections, nocturnal symptoms, e.g. asthma, eczema

Jayne is a healthy girl. She was toilet trained by day at 2½ years, but continued to wet the bed each night until she started school, when her mum felt that she should no longer wear nappies. Since then, she wets the bed four to five nights every week, usually on a Sunday and Monday night, although there is no pattern to the other nights. It's not quite clear when Jayne wets the bed because she doesn't usually waken. The family describe her as a deep sleeper, because nothing disturbs her once she is asleep. She hasn't had any daytime wetting or urgency.

Jayne is very embarrassed about her problem and doesn't want her friends or 10-year-old brother to know. She has her own bedroom, so it has been possible to keep the matter private. Mum wet the bed up until the age of 10. Jayne and her mum want the problem sorted so that, by the time Jayne gets invited to friend's houses for sleep-overs, she will be able to go without anxiety. Jayne goes to bed at 8 pm and her mum has tried lifting her at 11 pm, but with little success. Her mum has restricted fluids after 6 pm with no improvement. Dad has promised her a new bike when she stops wetting the bed – Jayne is very despondent that she will never get this reward.

Jayne is doing well at school and achieved above-average results in the standard assessment tests (SATs) – her reward was going to Disney World. She is popular, likes school and works hard. Her mother has no fears about possible bullying.

Interpretation of the history

A useful way of understanding enuresis is by thinking of it as a problem in one or more of the following three systems (the three systems approach):

- A lack of vasopressin release
- A problem of bladder instability
- An inability to waken in response to the sensation of a full bladder

This can be helpful in selecting the most appropriate treatment. Clinical signs indicative of each of the systems are:

- **Lack of vasopressin release:**
  - wets soon after going to sleep
  - large wet patches
  - dry nights only if the child wakes to go to toilet
  - weak urine concentration
- **Bladder instability:**
  - frequent daytime voiding
  - low voided volumes
  - multiple wetting at night
  - variable size of wet patch
  - wakes after wetting
- **Inability to waken from sleep:**
  - sleeping through wetting
  - an inability to wake from sleep

The nurse needs to consider:

- **Potentiating and associated factors:**
  - excessive fluid intake before bedtime (drinking a lot of fluid may be a habit, but diabetes mellitus needs to be excluded
  - fizzy drinks and caffeine
  - psychological stressors such as bullying, school failure or abuse
  - general immaturity or global developmental delay
  - restriction of fluids is ineffective in reducing bedwetting

Factors resulting in poor outcome:
  - adverse family reaction to a wet bed
  - failure with previously tried methods.
  - poor motivation: likely if several of the child's friends are enuretic or if there is a strong family history of enuresis, which occurs in 30–75 per cent of patients
  - behavioural difficulties and family stress
  - punishments in children who bedwet may be abusive and may prolong the wetting
- **Factors indicating a medical or anatomical cause:**
  - daytime urgency and wetting
  - poor urinary stream
  - recurrent urinary tract infections
  - poor bowel control

Bowel symptoms may have either a neurological or psychological cause, and management of the soiling rather than the wetting is usually a priority for the patient and family. It requires different clinical investigations from those recommended for enuresis alone.

Meaning of the history

The history has not identified any likely underlying organic cause for the enuresis. There is nothing in the history to suggest bladder instability or a lack of vasopressin release. Sleeping through the wetting and being a 'deep sleeper' suggest an inability to wake from sleep in response to a full bladder.

Jayne's mum's expectations seem appropriate, but the nurse felt that she might be putting too much pressure on Jayne to become dry. Wetting most Sundays may be related to Jayne being overtired if she has late nights at the weekend or possibly some anxieties about the next day at school. Jayne is said to be a conscientious pupil but her mum seems to place a lot of emphasis on academic achievement. Dad's promise to get her a bike when she becomes dry must seem totally unobtainable to Jayne and therefore is not a useful motivator.

Examination

A full examination is carried out:

- **Examination:**
  - height and weight, previous growth data
  - blood pressure
  - abdomen: palpable bladder? abnormal genitalia?
  - neurological examination of lower limbs, perineal sensation and reflexes
  - spine: sacral dimple? Sacral hairy patch?
- **Investigations:**
  - urinalysis
  - midstream urine for culture
  - measurement of urine output and fluid intake
- Jayne's height and weight are both on the 9th centiles
- Review of growth on the centile charts does not show any slowing of growth, which may indicate a chronic systemic disorder such as chronic renal failure
- Blood pressure is normal
- The anogenital area is of normal appearance
- Neurological examination normal
- Spine and overlying skin – no deformity or spina bifida

Self-test 2: Which abnormalities should be looked for in the anogenital area?

Answer: The position of the urethral opening should be checked for anomalous bladder drainage, and the anus for evidence of poor muscular tone indicative of a neurological abnormality. (A digital rectal examination, to assess tone and sensation, is not routinely carried out in children.) Findings of possible sexual abuse – refer to a paediatrician experienced in sexual abuse for further examination if indicated.

Self-test 3: What is the significance of a sacral pit or hairy patch?

Answer: Either may indicate an abnormality of the spinal cord requiring further investigation.

Self-test 4: Which nerve roots are responsible for bladder control and how do you test their function?

Answer: The roots of S1 and S2. Assess by testing ankle reflexes, looking for clawing of the toes and testing for sensation of the saddle area. A palpable bladder on abdominal examination may indicate a problem with bladder emptying as a result of impaired innervation.

The examination of Jayne was normal.

Interpretation of the examination

History and examination have not revealed any likely underlying pathology as a cause for the enuresis.

Jayne and her mother appear well motivated, with a positive attitude to treatment. There don't appear to be any negative factors.

Investigations

A clean catch midstream urine specimen taken in a sterile bottle is sent for examination and culture. The urine culture and examination for cells, blood and sugar were negative.

Jayne is asked to record her daily fluid intake on a couple of occasions, which is normal. She is also asked to measure urine output at each voiding over three to four 24-hour periods. Low or variable volumes of urine are found in bladder instability, because the bladder contractions lead to voiding before the bladder is full.

Children with daytime urinary symptoms and those with any congenital abnormality of the perineal region should be referred to a paediatrician or paediatric urologist for anatomical, functional and urodynamic investigation of the urinary tract.

Diagnosis

Nocturnal enuresis caused by an inability to wake from sleep in response to full bladder sensations.

Management and follow-up plan

General measures

- Regular review and supportive approach. Seeing the patient frequently helps with nocturnal bladder control, irrespective of the treatment used, and success is unlikely without it
- Give simple explanation of how the bladder works
- Provide reassurance and explanation about enuresis to the child and parents – will allay anxiety and adjust parental expectations
- Put problem in context: 15 per cent of 5 year olds are enuretic and 16 per cent of these remit each year
- Provide printed information from ERIC (Enuresis Resource and Information Centre)
- Assess parental expectations – intolerance worsens prognosis
- Assess family and child for functional pay-offs when wetting occurs
- Organize the keeping of a diary of wetting
- Use of alarm, desmopressin or bladder training as clinically indicated. The three systems approach provides an explanation of bedwetting that parents and children can understand. Compliance will be improved when families understand why a particular treatment is being used

Support
- Don't feel you're on your own
- Up to 20% wet at 5 years of age

Rewards
- Praise/reward improvements or progress towards becoming dry

Bladder control
- Encourage child to feel bladder sensations when full
- Encourage child to hold before toileting
- Measure functional bladder capacity

Fluids
- Increase daytime drinks
- Allow a small drink before bed
- Avoid fizzy drinks

Waking
- Stop lifting
- Ensure child is awake if you toilet him or her during the night

Expectation
- Try without nappies
- Look for any small signs of progress
- Expect progress

Your feelings
- Keep calm
- Don't feel guilty
- Don't lose your temper

Keep it positive
- Don't blame your child or yourself
- Don't think you've failed
- Focus on improvements, not wet nights

Toileting
- Make the toilet a pleasant place to be
- Encourage child to toilet last thing before sleep
- Praise child for waking at night to toilet

Figure 28.1 General strategies for the under-7s.

Children under 7 years of age

Children under 7 years of age who regularly wet the bed should be regarded as normal. However, this may cause or be a sign of considerable family distress. General management strategies are shown in Figure 28.1. Support from the health visitor or possibly social services may help.

Children over 7 years

Star charts and rewards may be used to change behaviour, such as compliance with treatment, while working towards the long-term goal of dryness. The reward has to be immediately obtainable and attempts should be made to change only one behaviour at a time. Children may feel guilty and responsible about wetting. Encouraging them to help strip the bed and remake it will make them feel that they are helping.

Alarms

Enuresis alarms (Figure 28.2) are indicated for children who don't waken in response to a full bladder. They can be effective even if they also have a lack of vasopressin and bladder instability. In motivated families, use of the alarm gives a success rate of 65–70 per cent.

How to use an enuresis alarm

- **Indication:** a child who doesn't waken in response to a full bladder
- **Case selection:** high degree of compliance and motivation from child and family required for success
- **Choice of alarm:** bedside unit or body worn unit, personal preference of child
- **How does it work:** conditioning therapy – the child learns to perceive the sensation of a full bladder while asleep and wake in time to go to the toilet. The principle consists of a detector mechanism, which becomes activated when wet. The sensor is connected to a battery and a loud buzzer. The buzzer goes off when the child wets, which wakes the child, who gets out of bed, turns off the buzzer and goes to the toilet. Initially the alarm sounds only after or during voiding, but gradually awakening and inhibition of voiding are associated with full bladder awareness
- **Preparation:** education of child and family in use of the alarm, forewarning of possible initial 'teething troubles'
- **Support:** weekly support from enuresis nurse initially and regular contact thereafter. Rewards or incentives for realistic goals

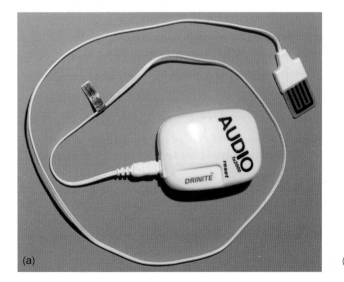

(a)

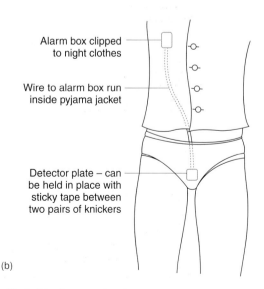

Alarm box clipped to night clothes

Wire to alarm box run inside pyjama jacket

Detector plate – can be held in place with sticky tape between two pairs of knickers

(b)

Figure 28.2 (a) Body-worn enuresis alarm; (b) diagram to show siting of body-worn alarm.

Desmopressin

The use of the synthetic analogue of the antidiuretic hormone desmopressin is the recommended intervention for young people who have a lack of vasopressin because it decreases urine production. It can be taken as tablets or a nasal spray. It is taken for 6 months and, if the child is dry and confident, it is gradually withdrawn over a period of 8 weeks. Control is rapid and therefore it can also be useful when a child spends nights away from home or for children for whom the alarm has been unsuitable.

Bladder training and oxybutynin

This is used to improve bladder stability and functional bladder capacity. It involves:

- Voiding as soon as there is a sense of urgency
- Regular fluid intake during the day
- Regular voiding during the day
- Relaxing when voiding

The anticholinergic drug oxybutynin relaxes the detrusor muscles around the bladder. The two combined have had a 70–100 per cent success rate in enuresis caused by bladder instability.

Self-test 5: How should Jayne be managed?

Answer: Use of enuresis alarm and general support.

Management of Jayne

The specialist nurse reassures Jayne and her mother that there is no pathological cause for the wetting. She provides an explanation of the working of the bladder and provides information leaflets on enuresis. Jayne is asked to continue to keep a diary of dry nights, to change herself when wet, to help mum change the bed and to put her wet things in the laundry basket. Her mum is asked to explore with school whether there are any issues that may be worrying Jayne.

The nurse discusses the enuresis alarm and trains Jayne and her mum in its use. It is agreed that Jayne will receive a reward for cooperating with the use of the alarm. The nurse asks Jayne's mum to ring her if there are any difficulties or should there be anything else she wishes to discuss. She does ring. There aren't any problems in school, but she realizes that she may have been putting some pressure on Jayne.

Jayne is seen 2 weeks later and she is coping well with the alarm. Jayne has been very cooperative with the treatments and has earned her reward of some Harry Potter stickers. The diary shows four dry nights in the previous week, which she is very proud of. Jayne has been asked to spend a night at her cousin's and is very anxious. The nurse arranges for the doctor to prescribe desmopressin and advises Jayne to use it first at home to check that it works.

After 3 months Jayne is dry most nights and dad has surprised her with the new bike. She hasn't been using the alarm for several weeks, but has continued with the other behavioural measures. She has decided to return the alarm, but wants to continue to use desmopressin for nights away from home. The nurse suggests that she try without it when she has a night with a trusted family member such as grandma, to see whether she still needs it. Jayne and her mum don't want to come back to clinic, but want the reassurance of keeping in touch by phone.

Background information

Epidemiology

About 15 per cent of 5 year olds, 10 per cent of 10 year olds and 1–1.5 per cent of adults bed wet. It is more common in boys and in social classes 4 and 5.

Aetiology

There are genetic, behavioural and cultural factors in its pathogenesis.

Lack of vasopressin release

Less urine is usually produced during sleep. This occurs via the release of arginine vasopressin (AVP) during sleep. AVP is produced by the hypothalamus, stored in the posterior pituitary gland and released in a pulsatile manner throughout sleep. AVP acts through the kidneys, increasing reabsorption of water and consequently reducing nocturnal urine production. Studies have shown that many children with enuresis have very low AVP production.

Bladder instability

The bladder remains stable when filling and has a reasonably large capacity. Research in Japan has shown that 32 per cent of a sample of children with enuresis had uninhibited bladder contractions during the filling phase, resulting in wetting before the bladder was full. It is suggested that this occurs only during sleep, so the child doesn't experience daytime wetting, although there may be some symptoms of bladder instability during the day.

An inability to waken in response to a full bladder

Sleep studies show that children with enuresis do not sleep more deeply; nor do wetting episodes occur in deep sleep any more than they do in light sleep. Enuretic children have problems in waking from sleep. They may fail to wake in response to external signals, such as an unexpected noise as well as the sensation of a full bladder.

Physiology

Micturition is a reflex action, initiated by the stretching of the bladder muscle as the bladder fills with urine (Figure 28.3). The afferent impulses pass up the pelvic splanchnic nerves and enter the second, third and fourth sacral segments of the spinal cord. Efferent impulses leave the cord from the same segments and pass via the parasympathetic preganglionic nerve fibres through the pelvic splanchnic nerves and the pelvic plexus to the bladder wall, where they synapse with postganglionic neurons. By means of this nervous pathway, the smooth muscle of the bladder wall is made to contract, and the sphincter vesicae (circular component of the muscle that is thickened at the base of the bladder) is made to relax. Efferent impulses also pass to the urethral sphincter via the pudendal nerve (S2, S3 and S4), and this undergoes relaxation. Once urine enters the urethra,

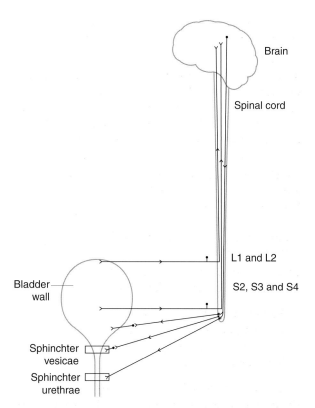

Figure 28.3 Diagram of nervous control of the bladder (sympathetic fibres have been omitted for simplification).

additional afferent impulses pass to the spinal cord from the urethra and reinforce the reflex action.

In young children, micturition is a simple reflex act and takes place whenever the bladder becomes distended. In the adult, this simple stretch reflex is inhibited by the activity of the cerebral cortex until the time and place for micturition are favourable. The inhibitory fibres pass downwards with the pyramidal tracts to the second, third and fourth sacral segments of the cord.

Further sources of information

Book

Butler RJ. *Understanding Nocturnal Enuresis, The Three Systems Approach*. Supported by an educational grant from Ferring Pharmaceuticals Ltd, Feltham, Middlesex

Article

Evans JHC. Evidence based management of nocturnal enuresis. *British Medical Journal* 2001; **323**: 1167–9

Website

www.eric.org.uk

Enuresis Resource and Information Centre.

Self-test 6: Phillip, aged 9 years, is seen in the enuretic clinic. He wets the bed most nights and doesn't want to talk about it. He is one of six children and shares a bedroom with two of his brothers. His mum says that she is fed up washing the sheets and his dad shouts at Phillip for wetting. They haven't tried any specific treatment other than taking him to the toilet at 11pm, which Phillip is now resisting.

A What is the likely success with the alarm?
B Indicate why the alarm is likely to be successful/unsuccessful
C What treatment would you try and why?

Answers:

A Poor
B Phillip shares a room, his family don't appear committed at present, and Phillip seems totally fed up and would be unlikely to cooperate
C Desmopressin: this would take the pressure off the mum, it would give Phillip a sense of achievement and raise his self-esteem, and get his dad off his back.

Chronic disorder

Pain and difficulty with passing stools

Age: 3 years

STEVEN RYAN

Presentation

A general practitioner referred Hannah with the following:

Please could you see this 3-year-old girl with constipation that has not responded to laxative treatment.

Self-test 1: What are the types of laxative commonly used?

Answer: Bulk forming, stool softener, stimulant, osmotic.

Initial considerations and action

- Normal human bowel habits are tremendously variable: in adults the expected range of stool frequency is from around once every 3 days to three times a day – a tenfold difference. In a population of Liverpool children, the whole gut transit time (which is mostly made up of colonic transit time) ranged from 7 to 90 hours
- Is the label of 'constipation' correct? A general definition of constipation is infrequent stools or hard painful stools and in children the condition is frequently associated with soiling – the involuntary passage of fluid stool. Voluntary soiling is known as encopresis and is always psychologically mediated. One definition of constipation in children is two of the following:
  - fewer than three stools a week
  - two episodes of soiling per week
  - a large stool every 7–30 days
  - palpable rectal or faecal mass
- Most constipation is functional but uncommonly may be the result of a structural abnormality or other pathological process
- However, many parents and grandparents believe that constipation in childhood is uncommon and must have a serious cause that requires investigation
- Childhood constipation is difficult to treat effectively but a variety of laxative treatments is available. Was the correct dose used in this case?
- Diet seems a much less important factor, at least in young children, compared with adults

History

The following history was obtained:

Hannah was passing one large hard stool every week. There was only intermittent slight soiling. She disliked defecation, finding it painful and on occasions she had also passed blood when passing a stool. Parents reported that her appetite became poor and abdomen mildly distended just before having her bowels opened. It had all started 6 months previously when she had been unwell with a cough and fever.

Her father in particular had thought she was being 'lazy' and had on occasions been upset with her. Once she was forced to sit on the toilet for 2 hours and was now scared to use the toilet or potty.

This seemed to have made the problem worse. Generally, she had a good range of foods in her diet including fruits and vegetables, but was a 'picky' eater. There was no excessive milk intake.

Hannah was currently on no drug treatment but had been tried on lactulose – an osmotic laxative – although she stopped taking it when a small dose seemed ineffective.

Self-test 2: List the possible maintaining factors in Hannah's case.

Answer: Recurrent anal fissure; fear of pain on defecation; negative association with toileting; possible poor diet; failure to use adequate treatment for long enough.

The history has several important components:

- **Confirming constipation:**
  - stool frequency
  - stool consistency
  - presence of soiling
  - symptoms on passing stool, e.g. abdominal or anal pain, rectal bleeding, posture, behaviour, effort involved
- Associated gastrointestinal symptoms, e.g. abdominal pain, distension, poor appetite
- **Consideration of initiating and maintaining factors:**
  - Illness: an acute illness can initiate constipation by, for example, causing dehydration and anorexia which leads to the formation of hard stools that can cause an anal fissure; the child is then afraid to defecate because of pain and this leads to persistent stool retention
  - Drugs: some drugs slow intestinal transit and are associated with constipation, the best known being opiates, e.g. codeine; these drugs may initiate the problem (as above) but persistent use can maintain constipation
  - Psychological including family:
    - the importance of these factors cannot be overestimated and for many children they become the most important maintaining factors
    - the interaction between the child and family may also exacerbate and maintain the problem by, for example, paying too much attention to stooling and toileting – it can become the centre of family life and tensions and the child may begin to use it to control the family
    - inappropriate chastisement or punishment
    - a lack of consistency within carers and between carers
    - child avoiding conflict and embarrassment by hiding soiled clothes
    - fear of the potty or the toilet because of association with pain, chastisement or humiliation
    - in the school setting: shame, bullying lack of privacy and confidentiality
  - Diet: although not usually a critical factor, the following dietary factors may be important:
    - low residue diet with few vegetables and fresh fruits
    - poor fluid intake
    - a high milk intake (usually associated with a poor intake of solid food) especially in toddlers and preschoolers
  - Established learning difficulties:
    - constipation is frequent in this situation and usually has a multifactorial basis; encopresis is also much more common in this group and both are very persistent
    - in children with Down's syndrome, it may result from hypothyroidism
  - Neurological disorder: a severe neurological disorder, such as spastic quadriplegic cerebral palsy, is almost always associated with constipation; important factors in these patients are:
    - poor, milk formula-based diet
    - inability to strain at stool
    - spastic muscle of defecation unable to relax
    - poor posture – unable to sit upright
    - dehydration
- **Consideration of other aetiologies:**
  - Congenital abnormalities of the lower bowel usually present in the newborn period but occasionally can present later. Late-onset Hirschsprung's disease (aganglionosis of the colon) is rare, but features suggesting its presence would include constipation from the

first day or two of life, and the absence of pain on defecation and the persistent passage of small pellets rather than large stools. Hypothyroidism can cause constipation but is usually associated with other features (see Chapter 39). Lower spinal neurological abnormality is also rarely associated with constipation and an important part of the examination is directed to this area. Features in the history suggesting this possibility include urinary incontinence and problems of gait. Note, however, that there is a strong association between constipation and recurrent urinary tract infections

– Treatment offered so far: in order to plan future treatment

---

Self-test 3: List the reasons why a child with cerebral palsy is more prone to constipation than other children.

Answer: Lack of voluntary muscle contraction or spastic muscles; poor diet – low in fibre and fruit; poor fluid intake; lack of gravity aiding defecation.

Examination

The purpose of the examination is to:

- Look for signs of chronic illness
- Seek signs of constipation, i.e. abdominal distension or faecal loading
- **Examine the anus (subject to consent) for:**
  - abnormal placing
  - fissures
  - anal tone
- **Exclude neurological disorders by:**
  - inspecting and palpating the lower vertebral column
  - observing gait
  - testing lower limb deep tendon reflexes and plantar reflexes
- Look for features of hypothyroidism including goitre, short stature, obesity, hair and skin in poor

condition, hoarse voice, bradycardia, cold peripheries, slow-relaxing deep-tendon reflexes

Rectal examination

Although inspection of the anus, subject to the child's consent, should always be undertaken, the same cannot be said of rectal examination. Whereas in adult anorectal disorders it is almost mandatory to undertake this examination, children are generally spared. The reasons include the lack of additional useful information that is obtained and the psychological trauma that may be involved. These factors need to be considered before undertaking rectal examination.

Hannah was an appropriate weight and height for her age and there were no signs of chronic disease, including hypothyroidism, or a neurological disorder. The diagrams show the findings on examination of the abdomen and anus. Her gait was normal as was her lower limb tone, power, and knee and ankle reflexes. Her plantar reflexes were down going. There were no features of hypothyroidism and no goitre. Inspection of her lumbar spine and sacrum revealed no abnormality. Rectal examination was not undertaken. Figure 29.1 shows the examination findings.

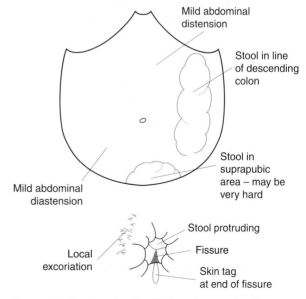

Figure 29.1   Examination findings in constipation.

Investigations

Although most children with constipation or soiling do not require any investigations, occasionally they are required.

- **Abdominal radiograph (Figure 29.2):** confirms stool retention; may be useful if primary problem is soiling caused by spurious diarrhoea
- **Lumbosacral radiograph:** if abnormality on inspection of lumbosacral spine
- **Magnetic resonance imaging (MRI) of lower spinal column and nerve roots:** if neurological deficit detected

- **Urinary tract ultrasonography:** if associated urinary symptoms
- **Thyroid function tests:** if clinical evidence of hypothyroidism
- **Rectal biopsy:** if Hirschsprung's disease is suspected

Hannah had no investigations undertaken.

Diagnosis

Simple functional constipation.

Self-test 4: For each of the percentages below, which of the subsequent descriptions about faecal continence is appropriate?
A 1 per cent
B 3 per cent
C 50 per cent
D 90 per cent
E 95 per cent
1 Children aged 3 who are continent
2 Children aged 21 months who are continent
3 Children aged 5 who occasionally soil
4 Children aged 5 who soil regularly
5 Children aged 5 who are clean night and day

Answers: 1D, 2C, 3B, 4A, 5E.

Management and prognosis

Hannah's mother had thought that Hannah must have a physical obstruction within the bowel, and had wanted investigations leading to its identification and treatment. The doctor understood why she had considered this possible cause, but then explained how Hannah's constipation had arisen. It was also reassuring to know that this was a very common problem. The model the doctor proposed was that a viral infection with fever and dehydration had led to stool hardening, which had caused a painful anal fissure. Consequently, Hannah had retained stool because of continuing fear of pain on defecation. This had led to an increase in the capacity of the rectum and a vicious circle of hard stool retention and recurrent anal fissure.

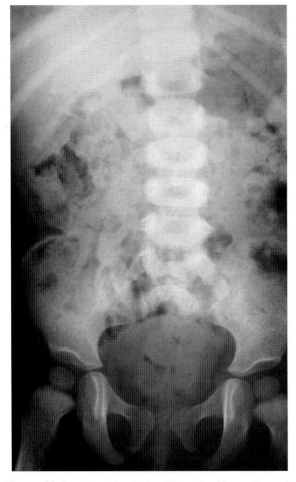

Figure 29.2 An abdominal radiograph with much stool, demonstrating constipation.

Communication

Probably the most important element of the first consultation at hospital is communication. It is important that, before initiating or changing treatment, the child and family understand the nature of functional constipation and its management. Medical treatment – with laxatives, for example – is often required for many months and compliance is an important issue. It is known that compliance is improved if patients have a good understanding of their condition. Specific points that should be covered are:

- Find out the parent's/child's current understanding and beliefs, to reinforce correct beliefs and negate erroneous ones (e.g. 'there must be a twist or blockage in the bowel)
- Explain in simple terms the normal function of the lower bowel, how constipation is initiated and how it is maintained
- Explain how treatments work and the time course over which they are effective (e.g. lactulose works by softening the stools, consistently, until the child is no longer fearful of passing hard painful stools)

- Explain that negative reinforcement (telling off, getting angry) is counterproductive
- The control of defecation is voluntary and behaviour modification using psychological techniques can be helpful – varying from simple reward systems (star charts) to detailed psychological intervention

Treatments

It was advised that Hannah recommenced treatment with lactulose, an osmotic stool softener. The advised dose was that which caused her stools to become persistently softer but without causing fluid diarrhoea. Her mother was asked to titrate the dose.

There is currently no systematic review comparing the efficacy of constipation treatments on long-term outcome. Treatment is therefore based on other evidence – basic physiological principles, single controlled trials – often looking at short-term outcomes and custom and practice. A range of interventions is possible (Table 29.1).

Lactulose and senna are the most frequently used medications in the UK and rectal administration is

Table 29.1   Interventions used in constipation

Intervention	Mechanism	Example
Medications		
Administered orally	Osmotic laxatives	Lactulose
	Stimulant laxatives	Senna
	Bulk laxatives	Bran fibre
	Stool softeners	Docusate, paraffin
Administered rectally	Osmotic laxatives	Sodium citrate
	Stimulant laxatives	Glycerol suppository
Psychological	Biofeedback training	
	Reward training	
	Regular toileting	
Dietary		
Foods	Increased fruits and vegetables	
	Increased intake of fruit juice	
Water	Increased water intake	

used as a last resort. This route is more commonly used in children with severe neurological impairment. Dietary adjustments are usually disappointing and this echoes the fact that dietary factors are less important in childhood constipation. In general, simple laxatives are used first and psychological interventions are reserved for later. However, if there is soiling with little constipation, i.e. encopresis, then this is the preferred route.

How to toilet train a child with constipation and soiling

- Sit him or her on the toilet regularly – three to four times a day
- Reward him or her for doing this (e.g. star chart)
- Particularly useful after meals – take advantage of the gastrocolic reflex

- Regularly check pants through the day – reward for cleanliness
- Especially reward for opening bowels in toilet
- Give him or her responsibility for aspects of cleanliness, e.g. 'new for old' underwear exchange
- General rules: be consistent, be positive, never punish

Normal defecation

Figure 29.3 shows the normal anatomy of the anorectum and associated pathways. The mechanism of normal defecation is:

- Stool arrives in the rectum and distends it – it contracts in response

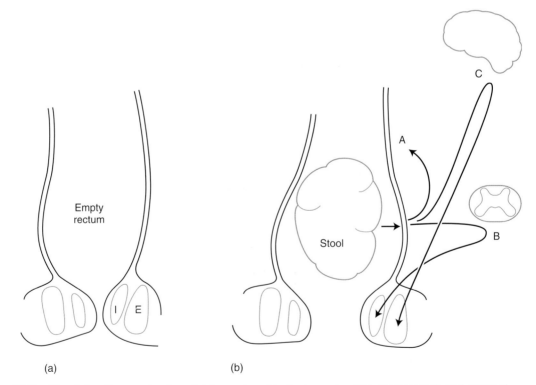

(a)   (b)

Figure 29.3 The defecation mechanism. (a) Anus closed by tonic contraction of internal (I) and external (E) sphincters; (b) stool stimulates stretch receptors, which: (A) intrinsically stimulates colonic contraction; (B) relaxes internal sphincter by reflex; and (C) initiates voluntary relaxation of the external sphincter and other voluntary muscle actions, e.g. straining.

- Stretch receptors are activated
- These receptors stimulate intramural neurons via synaptic connections
- These neurons inhibit muscle tone in the internal anal sphincter, causing relaxation
- Stool is now forced into the anal canal, stimulating receptors of sensory neurons under the epithelium
- A reflex then relaxes the external anal sphincter and allows defecation
- The action of the external sphincter is also under voluntary control so that the relaxation may be assisted or opposed
- Voluntary increase of intra-abdominal pressure by the Valsalva manoeuvre also assists defecation

Figure 29.4 shows situations in which normal defecation is prevented or inhibited as a result of problems with the normal mechanism.

Further sources of information

Articles

Brooks RC, Copen RM, Cox DJ, Morris J, Borowitz S, Sutphen J. Review of the treatment literature for encopresis, functional constipation, and stool-toileting refusal. *Annals of Behavioral Medicine* 2000; **22**: 260–7

Loening-Baucke V. Modulation of abnormal defecation dynamics by biofeedback treatment in chronically constipated children with encopresis. *Journal of Pediatrics* 1990; **116**: 214–22

Loening-Baucke V. Constipation in children. *Current Opinion in Pediatrics* 1994; **6**: 556–61

Loening-Baucke V. Management of chronic constipation in infants and toddlers [see comments].

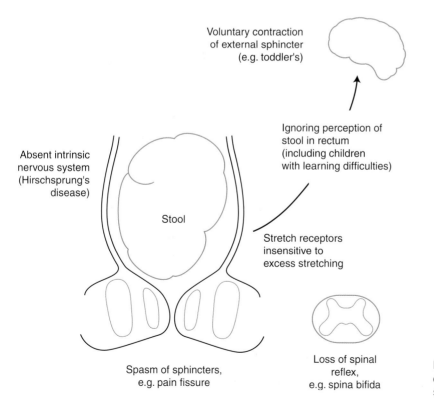

Figure 29.4 Abnormalities in the defecation mechanism. E, external sphincter; I, internal sphincter.

American Family Physician 1994; **49**: 397–400, 403–6, 411–13

Staiano A, Tozzi A. Diagnosis and treatment of constipation in children. *Current Opinion in Pediatrics* 1998; **10**: 512–15

Websites

www.jr2.ox.ac.uk/bandolier/band46/b46-3.html

Review of treatment of adult constipation.

Self-test 5: A 4-year-old boy is reviewed. He has constipation, passing a formed motion only about once a week. The stools are hard but, despite blood being passed from anal fissures, he has had little pain on defecation. He suffers from severe soiling and dirties several pairs of pants each day. He also suffers from bedwetting and daytime urinary incontinence. Examination shows that he has wasting of the calf muscles, and brisk knee and ankle reflexes.

A What underlying abnormality accounts for his symptoms?

B What further examination is required?

C Why does he suffer little pain on defecation despite anal fissures?

D What imaging investigations would be helpful?

E Is bedwetting, by itself, usually abnormal in a 4-year-old boy?

Answers:

A A lower spinal abnormality

B Examination of the lumbosacral vertebral area and of anal tone

C The neurological abnormality reduces sensation

D Radiograph of lumbosacral spine or MRI

E No, it's very common

Recurrent attacks of abdominal pain

Age: 7 years

STEVEN RYAN

Presentation

Kevin was being reviewed in outpatients by a paediatrician. He had already been reviewed twice and this was a follow-up visit. The paediatrician had not yet come to a conclusion on the nature of the pain and had been asking Kevin through his mother to keep a diary of the pain.

Initial considerations and action

The consultant had some medical students with him and he summarized as follows:

- Recurrent abdominal pain is very common
- Perhaps only 1 in 20 children presenting to him have a significant 'medical' condition
- It is important to identify such children so that they can be appropriately treated
- Important clues to this include the site and pattern of the pain, coexistent symptoms and abnormalities on physical examination
- Functional disorders such as constipation and migraine are responsible for many cases
- Very frequently no specific diagnosis or classification is possible and the term 'non-specific abdominal pain' may be applied
- Abdominal pain is also frequently a consequence of psychological problems (here the students agreed, remembering the mild abdominal discomfort they suffered before entering the examination hall!)
- Consequently, a holistic approach to the diagnosis and management of such children is necessary.

Other workers such as those in the child and adolescent mental health team may need to be brought in. Patience may be required to collect the necessary information and, in the absence of clues to 'organic' disease, this may be needed over several appointments

History

The consultant reviewed the history at presentation:

Kevin, aged 7, had been referred by his GP. He had been suffering from abdominal pain for about 6 months. The pain was intermittent, central periumbilical, colicky, each episode lasting about 1–2 hours. He felt nauseous through the attack and on three occasions had vomited. At that time there seemed to be no provoking factors in the environment, life or diet of Kevin. The family were not able to define the timing of attacks clearly, but they were as frequent as four to five times per week, and he was missing a significant amount of school with them. He was noted to be pale (his mother described him as looking 'green') during the episodes.

He was the first child of Sarah (28), a housewife, and Colin (32), a salesman who was on the road a lot and consequently spent a lot of time away from home. Sarah was therefore lonely and enjoyed Kevin's company. Indeed, sometimes when he had not gone to school because of his abdominal pain, and he felt better later in the day, he and his mother would go out together to the park or the shops. The family had moved into the area about 10 months ago. Kevin said he enjoyed his new school when asked directly by the doctor, but his mother said that he'd been a lot happier at his old school and thought it just needed time for him to settle in. His mother was in good health but, 1 year ago, had had a miscarriage which had been very upsetting, although they had not mentioned it to Kevin.

Self-test 1: What psychological factors might be responsible for Kevin's symptoms?

Answer: Worries about school; father being away from the home; attachment to mother; moving into a new area; mother's reaction to her miscarriage.

Kevin had otherwise had no health problems. In particular, he had a good appetite, no disorder of bowel habit and no urinary symptoms.

His father had irritable bowel syndrome. There was no family history of migraine.

The history is compatible with a functional cause of pain perhaps with psychological factors. To help exclude organic disease examination is required, even though it might be considered unlikely to reveal an abnormality. A normal examination is also useful for the purposes of reassurance.

> **How to differentiate organic and non-organic abdominal pain**
>
> See Table 30.1.

Examination (Figure 30.1 and Table 30.2)

The examination was unremarkable:

- Normal height and weight
- No sign of nutritional compromise
- Kevin looked at ease
- No signs of chronic disease – such as clubbing of the nails
- Kevin was not clinically anaemic
- Mouth, tongue and dentition were healthy
- Abdomen was soft, non-distended and there was no tenderness, either superficially or deeply

Table 30.1 Differentiating organic and non-organic pain on history

Feature	Organic pain	Inorganic pain
Time of day	Can wake from sleep	When awake
Time of week	Any time	Preschool is classic 'Monday morning' or better at weekends
Sites	Loins – renal Epigastric – stomach Right upper quadrant – liver Pelvis – ovarian pain	Central periumbilical
Degree of localization	May be very localized	Vague
Persistence	Yes	More intermittent
Family history	Not usually	Commonly chronic pain conditions such as irritable bowel or migraine
Other symptoms	Frequently, e.g. diarrhoea in bowel disease; vomiting with gastric disease	Not usually
Nutritional status	More likely to be compromised	Normal

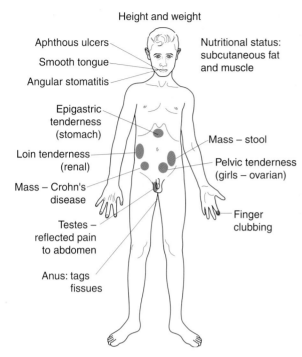

- Height and weight
- Aphthous ulcers
- Smooth tongue
- Angular stomatitis
- Nutritional status: subcutaneous fat and muscle
- Epigastric tenderness (stomach)
- Mass – stool
- Loin tenderness (renal)
- Pelvic tenderness (girls – ovarian)
- Mass – Crohn's disease
- Testes – reflected pain to abdomen
- Finger clubbing
- Anus: tags fissues

Figure 30.1 Features to seek in the examination of the child with recurrent abdominal pain.

- The liver and spleen were not palpable
- The lower pole of the right kidney was felt
- There were no faecal masses, especially in the left lower quadrant and suprapubically
- On inspection the anus was healthy with no evidence of fissure or anal tags
- Rectal examination was not performed
- His genitalia were healthy and both his testes were fully descended in the scrotum

Self-test 2: What could a finding of severe persistent mouth ulcers, anal fissure and a mass in the left iliac fossa indicate in a 14-year-old boy with weight loss?

A Constipation
B Crohn's disease
C Ulcerative colitis
D Coeliac disease
E Irritable bowel syndrome

Answer: B.

Self-test 3: What sign might be present in his hands?

A Splinter haemorrhages
B Clubbing of nails

Table 30.2 Clinical examination findings and their potential meaning in children with recurrent abdominal pain

Findings on examination	Potential meaning
Malnutrition	Underlying organic disease, especially malabsorption
Mouth ulcers	Inflammatory bowel disease
Smooth tongue, pale conjunctivae, angular stomatitis	Iron deficiency caused by iron malabsorption from small bowel disease
Anal tags	Recurrent anal fissures or Crohn's disease
Anal fissures	Constipation
Indentable mass in left iliac fossa	Constipation
Tenderness in loins	Renal disease, e.g. calculi, pyelonephritis
Epigastric tenderness	Dyspeptic disease, especially *Helicobacter pylori* infection
Mass with or without tenderness in right iliac fossa	Crohn's disease
Vesicular rash especially on buttocks	Coeliac disease (rash is dermatitis herpetiformis)
Pelvic tenderness or mass	Ovarian cyst, pelvic inflammatory disease

C Palmar erythema

D Dupuytren's contracture

Answer: B.

Most children presenting with abdominal pain have no abnormality on examination and therefore normal examination findings are reassuring. However, abnormal findings can indicate underlying disorders.

Investigations

No investigations were performed.

As there were no indications from the history and examination that there was a specific organic cause, no investigations were ordered. Investigations can be ordered to provide reassurance and some parents are very keen to have some tests done. This is reasonable provided that the tests are not too invasive and not too extensive. Some tests such as abdominal radiography are very insensitive and non-specific and, in view of the radiation dose involved, are disappearing from routine practice. Ultrasonography seems to be a reasonable alternative. Urine culture and microscopy are worthwhile and a simple blood count and inflammatory marker test (such as C-reactive protein or CRP) are reasonable. A sensitive and specific marker for coeliac disease (e.g. tissue transglutaminase) may be indicated because coeliac disease may not always present with other gastrointestinal symptoms. Table 30.3 shows a list of investigations to be undertaken in specific circumstances.

Further history

At the end of the first appointment the doctor said that he needed further information. He was pretty sure that there was no serious organic disease and he thought that Kevin had functional abdominal pain. He used the medical students' earlier comment to show how psychological factors can be responsible for physical symptoms, and asked Kevin's parents to reflect on this. He also asked them to keep a diary (Figure 30.2), which timed the episodes and also set them in the context of Kevin's life. In addition he suggested talking to Kevin's teacher.

School

Mrs Foster met Kevin's parents and said that he was a bit of a loner – he was very much seen as the new boy and she did wonder if there was 'something going on'. She would now keep a closer eye.

Rather than tell the family how he would summarize the evidence, the doctor asked Kevin's parents to say what

Table 30.3 Investigations of abdominal pain

Symptoms	Investigations
Urinary symptoms – frequency, dysuria, loin pain	Urine microscopy and culture, renal ultrasound
Dyspeptic symptoms and epigastric tenderness, heartburn	*Helicobacter pylori* serology, endoscopy with biopsy, urease test for *Helicobacter pylori* and culture
Features of inflammatory bowel disease	Full blood count, C-reactive protein, erythrocyte sedimentation rate, contrast study, endoscopy
Features of coeliac disease	IgA anti-endomysial antibodies in blood, endoscopy and biopsy of gut mucosa
Renal or ureteric colic	Renal ultrasonography, plain radiograph of abdomen
Recurrent pain and diarrhoea, bloating	Stool microscopy for ova, cysts and parasites (e.g. *Giardia lamblia*)
Pelvic pain, dyspareunia	Pelvic ultrasonography
Severe recurrent episodes of pain with vomiting	Amylase

they felt. This is an example of enhanced communication skills. By doing this he was able to find out what their knowledge, understanding and questions were. He listened actively and then he was able to summarize what was said:

- Kevin had pains at all sorts of time
- They were much more likely to occur before school and especially on Sunday night and Tuesday morning
- They were more likely to happen when his father was away
- He did worry about the change that came over his mother when she had her miscarriage, although of course he knew nothing about it. He just assumed it was something he'd done wrong and he just did his best to please her

Diagnosis

Non-organic abdominal pain with a significant psychological component.

Management

It was important that the parents understood the psychological factors that were promoting their son's symptoms. Allowing them to come to that understanding is more effective than 'telling them'. The consultant also used the same technique in terms of management. Instead of initially proposing a management plan, he asked the parents how they thought the situation could be improved. They proposed:

- School: to talk to Kevin's teachers to explain his symptoms; to look for evidence of bullying
- Home life: Kevin's father to ask his company to try to change his schedule. The consultant wrote a supportive letter
- Talking to Kevin: Kevin's mother was going to talk about her miscarriage and the couple realized the problem with not discussing important family issues
- Act sick – be sick!: if Kevin was unwell and off school he was to go to bed without entertainment. It was

Date	Time	Symptoms	Comments
Saturday	—	No pain	
Sunday evening	18:30	Tummy ache Feels sick	Went to bed, had paracetamol
Monday morning	07:15	Pain when wokeup	Settled by mid-morning
Tuesday	—	No pain	
Wednesday	14:00	At school – pain then pale vomited	Sent home. Paracetamol helped
Thursday	08:00	Very bad episode	Stayed at home Better by 11:30
Friday	—	No pain	
Saturday	11:00	In car Felt sick Tummy ache, vomited	Pain only 20 minutes
Monday	10:00	Mild tummy ache in class	Stayed at shool

Figure 30.2 Symptom diary for the patient.

important that being sick was a less rewarding experience than being at school

When Kevin was reviewed 3 months later he was making good progress. Some bullying had been identified at school and dealt with, and Kevin was developing some new friends. His consultant discharged him from follow-up. This is important even before complete resolution of the symptoms. It's very easy to over-medicalize functional symptoms and prolong them.

Background knowledge

Psychosomatic symptoms in children

Traditionally, as doctors, we are trained to seek out, identify and treat 'organic' diseases, and those children who are left are deemed to be suffering from non-organic disease. The symptoms are generally described as functional (Figures 30.3 and 30.4), in that no structural abnormality is associated with them. However, there is a range of these functional disorders from classic migraine with well-defined criteria for assignment to vague symptoms of intermittent dizziness that are not well characterized in the medical literature. Health culture in the UK has followed this trend, so that it has become unfashionable, if you like, to have a psychological component in the cause of such a functional disorder. Consequently, it becomes difficult to engage families in an area that may be therapeutically rewarding. In headaches, for example, psychologically mediated therapeutic interventions are known to as effective as drug treatments, but many families shy away from this area. Given the general interest in more alternative and holistic treatments (in often quite serious organic disease), this reluctance to consider the mind in health is paradoxical.

> ### How to raise psychological issues in a consultation
>
> Part of the reason for this reluctance is that, in many people's minds, a psychological reason for illness suggests blame and fault, and this is a great barrier.

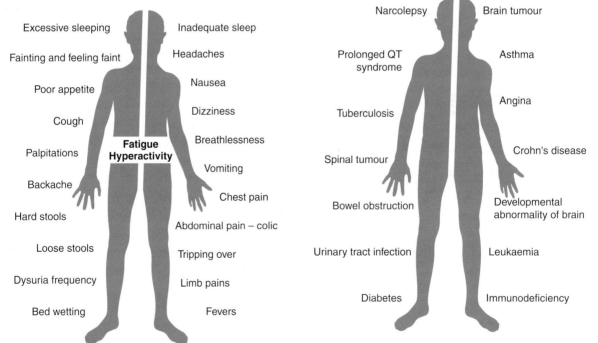

Figure 30.3 Common functional symptoms in children.

Excessive sleeping — Inadequate sleep
Fainting and feeling faint — Headaches
Poor appetite — Nausea
Cough — Dizziness
Palpitations — Breathlessness
Backache — **Fatigue Hyperactivity** — Vomiting
Hard stools — Chest pain
Loose stools — Abdominal pain – colic
Dysuria frequency — Tripping over
Bed wetting — Limb pains
— Fevers

Figure 30.4 Possible causes of symptoms that are usually functional.

Narcolepsy — Brain tumour
Prolonged QT syndrome — Asthma
Tuberculosis — Angina
Spinal tumour — Crohn's disease
Bowel obstruction — Developmental abnormality of brain
Urinary tract infection — Leukaemia
Diabetes — Immunodeficiency

Therefore, when raising these concepts some useful principles to discuss are:

- All diseases have a psychological component, e.g. terminal cancer
- Psychological treatments are known to improve organic conditions, e.g. hypnosis to control pain
- Try to discover what psychological adaptations the family has already undertaken (without 'knowing') to show that it's a common approach, e.g. a reward system is a basic psychological technique
- By using the term 'psychology' we are not suggesting blame, fault or psychosis
- Give and share examples of common psychological symptoms, e.g. nausea, abdominal discomfort when anxious before an exam
- Explain that drug therapies are frequently ineffective at controlling symptoms

Reassurance is a key skill in dealing with these conditions and a good history, thorough examination and some relevant investigations can help. Good listening skills and good understanding and acknowledgement of parental and child concerns are important. If a family really think that you understand their concerns, they will be more likely to accept your reassurance.

Further sources of information

Articles

Alfven G. Recurrent abdominal pain. A worldwide problem of organic, functional and psychosomatic aetiology. *Acta Paediatrica* 2001; **90**: 599–601

Anbar RD. Self-hypnosis for the treatment of functional abdominal pain in childhood. *Clinical Pediatrics* 2001; **40**: 447–51

Hunnicutt KL, Benjamin JT. A 6-year-old child with abdominal pain. *Clinical Pediatrics* 2001; **40**: 563–4

Simpson M, Buckman R, Stewart M, Maguire P, Lipkin M, Novack D, Till J. Doctor-patient communication: the Toronto consensus statement. *British Medical Journal* 1991; **303**: 1385–7

Stordal K, Nygaard EA, Bentsen B. Organic abnormalities in recurrent abdominal pain in children. *Acta Paediatrica* 2001; **90**: 638–42

Zeiter DK, Hyams JS. Recurrent abdominal pain in children. *Pediatric Clinics of North America* 2002; **49**: 53–71

Websites

www.doctorupdate.net/du_toolkit/s_sorters/s68.html

www.keepkidshealthy.com/symptoms/abdominalpain.html

www.aafp.org/afp/990401ap/1823.html

Self-test 4: Helen is 14 and has a 2-year history of intermittent periumbilical abdominal pain. She has lost a lot of weight and there has been some vomiting. She says she feels awful. It is suspected that she has anorexia nervosa. She has also had intermittent diarrhoea. Examination shows that she is very thin, but she also has finger clubbing, mouth ulcers and perianal skin tags.

A What is the most important underlying condition to rule out?

B What tests are appropriate?

Answer:

A Inflammatory bowel disease, such as Crohn's disease

B Blood count, C-reactive protein and contrast study of bowel

Delay in puberty

Age: 14 ½ years

LEENA PATEL

Presentation

A referral letter from the GP to a paediatrician about Oliver:

This young man came to see me today with his mother. They are concerned that, although he is 14 ½, he is not yet showing any signs of pubertal development. He has no significant past medical history. I have not examined his testicles. I think that he is almost certainly a normal boy. However, his mother is very keen for a specialist opinion. Please could you see him.

Self-test 1: What is the first sign of puberty in boys and in girls?

Answer: In boys it is enlargement of the testes to ≥4 mL volume and indicates normal gonadotrophin secretion. In girls, the size of the ovaries cannot be assessed clinically and the first sign of puberty is development of breast buds as a result of oestrogen secretion from the ovaries.

Initial considerations and action

The age of onset of puberty is influenced by a number of physiological factors and varies considerably among healthy children (Tables 31.1 and 31.2).

Delayed puberty is a clinical condition in which pubertal events:

- Start late – defined as absence of signs of puberty by age:

  - 15 years in boys
  - 14 years in girls or
- Are attenuated in progression

However, at this sensitive time of their life, teenagers often present earlier with concerns about their lack of development. For Oliver, significant anxiety is indicated by:

- The consultation with the GP
- His mother requesting a specialist opinion despite the GP's impression that Oliver is a normal boy

The paediatrician requests a non-urgent appointment for Oliver to be seen in the outpatient clinic.

Table 31.1 Age of onset of puberty

	Boys	Girls
Average age (years)	12	11
Range (years)	9.5–13.5	8.5–13.0

Table 31.2 Physiological factors influencing the timing of puberty

Gender: later in boys
Race: earlier in African and black American children
Genetic potential: later if parent(s) late
Nutrition: later in thin than in obese children
Physical activity: later in athletes, gymnasts and ballet dancers
Climate: later in cold temperate
Vision: earlier in blind children

History (Tables 31.3 and 31.4)

Oliver attends the outpatient clinic with his parents at 14.7 years of age:

Oliver's parents reveal that they had not been worried about Oliver until an episode at school a few months ago. That day Oliver came home upset because one of the lads had made a nasty comment about his 'privates' in the changing room. Oliver believes that he is not yet in puberty. Initially he had not let it bother him because his father had told him that he had been a 'late developer'. But the episode at school was humiliating and Oliver has given up football despite the fact that he really enjoyed it.

Neither Oliver nor his parents are particularly worried about his height and weight. They feel that he has been growing despite always having been small. Oliver's height had been measured twice at the GP's surgery and they had been told that he was growing normally. The paediatrician makes a note of obtaining these measurements from the GP. Father remembers being short when he started secondary school and only began shaving when he was in his 20s. Mother started her periods when she was 16 years old. Oliver's two younger sisters are 5 and 8 years old and healthy.

Oliver is also described as healthy by his parents. He does not have asthma or any other illnesses, has not been on any medication and has not required any operations on his testes. There has been no recent change in his energy level or appetite. He loves his food, is usually the first to smell what's cooking and his bowels are regular. His birth-weight was 3.2 kg and there were no perinatal problems. He was not slow with walking or talking. His schoolwork remains above average.

Interpretation of the history

Oliver believes that he has not yet started puberty and this will need to be confirmed during the examination.

The family history reveals that both mother and father were late maturers. The mean age at menarche is 13½ years (standard deviation 1.0 year). Facial hair in

Table 31.3 Classification of delayed puberty according to main clinical features and gonadotrophin levels

Gonadotrophin levels	Clues from the history	Clues from stature	
		Normal stature	**Short stature**
Normal or lowish	Chronic systemic disease, e.g. inflammatory bowel disease, uncontrolled asthma		Constitutional delay in growth and puberty Glucocorticoid excess Noonan's syndrome Skeletal dysplasia
Low (hypogonadotrophic hypogonadism)	Anorexia nervosa Female athlete Gonadotrophin deficiency from cranial tumour, radiotherapy or surgery	Isolated gonadotrophin deficiency (Kallman's syndrome)	Hypothyroidism Hypopituitarism Prader–Willi syndrome
High (hypergonadotrophic hypogonadism)	Gonads damaged by radiation or chemotherapy	Primary testicular failure, e.g. Klinefelter's syndrome, cryptorchidism	Primary ovarian failure, e.g. Turner's syndrome

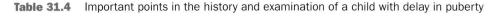

Table 31.4   Important points in the history and examination of a child with delay in puberty

History

Growth in height and weight

Undescended testes, orchidopexy, torsion of testes (primary gonadal failure)

Endocrine disorder

Chronic systemic illness

Treatment: glucocorticoids, chemotherapy, radiotherapy, cranial surgery

Family history: delayed puberty (delayed menarche, late development as a teenager, delayed growth spurt), hypogonadism, infertility, short stature

Anosmia or hyposmia (Kallman's syndrome)

Intelligence and learning difficulties (Klinefelter's syndrome, Noonan's syndrome)

Psychological impact of physical appearance

Examination

Pubertal assessment:
    Undescended testes (primary gonadal failure, gonadotrophin deficiency)
    Testes size, location, consistency
    Breast development
    Pubic hairs, axillary hairs

Height in relation to stage of puberty, previous heights, height velocity and parents' heights – normal or short (see Table 31.3)

Sitting height to subischial leg length ratio (eunuchoid proportions in primary gonadal failure, disproportion in skeletal dysplasia)

Weight: overweight (Prader–Willi) or underweight (anorexia nervosa)

Gynaecomastia (physiological, Klinefelter's syndrome)

Sense of smell (Kallmann's syndrome)

Signs of a lesion affecting the anterior pituitary: vision, visual fields, fundi

Signs of specific syndromes such as Turner's, Noonan's or Klinefelter's syndrome

Signs of hypothyroidism

---

boys develops well after the appearance of other secondary sexual characteristics, and most boys need to shave by 18 years of age.

Although Oliver is described as 'small', he was not growth retarded at birth and the history suggests that he has a normal growth rate and good general health. This, along with delayed puberty and family history of delayed puberty, raises the possibility of constitutional delay in puberty and growth.

Oliver's history does not suggest the following:

- Endocrine conditions such as hypothyroidism (see Chapter 19)
- Chronic systemic disorders such as asthma, which may be associated with delayed puberty and poor growth
- Learning difficulties which might be expected with Noonan's syndrome and Klinefelter's syndrome

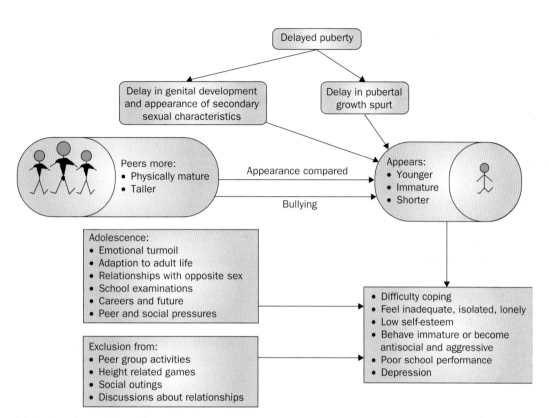

Figure 31.1 Psychosocial problems associated with delayed puberty.

The history reveals the psychological impact of lack of sexual maturation, at a time when other teenagers are maturing, on Oliver and his parents (Figure 31.1). Unpleasant comments from peers have made Oliver unhappy about his appearance. To avoid being seen by his peers and to avoid further humiliation, he has given up a favourite activity. Teenagers with delayed puberty may feel worse if a younger sibling overtakes them, but this is not the case with Oliver. Oliver's parents appear to have had a sensible attitude as a result of his father's experiences of 'late development'. Their recent anxiety stems from Oliver's emotional distress and they may wish to have reassurance about his future sexual maturity, fertility and adult height.

Examination (Table 31.4)

The paediatrician starts with the general examination and leaves pubertal assessment until the end because Oliver may not like being completely undressed right at the beginning.

- Oliver's growth measurements are plotted on growth charts
- Standing height: 152.5 cm (between 2nd and 9th centiles)
- Weight: 38.2 kg (between 2nd and 9th centiles)
- His spine does not appear obviously short compared with his limbs
- Mother's and father's heights are measured as 160 cm and 173 cm respectively.

The following are also noted:

- Nervous during the consultation but does reply sensibly to questions
- Appears much younger than 14.7 years from his face and stature
- No acne, no facial, axillary or pubic hairs, and no gynaecomastia
- Genitalia are normal but underdeveloped

- Both testes are palpable in the scrotum and their volumes are 2 mL with a Prader orchidometer
- Pulse is 82/minute and regular
- No dry skin, no goitre
- Normal distribution of fat and no truncal adiposity
- Visual fields and fundus examination are normal
- No dysmorphic features

Self-test 3: Obtain a growth chart and plot Oliver's height and weight, and his parents' heights (see Chapter 19). What centile positions are they on and what is the mid-parental height?

Answer: On a boy's chart from the UK 1995 reference data:
Oliver's:
   Height: between 2nd and 9th centile
   Weight: just above the 2nd centile
Father's height: just above the 25th centile
Mother's height: between 25th and 50th centiles
(plotted at 160 + 14 = 174 cm)
Mid-parental height: 173.5 cm

Interpretation of the examination

Oliver is assessed to be pre-pubertal from the size of his testes and penis, and absence of secondary sexual characteristics.

Gynaecomastia is physiological in many boys during puberty, but regresses after 18–24 months. Gynaecomastia in a boy with no signs of puberty raises the possibility of Klinefelter's syndrome.

Oliver's growth chart shows that he is inappropriately short compared with his parents. The previous measurements at the GP's surgery will reveal whether his height velocity is appropriate for his pre-pubertal status. Short stature in comparison to parents' heights, but normal height velocity in the absence of specific pathological features, will favour constitutional delay in puberty and growth and exclude conditions associated with poor height velocity (hypothyroidism, hypopituitarism and Noonan's syndrome – see Chapter 19).

Hypogonadotrophic hypogonadism and gonadal failure are also less likely as explanations for Oliver's lack of pubertal development because they are associated with normal stature, relatively short spine and long legs (eunuchoid proportions). Gonadotrophin deficiency may be isolated or secondary to a space-occupying lesion affecting the anterior pituitary – hence the importance of examining the visual fields and fundi.

Oliver appears to be a bright boy and his nervousness is possibly related to embarrassment and anxiety about his appearance and the anticipation of being examined.

Investigations and results

The history and examination findings suggest that the most likely explanation for Oliver not yet showing signs of puberty is constitutional delay (Table 31.5). The diagnosis is clinical and supported by a delayed bone age. A bone age from a radiograph of the left hand and wrist is therefore requested. Constitutional delay in growth and puberty is one extreme of the normal variation in the rate of maturation.

Oliver does not require any other investigations at this stage (Table 31.5).

Self-test 4: What is the use of bone age estimation and how is it estimated?

Answer: Bone age helps in assessing:
- Variation in the rate of maturation and maturational change throughout the growing period
- Linear growth potential

Although linear growth potential is mainly determined by maturation of the bones in the lower limbs and back, the radiograph of the left hand and wrist is used for ease of positioning and large number of bones in a small area. To assess the bone age, ossification in the bones (distal radius and ulna, carpals, metacarpals and phalanges) from the radiograph are compared with reference standards ('atlases') derived from healthy children using either the:
- Whole hand atlas approach (Greulich and Pyle method) or
- Bone by bone approach (Tanner TW2 method)

Table 31.5 Features pointing to pathological delay in puberty in a boy and investigations

Clinical features

Testes: absent, rudimentary, small and firm, or pre-pubertal when other secondary sexual characteristics present

Gynaecomastia

Normal or tall stature

Short stature with poor growth rate

Eunuchoid proportions, disproportion between spine and limbs

Anosmia

Low intelligence

Dysmorphic features

Investigations to consider

Karyotype for Klinefelter's syndrome

Basal serum luteinizing hormone (LH) and follicle-stimulating hormone (FSH) and after stimulation with LHRH (LHRH stimulation test): differentiates gonadotrophin deficiency from primary gonadal failure (see Table 31.3)

Human chorionic gonadotrophin (hCG) stimulation test if LH and FSH levels are not high and a testicular defect is suspected: rise in testosterone demonstrates adequate Leydig cell function

Magnetic resonance imaging of head for space-occupying lesion affecting anterior pituitary

Skeletal survey for skeletal dysplasia

Diagnosis

Oliver is a 14.7-year-old boy with:

- Constitutional delay in growth and puberty, suggested by:
  - good general health
  - normal birthweight
  - inappropriately short for his parents
  - height velocity normal for pre-pubertal stage
  - family history of delayed puberty
  - delayed bone age

- Considerable emotional distress about his delay in puberty.

Constitutional delay in growth and puberty can occur in boys and girls, but more commonly presents as a problem in boys. It is the most common reason for boys presenting with concerns about delay in puberty, short stature or both:

- Onset of puberty is delayed
- Puberty is normal (the sequence of appearance of sexual characteristics is normal)
- Progress through puberty may be slow
- There is a delay in the pubertal growth spurt
- There is a delay in attaining normal adult height

The onset of puberty may be physiologically delayed irrespective of height. At presentation, boys with CDGP are inappropriately short for their parents but not necessarily short as defined by height less than the 2nd centile (Figure 31.2). They also appear short compared with most of their peers, who will be taller as they go through a pubertal growth spurt. This relative short stature is temporary, corrects itself with the delayed pubertal growth spurt and adult height attained is appropriate for the parental target.

Constitutional delay in growth and puberty commonly results in extreme anxiety:

- Boys tend to be concerned about their physical appearance
- Parents may be more concerned about their son's:
  - psychological well-being
  - future sexual maturity
  - fertility
  - adult height

Management

Constitutional delay in growth and puberty is a physiological condition and as such does not require any treatment. However, the anxiety and psychological effects from it need to be addressed by:

- Explanation and reassurance about the condition
- Discussion about treatment options – not caused by growth hormone deficiency and growth hormone treatment is not indicated

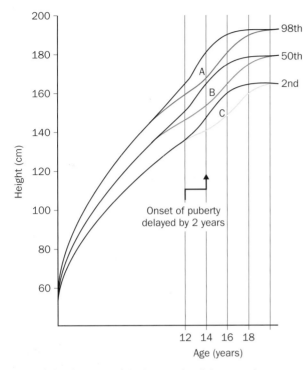

Figure 31.2 Theoretical example of the growth pattern of three boys (A,B,C) with delay in puberty. Although their heights are on the 98th, 50th and 2nd centiles in childhood, they have the same pattern of growth: onset of puberty delayed by 2 years (at age 14 years instead of 12 years); pubertal growth spurt therefore delayed and relative short stature (compared with peers) during adolescence; and expected adult height attained but at an age later than average.

How to reassure a boy with CDGP

The paediatrician explains the following to Oliver and his parents:

● He is a normal boy who is simply taking after his parents
● There is nothing to suggest that he has a disease or deficiency of the hormones that control puberty
● The age at which puberty starts varies considerably: it can be early for some and late for others like Oliver
● He looks different compared with other boys his age because they will:
 – have started puberty around the average age
 – be going through their growth spurt
● Oliver will start pubertal development at some stage in the future
● Until he starts puberty, he will continue to grow at a steady pace – Oliver's likely pattern of growth is illustrated to him on his growth chart
● His delay in starting puberty is an advantage in terms of the adult height he will attain because it gives him a longer time to grow
● When puberty does start:
 – his development will be normal
 – he will have a growth spurt
 – his adult height will be normal and in keeping with his parents' heights
● He will not be short as an adult
● His sexual drive, sexual function and fertility will be normal

Treatment option for CDGP

The paediatrician also explains the treatment options:

● Puberty can be artificially 'kick started' with hormone treatment if Oliver does not wish to wait for his puberty to start naturally
● Treatment should be considered only if Oliver has major psychosocial problems and feels he cannot cope with them
● Treatment will bring forward the timing of the start of puberty and therefore progress with sexual development and the growth spurt
● Treatment will not make him taller or shorter than what he is destined to be as an adult

Oliver finds the explanation about his future pubertal development and growth reassuring. With his parents he decides that he does not wish to have any treatment that 'tinkers with nature'.

Most patients like Oliver are reassured by proper explanation about their different but normal pubertal development and growth pattern, final development and height prognosis. For those with major psychosocial problems, treatment is indicated with low-dose oxandrolone (age 11–13 years) or testosterone (age >13 years) for 3–6 months and supervised by a specialist. Exceptionally boys may require psychological counselling.

A follow-up appointment after 3 months is made to assess:

- Signs of pubertal development
- Height increment
- Oliver's emotional state

If Oliver wishes to have treatment at that stage or has major psychological problems, he will need to be referred to a specialist in paediatric endocrinology.

Follow-up

At follow-up 3 months later, Oliver and his parents feel that he has 'not grown at all'. His measurements show that he has grown 0.7 cm since the last visit.

The paediatrician explains:

- That Oliver is still pre-pubertal and the growth rate is characteristically poor before the onset of puberty
- The bone age result: Oliver's bone age is delayed by about 3 ½ years compared with his calendar age:
  - this is expected in CDPG
  - height is determined by the size of the bones that sit one on top of another
- The delayed bone age indicates that:
  - Oliver's bones are maturing and growing slowly
  - his height and development are more appropriate for his bone age
  - there is considerable growth potential and Oliver will indeed grow to be much taller than might seem possible at present

The paediatrician repeats the information about Oliver's pubertal development and growth being normal but different as a result of delayed timing.

Oliver maintains that he does not wish to have any treatment if he is going to 'develop and grow naturally with time'. He has further follow-up at 3- to 4-monthly intervals. At 15.7 years of age, his testes volumes are 4 mL each and indicate that he has started puberty. He subsequently makes normal progress through puberty and goes through a growth spurt.

At 17.3 years his testes are 12 mL in volume and his height velocity is at its peak. Oliver is discharged at 18.3 years of age because he is very pleased that he is as tall as his father (Figure 31.3). He is now shaving twice a week and is aware that his growth rate is slowing down.

The height velocity chart illustrates that peak height velocity (Figure 31.3) is delayed by approximately 3 years.

Background information

Normal puberty

Puberty is the period of:

- Growth and maturation of primary sexual characteristics (gonads and genitals)
- Appearance of secondary sexual characteristics (breast development, pubic and axillary hair, voice change)

The neuroendocrine system that controls GnRH (gonadotrophin-releasing hormone) secretion is described as the GnRH pulse generator. It is restrained by inhibitory influences during infancy and the pre-pubertal period, so that pulsatile release of GnRH is suppressed. The onset of puberty is initiated by pulsatile release of GnRH from the hypothalamus, when inhibitory influences on the GnRH pulse generator are disrupted. This stimulates pulsatile secretion of follicle-stimulating hormone (FSH) and luteinizing hormone (LH) from the anterior pituitary, which in turn stimulate gonadal activity (Figure 31.4).

The development of secondary sexual characteristics (pubic hair, axillary hair, apocrine gland development and body odour, acne) is the result of androgens.

The pubertal growth spurt

The pubertal growth spurt is dependent on:

- Sex steroids
- Growth hormone

  It commences:

- Early in puberty (peak height velocity between B2 and B3) in girls

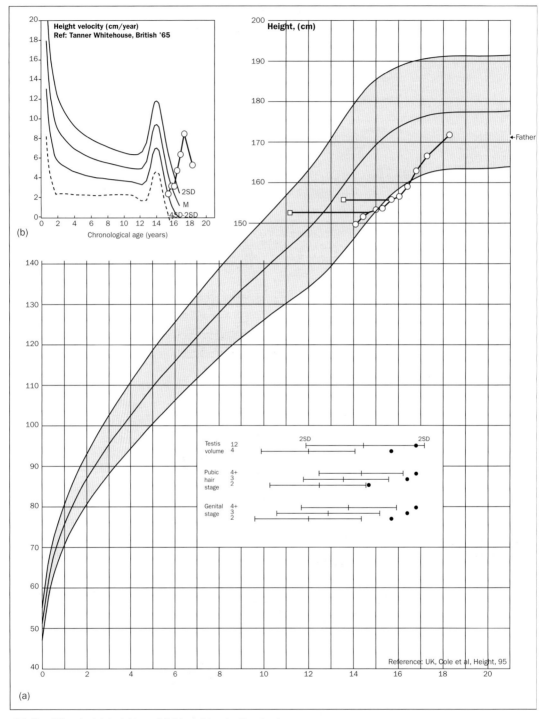

Figure 31.3 Oliver's (a) height and (b) height velocity charts.

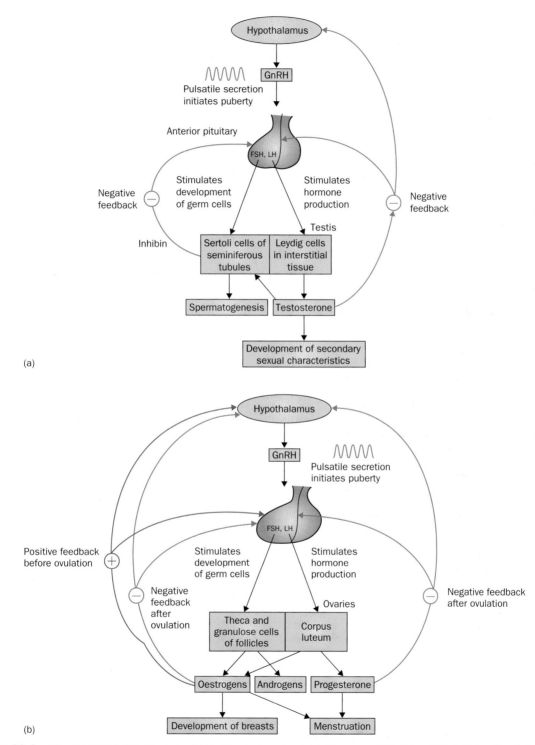

(a)

(b)

Figure 31.4   The hypothalamic–pituitary–gonadal axis in pubertal (a) boys and (b) girls. FSH, follicle-stimulating hormone; GnRH, gonadotrophin-releasing hormone; LH, luteinizing hormone.

- Relatively later in boys (peak height velocity at testes volumes of 12 ml, G4–G5). The relatively late spurt explains why CDGP is a problem that predominates in boys

The harmony of puberty and timing of the pubertal growth spurt

The development of various secondary sexual characteristics and the timing of the growth spurt occur in a fixed order (Figure 31.5). This is irrespective of the age of onset of puberty. Absence of this normal pattern suggests an endocrine abnormality. Adult development is generally attained 3–3.5 years after the onset of puberty. Table 31.6 shows the differential diagnosis of delayed puberty.

Gonadotrophin deficiency – a snapshot

Lack of pubertal development caused by gonadotrophin deficiency may be difficult to distinguish from CDGP when there is no family history of late development and no anosmia.

Basal LH and FSH levels and the LHRH (LH-releasing hormone) test are of limited value. Normal levels and a good response to LHRH exclude gonadotrophin deficiency. However, low gonadotrophin levels do not exclude CDGP because it is a state of physiological gonadotrophin deficiency, albeit temporary. When there is uncertainty, short-term treatment with testosterone to induce puberty followed by a period of observation is helpful:

- Further pubertal development suggests CDGP
- Lack of further development suggests gonadotrophin deficiency – treatment with testosterone is required to induce, complete and maintain pubertal development. Spermatogenesis and fertility may be possible with human chorionic gonadotrophin (hCG) treatment

Primary gonadal failure – a snapshot

Primary testicular failure may be the result of:

- Klinefelter's syndrome – therefore, boys with delayed puberty and small firm testes should have a karyotype done

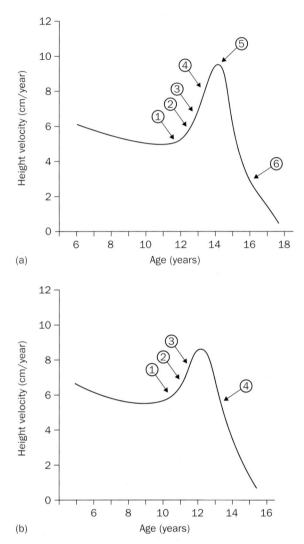

Figure 31.5 The sequence of sexual characteristics in relation to peak height velocity in (a) boys and (b) girls. In boys (a) the stages are: (1) onset of puberty with testes volume 4 mL; (2) pubic hair develops; (3) growth of penis; (4) axillary hair appears; (5) voice breaks; and (6) facial hair appears (when growth rate slows). In girls (b) the stages are: (1) onset of puberty with development of breast buds; (2) pubic hair develops; (3) axillary hair appears; and (4) menarche when growth rate slows, usually at breast stage 3–4.

- Absent or rudimentary testes
- Testicular atrophy from torsion or surgery for cryptorchidism
- Testicular damage from chemotherapy or radiotherapy

Table 31.6   Differential diagnosis of delayed puberty

	Constitutional delay	Isolated hypogonadotrophic hypogonadism	Primary gonadal failure	Skeletal dysplasia
Occurrence	Common	Rare	Klinefelter's syndrome: 1 in 750 newborn males	
Stature	Short	Normal	Normal or tall, slim	Short
Spine and limb proportions	Relatively short spine	Relatively short spine	Relatively short spine and long legs	Disproportionate
Specific features	Family history of delayed puberty	Kallmann's syndrome: Anosmia Cryptorchidism Small penis	Klinefelter's syndrome: Karyotype 47 XXY Low intelligence Small firm testes Small penis Gynaecomastia Female fat distribution	
Bone age	Delayed	Delayed	Delayed	Appropriate or advanced
Basal serum LH and FSH	Low or normal and response to LHRH may be poor or normal	Very low to normal and response to LHRH poor	Very high and supranormal response to LHRH stimulation	Normal or low
hCG test in boys	Significant rise in testosterone to hCG	Subnormal	Testosterone low and no response to hCG	Significant rise in testosterone to hCG
Treatment with low dose testosterone for 3–6 months in boys	Testicular volume increases, testosterone level increases to pubertal range	Testes remain small, testosterone level remains low	Testes remain small	Treatment with testosterone is not indicated

FSH, follicle-stimulating hormone; hCG, chorionic gonadotrophin; LH, luteinizing hormone; LHRH, luteinizing hormone-releasing hormone.

The two basic functions of the testes are to produce male hormones and sperms. Both are affected in testicular failure. Treatment with testosterone is required to induce, complete and maintain pubertal development. The testes remain small and cannot produce sperms. A relatively empty scrotum has psychological effects and prosthetic testes can be implanted for appearance.

Primary gonadal failure is also a feature of Turner's syndrome and girls with delayed puberty should have a karyotype done.

Precocious puberty – a snapshot

Definition

Onset of puberty: <8 years in girls and <9 years in boys.

Classification of conditions associated with precocious puberty according to gonadotrophin levels

- Gonadotrophin dependent or central – gonadotrophin levels high: idiopathic (almost exclusively girls)
  secondary (equal sex distribution) to central nervous system lesions, e.g. tumour, trauma, hydrocephalus
- Gonadotrophin independent – gonadotrophin levels suppressed:
  – congenital adrenal hyperplasia
  – exogenous oestrogens or androgens
  – McCune–Albright syndrome

Further sources of information

Articles

Argente J. Diagnosis of late puberty. *Hormone Research* 1999; **51**(suppl 3): 95–100

Sedlmeyer IL, Palmert MR. Delayed puberty: analysis of a large case series from an academic center. *Journal of Clinical Endocrinology and Metabolism* 2002; **87**: 1613–20

Self-test 5: The following are true of normal puberty:
A Peak height velocity in girls occurs after menarche
B Peak height velocity in boys occurs at testicular volumes of 12 ml
C Its onset coincides with pulsatile release of LH and FSH
D Onset can be as early as 7 years of age
E Adult height is attained by age 18 years

Answers: True: B and C.
False:
A It occurs at B2–3

D Onset of puberty <8 years in girls and <9 years in boys is precocious
E It depends on the age of onset of puberty and may be delayed

Self-test 6: What is the consequence of rapid induction of puberty with high doses of testosterone in a boy?

Answers:
- May progress through puberty abnormally fast
- Inadequate growth spurt and therefore adult height compromised
- Difficulty adjusting emotionally
- Frequent uncontrollable and embarrassing erections

Note: a similar situation in girls affects the quality of breast development.

Self-test 7: Explain why the testes remain small in hypogonadotrophic hypogonadism when puberty is induced with testosterone treatment.

Answer: The testes fail to grow as a result of gonadotrophin deficiency. Normal testicular enlargement is controlled by:
1 LH secretion which stimulates the Leydig cells to grow and produce testosterone,
2 FSH and testosterone, which cause growth of the seminiferous tubules and spermatogenesis

Self-test 8: Why are undescended testes a feature of gonadotrophin deficiency and primary gonadal failure?

Answer: Testes develop from genital ridges and lie below the developing kidneys in early fetal life. Chorionic gonadotrophins from the maternal circulation stimulate the growth of the testes. They remain in their abdominal position close to the inguinal canal until around 7 months of gestation. Thereafter, they descend into the scrotum under the influence of gonadotrophins and testosterone. Imperfect development of the testes, gonadotrophin deficiency and failure to secrete testosterone result in incomplete descent of the testes, which is associated with the following complications:

- Atrophy
- Infertility in bilateral cases
- Torsion

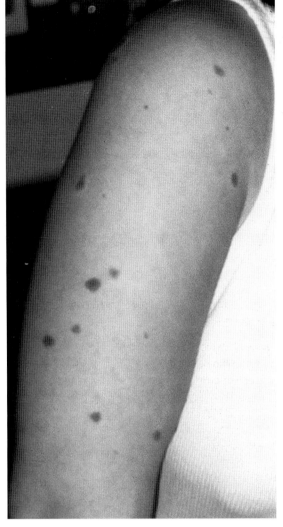

Figure 31.6   The arm of the girl in Self-test 10.

- Development of malignant tumour
- Psychological effects of an empty scrotum

Self-test 9: A delayed bone age is expected in children with:

A **Hypochondroplasia**

B **Hypothyroidism**

C **Hypopituitarism**

D **Familial short stature**

E **Congenital adrenal hyperplasia**

Answers: True: B, C.

Delayed bone age is seen with:

- Any condition where puberty is delayed, e.g. CDGP
- Endocrine deficiency – hypothyroidism, growth hormone deficiency
- Chronic disease, e.g. asthma, inflammatory bowel disease
- Long-term corticosteroid treatment

Bone age is appropriate for chronological age in hypochondroplasia and familial short stature (see Chapter 19).

Bone age is advanced with congenital adrenal hyperplasia and precocious puberty.

Self-test 10: Figure 31.6 shows the arm of a girl who presented at age 15 years with delayed puberty and height well below 0.4th centile. What investigation will you arrange first?

Answer: Karyotype for Turner's syndrome. Turner's syndrome should be considered foremost in girls with short stature and delayed puberty. Multiple pigmented naevi are a common feature.

A child who is overweight

Age: 15 years

STEVEN RYAN

Presentation

Letter from general practitioner:
Please would you review 15-year-old Louise. She is overweight. At 15 years and 1 month of age she weighs 88 kg and her height is 165 cm. Her food intake does not appear excessive, based on the history given. However, she has not responded to my advice to reduce her calorie intake and her excessive weight seems to be increasing. She is now being teased and bullied at her school and is desperate to lose weight. Her mother, who is also incidentally overweight, is concerned that Louise has an underlying metabolic disorder causing her excessive weight.

Self-test 1: Calculate the body mass index (BMI) of Louise.

Answer: $88/1.65^2 = 32.2\,\text{kg/m}^2$

Initial considerations and action

Obesity – excessive fat deposition – is predominantly caused by a food energy intake beyond the energy expended. This imbalance may be very moderate but cumulatively, over long periods, it may lead to very excessive fat storage. Obesity is now a worldwide epidemic with massive health implications, predominantly manifest in adulthood but with its roots in childhood. Obesity is now increasingly seen before the age of 5 years in the UK (Figure 32.1).

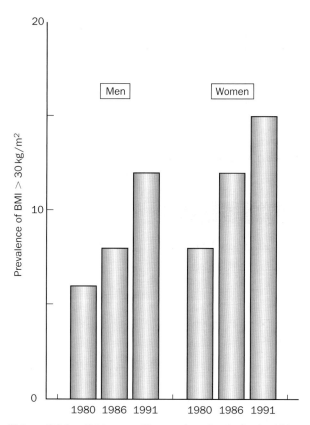

Figure 32.1 Evidence of increasing obesity in the UK. BMI, body mass index.

A very small number of overweight children have a specific disorder to account for their obesity. Clues to there being an underlying disorder are:

- Short stature and obesity
- Slow rate of height gain and obesity
- Dysmorphic features and obesity

- Features of corticosteroid excess
- Features of thyroid hormone deficiency

Self-test 2: For each description (A–E), give the underlying diagnosis (1–5):

A **Short stature and obesity in a 9-year-old boy who appears infantile**

B **Severe learning difficulties and obesity**

C **Severe asthma on maximum treatment**

D **An overweight teenage girl with a deep voice who dislikes the cold**

E **A boy with undescended testes at birth and floppiness, who is now grossly obese**

1 **Cushing's syndrome**

2 **Hypothyroidism**

3 **Growth hormone deficiency**

4 **Prader–Willi syndrome**

5 **Down's syndrome**

Answer: A3, B5, C1, D2, E4.

History

The history can be divided into a number of key areas:

- Review of previous and current growth including pubertal development
- Dietary history
- Symptoms of underlying causes: endocrine and other
- Health consequences of obesity: physical and psychological (including degree of physical activity)
- Family history of obesity
- Previous interventions to deal with the problem and their effectiveness

Louise and her mother give the following history.

Review of previous and current growth

Louise's mother shows the growth chart she and health professionals have been keeping. It shows that the excess weight that Louise has accumulated has been steadily increasing but seems to have accelerated in the last 2 years. Louise had a normal height and birthweight. She is clearly taller than average.

Louise had her first signs of breast development at 9 years of age and her first pubic and axillary hair were noted when she was early in her tenth year. Menarche was at the age of 12.

Dietary history

Quantity of intake: Louise did not at first have an increased appetite and her mother did not report her taking large quantities of food. However, Louise did admit to 'grazing', i.e. eating modest quantities of food and snacks through the day. As an example, on the way home from school she would generally eat a chocolate snack bar.

Quality of intake: Louise ate very little in the way of fresh fruit. Most of her snack foods were heavily processed with high-energy density and she was not keen on vegetables.

Self-test 3: For each food item select the appropriate calorie content:

A **Medium apple**

B **Medium banana**

C **Medium orange**

D **Cola 6 fl oz**

E **One slice wholemeal bread**

F **Six chicken nuggets**

G **Regular hotdog**

H **12-inch cheese pizza**

I **Large French fries**

1 **360 calories**

2 **60 calories**

3 **900 calories**

4 **80 calories**

5 **50 calories**

6 **240 calories**

7 **80 calories**

8 **300 calories**

9 **70 calories**

Answer: A2, B4, C5, D7, E9, F8, G6, H3, I1.

Symptoms of underlying causes: endocrine and other

There had been no significant past medical history of note. On specific questioning there were no symptoms compatible with hypothyroidism (constipation, intolerance of cold, change in voice, poor hair or skin condition, deterioration in school work). Her good growth was against Cushing's syndrome and this, her normal development and lack of dysmorphic features made a genetic disorder very unlikely.

Health consequences of obesity: physical and psychological (including degree of physical activity)

Louise said that she felt tired easily and she had poor exercise tolerance. She had almost stopped taking part in organized physical activities at school – she became breathless and sweaty when any intensity of activity was involved. Louise undertook very little physical activity. She took public transport to school and spent little time away form the home. Her favourite activity was watching the television in her bedroom.

Louise was also being teased and occasionally bullied at school because of her weight. Consequently she had few close friends.

Family history of obesity

She is an only child. Both her parents are overweight and her mother (aged 43) had some knee pain, which was said to be related to her weight. Her father, aged 48, had just been diagnosed with type 2 diabetes. He was obese and had just started a diet.

Previous interventions to deal with the problem and their effectiveness

Several attempts at dieting had been undertaken with sudden drastic restriction of food intake at home. However, Louise said she'd found the whole thing overwhelming and had continued eating snack foods out of the house.

Interpretation of the history

This history is entirely compatible with environmental obesity, i.e. excess energy intake over requirements. Louise is a tall girl who had a relatively early puberty, and this alone makes other causes unlikely. She does not feel that she is a 'greedy' person, but her persistent calorie intake throughout the day is quite substantial. Her selection of high-energy density and accompanying low-satiety value foods exacerbates the problem. Her physical activity level, and therefore her energy requirements, are also low, both of which cause the problem but are also now partly a result of the problem – a vicious circle if you like. Both her parents are overweight and suffering the consequences of it. This finding is not atypical. Both genetic factors (determining appetite and metabolic rate) and sharing the same nutrient-rich environment that is low in physical activity are likely to play a part (Figure 32.2).

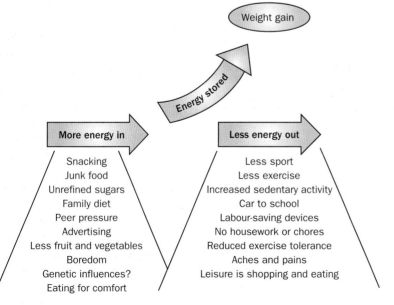

Figure 32.2 Factors influencing energy balance in modern life.

Examination

The purpose of the examination is to:

- Confirm the presence and degree of obesity
- Look for dysmorphic features
- Look for features of hypothyroidism
- Exclude short stature
- Look for features of corticosteroid excess
- Check blood pressure
- Check genitalia and pubertal status

Louise was examined and these were the findings:

- Height: 166 cm
- Weight: 89 kg
- BMI: 32 kg/cm^2
- Blood pressure (adult cuff): 118/76 mmHg
- Pubertal status: adult
- Appearance: obese with general increased subcutaneous fat; round face, flushed cheeks, striae on thighs, no dysmorphic features
- Features of hypothyroidism: no goitre (Figure 32.3), pulse 88/minute, warm peripheries, limb reflexes normal, healthy skin

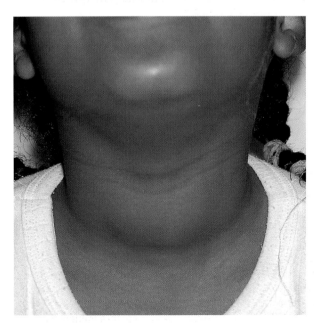

Figure 32.3　Goitre in a child with hypothyroidism.

Interpretation of the examination

Louise is confirmed as being obese (definition BMI > 30 or > 95th centile for age – Figure 32.4). She is tall and there is no dysmorphism, so a genetic cause is unlikely. Nor are there any signs of hypothyroidism. Some of her features (round face, flushed cheeks and striae) are found in Cushing's syndrome (corticosteroid excess), but they are also commonly observed in environmental obesity. The absence of short stature and the family history of obesity make such a problem very unlikely.

Investigations

Routine investigations are not required for environmental obesity. Investigations are indicated if another cause is suspected. Louise was not investigated but Table 32.1 shows when tests, and what investigations, are indicated.

Diagnosis

Environmental obesity.

Management and prognosis

The principles of management of obesity are well understood, but unfortunately the effectiveness of delivering these principles are not and outcome in terms of sustained weight loss is disappointing. The basic principle is to make energy balance negative. This is achieved with a combination of dietary advice and advice on increasing physical activity. The principle is to allow for a slow reduction in weight over many months – if not years. It is also to establish a permanent change in behaviour rather than a quick fix, which is likely to result in a rebound effect. Regular review and support seem to be important in maintaining weight loss.

The main burden of obesity is felt in adulthood, but increasingly consequences are being seen in childhood – and since the onset of environmental obesity seems to be occurring earlier this trend may continue. Musculoskeletal strain and psychological problems are relatively common, and adult-type (type 2) diabetes is now being reported.

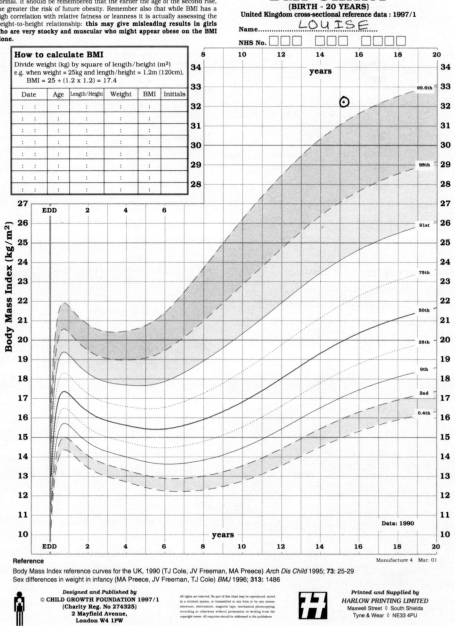

Referral guidelines

Refer a girl whose BMI falls above the 98th centile as obese. Consider referral, as overweight, a girl whose BMI falls above the 91st centile even on the basis of a single measurement. Consider for referral a girl whose BMI falls below the 2nd centile as being significantly underweight even on the basis of a single measurement. During infancy large but transient changes in centile may occur due to the shape of the charts, and these changes are normal. It should be remembered that the earlier the age of the second rise, the greater the risk of future obesity. Remember also that while BMI has a high correlation with relative fatness or leanness it is actually assessing the weight-to-height relationship: **this may give misleading results in girls who are very stocky and muscular who might appear obese on the BMI alone.**

How to calculate BMI

Divide weight (kg) by square of length/height (m^2)
e.g. when weight = 25kg and length/height = 1.2m (120cm),
  BMI = $25 \div (1.2 \times 1.2) = 17.4$

Date	Age	Length/Height	Weight	BMI	Initials
: :	:	:	:	:	
: :	:	:	:	:	
: :	:	:	:	:	
: :	:	:	:	:	
: :	:	:	:	:	
: :	:	:	:	:	
: :	:	:	:	:	

GIRLS
BMI CHART
(BIRTH - 20 YEARS)
United Kingdom cross-sectional reference data : 1997/1

Name.. LOUISE

NHS No.

Body Mass Index (kg/m²)

Data: 1990

Manufacture 4   Mar. 01

Reference

Body Mass Index reference curves for the UK, 1990 (TJ Cole, JV Freeman, MA Preece) *Arch Dis Child* 1995; **73**: 25-29
Sex differences in weight in infancy (MA Preece, JV Freeman, TJ Cole) *BMJ* 1996; **313**: 1486

Designed and Published by
© CHILD GROWTH FOUNDATION 1997/1
(Charity Reg. No 274325)
2 Mayfield Avenue,
London W4 1PW

Printed and Supplied by
HARLOW PRINTING LIMITED
Maxwell Street ◊ South Shields
Tyne & Wear ◊ NE33 4PU

Figure 32.4   Louise plotted on a body mass index (BMI) chart. © Child Growth Foundation. The chart shown here is intended for illustrative purposes only. The range of UK growth reference charts may be purchased from Harlow Printing, Maxwell Street, South Shields, NE33 4PU.

Table 32.1 Investigtions for causes of obesity

Condition	Features	Tests
Hypothyroidism	Goitre, slow pulse, cold skin, Hair poor condition, constipation Reduced height velocity	Blood thyroxine, T_3 and thyroid-stimulating hormone Thyroid autoantibodies
Cushing's syndrome	Short stature, central adiposity, 'moon face', cervical hump, striae, hypertension, osteoporosis	Urinary cortisol excretion Dexamethasone suppression test
Growth hormone	Short stature, infantile appearance, lack of energy, poor sleep pattern	Growth hormone stimulation test
Prader–Willi syndrome	Growth retarded and floppy, at birth, undescended testes, short stature, small genitalia, obsessive relentless consumption	Chromosomes: deletion of chromosome 15 or uniparental disomy

T_3, triiodothyronine.

In fact Louise was referred through to a specialized multidisciplinary obesity team who administered dietary advice and a specialized exercise programme. Over a period of 6 months she lost 4.8 kg in weight and increased in height by 2 cm. Her BMI was now <30.

How to measure energy balance

- **Energy input:** use a food energy table to determine the total calorie intake:
  - these tables are usually based on calorimetry – measuring the heat output caused when food is burnt
  - you then need to use a diary, but remember that people tend to underestimate their food intake
  - work out the total intake of protein, carbohydrate and fat, then calculate the energy intake by multiplying each gram of these as follows:
    - fat: 9 kcal/g
    - carbohydrate: 4 kcal/g
    - protein: 4 kcal/g
  - bring the patient into a completely enclosed secure environment and measure what he or she eats

- **Energy output:** measure the amount of oxygen consumed – called indirect calorimetry:
  - doubly labelled isotopes: a form of indirect calorimetry based on the elimination of deuterium (hydrogen-2) and oxygen-18 from urine
  - the technique measures the turnover of hydrogen and oxygen into water and carbon dioxide; energy expenditure is calculated from the difference
  - children being tested can continue their normal activity
  - estimate energy expenditure outside clinical situations by monitoring heart rate and maintaining an activity diary

Background information

Physiology: energy balance

Put quite simply:

Energy in = Energy used + Energy stored

The energy stored, as fat, is the cause of obesity. Energy intake can be calculated by a dietary assessment

Table 32.2 Expected energy intakes in boys and girls

| Age (years) | Energy intake (MJ)[a] | |
	Boys	Girls
1	3.9 (900)	3.6 (870)
5	5.2 (1200)	3.6 (1150)
10	8.3 (2000)	7.3 (1750)
15	11.5 (2800)	8.8 (2100)

[a]Values in parentheses are kilocalories.

in which the energy content of all nutrients taken in is summated. In real life this is a difficult area and many obese individuals under-report their energy intake – giving rise to the false notion that abnormally low basic energy requirements are responsible for excess weight gain. This fallacy has been disproved by careful research. The energy content of most food products can be worked out from food tables. Dieticians calculate nutrient intakes from these tables.

The approximate estimated average daily energy requirements of children living in the UK have been calculated and can be summarized as shown in Table 32.2.

Obesity occurs when intakes in excess of these requirements are consumed. The other factor that can be modified is obviously energy use. Energy use itself can be divided into different categories:

$$\text{Energy used} = \text{Basal metabolic rate} + \text{Energy used to digest food} + \text{Physical activity}$$

In clinical practice it is not usual to change basal metabolic rate, although theoretically this can be undertaken with drugs such as thyroxine. Significant side effects and risks preclude this approach. It can be seen that hypothyroidism and growth hormone deficiency contribute to obesity by diminishing the basal metabolic rate. Physical activity can readily be modified and successful research programmes have demonstrated that sustained reduction in weight in children can occur.

Physiology of thyroid function

Figure 32.5 shows the mechanisms controlling the levels of thyroid hormones and the situation in disturbances of thyroid function.

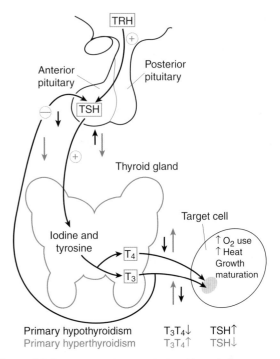

Figure 32.5 Thyroid function in health and disease. T_3, triiodothyronine; T_4, thyroxine; TRH, thyroid hormone-releasing hormone; TSH, thyroid-stimulating hormone.

Further sources of information

Books

Holland B, Welch AA, Unwin ID, Buss DH, Paul AA, Southgate DAT. *McCance and Widdowson's The Composition of Foods*, 5th edn. Cambridge: Royal Society of Chemistry, 1991

Department of Health. Dietary reference values for food energy and nutrients for the United Kingdom. *Report of the Panel on Dietary Reference Values of the Committee on Medical Aspects of Food Policy.* London: HMSO, 1991

Articles

Dietz WH, Gortmaker SL. Preventing obesity in children and adolescents. *Annual Review of Public Health* 2001; **22**: 337–53

Epstein LH, Paluch RA, Gordy CC, Dorn J. Decreasing sedentary behaviors in treating pediatric obesity. *Archives of Pediatrics and Adolescent Medicine* 2000; **154**: 220–6

Reilly JJ, Wilson ML, Summerbell CD, Wilson DC. Obesity: diagnosis, prevention and treatment; evidence-based answers to common questions. *Archives of Disease in Childhood* 2002; **86**: 392–5

Websites

www.aafp.org/afp/990215ap/861.html

An excellent review article.

www.ed.gov/databases/ERIC_Digests/ed328556.html

Another excellent review article.

Self-test 4: Fourteen-year-old Angela was referred for being overweight; she had a BMI of 32 and her weight had increased significantly over the past 2 years. She also complained of feeling the cold, her hair was in poor condition, and teachers had reported that her school performance had slipped – they felt she was being teased by her peers. She had not yet started her menstrual periods. She was examined and some specific features were noted. She had a single blood test, which confirmed the diagnosis. And treatment was started.

A What is the likely diagnosis?

B What other features might exist in the history?

C What specific abnormalities might have been found on examination?

D What tests were done and what results were seen?

E What treatment was commenced and for how long?

Answer:

A Autoimmune thyroiditis causing hypothyroidism

B Constipation, dry skin, puffy eyes, eyebrow loss, constipation, hoarse voice

C Goitre, bradycardia, slow relaxing reflexes

D Thyroid function – raised TSH (thyroid-stimulating hormone), reduced thyroid hormone (thyroxine or T_4), and thyroid autoantibodies could be present

E Thyroxine – life long

Community

A sudden pain in the hip and difficulty walking

Age: 8 years

JACKIE GREGG

Presentation

Eight-year-old Patrick presents to the accident and emergency department (A&E) with a 24-hour history of a limp and pain in his right hip. Patrick is a healthy lad, apart from having a recent viral throat infection. There is no history of trauma.

Self-test 1: What is the most common cause of acute pain in the hip in children?

Answer: Transient synovitis.

Initial considerations and action

Hip pain is a common presenting symptom in childhood and adolescence. A toddler may not be able to articulate his or her pain and is more likely to present with refusal to weight bear, whereas an infant moves the limb less than its fellow. Conditions affecting the hip may initially present with referred pain to the knee; it's important therefore to examine both joints.

The most common causes of limp and pain in the hip are:

- Transient synovitis (irritable hip)
- Perthes' disease
- Infection – osteomyelitis, septic arthritis, tuberculosis (TB), viral, e.g. mumps
- Slipped upper femoral epiphysis (SUFE)
- Trauma
  - severe
  - mild, may exacerbate slipped femoral epiphysis
  - non-accidental injury

Figure 33.1 shows an immature joint.

Rarer causes of hip pain:

- **Haematological:** sickle-cell disease, haemophilia, leukaemia
- **Malignancy:** simple bone cysts are the most common benign tumour found around the hip. The most common malignant tumours are osteosarcoma, Ewing's tumour and lymphoma
- **Congenital dislocation of the hip:** pain in untreated cases is rare and is usually secondary to failed treatment
- **Tendinosis:** usually occurs in active, athletic adolescents
- **Bone dysplasias and metabolic disorder:** conditions such as multiple epiphyseal dysplasia, Gaucher's disease and hypothyroidism may result

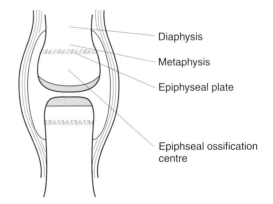

Diaphysis

Metaphysis

Epiphyseal plate

Epiphseal ossification centre

Figure 33.1 Immature joint.

in hip pain because they interfere with normal development of the epiphysis or hyaline cartilage. However, they are usually bilateral and involve other joints

- **Iatrogenic:** drug reaction, fractures from steroids
- **Referred pain:** pain in the lumbar spine, ureters, pelvic organs and appendix may be referred to the hip
- Non-organic

Self-test 2: What is the most common cause of acute pain in the lower limb?

Answer: Trauma.

Patrick and his mother are seen by the senior A&E doctor.

History

Patrick is a healthy active boy. His mum had noticed a slight limp when he returned from school the previous day. This had worsened over the evening when he suddenly started to complain of pain in his right hip. Patrick had a dose of paracetamol; the pain eased while he rested and he had a reasonable night's sleep. However, the pain returned when he got out of bed next morning and tried to walk on it.

Patrick is a member of the Cub football team. He had played a match 3 days ago, but hadn't sustained any trauma.

Patrick had had a sore throat for a few days and his GP had diagnosed a viral upper respiratory tract infection.

There is no family history of bone or joint disease. Patrick's mother described him as an outgoing boy who has lots of friends. He is not on any medication.

Interpretation of the history

Points to consider in the history:

- Age of the child
- History of trauma
- Involvement of other joints
- Fever and systemic upset, including a rash
- Pain: aggravating/relieving factors, site, timing
- Emotional problems

Age of the child

This is important when considering the differential diagnoses, e.g.

- **Transient synovitis:** most common condition in 3–8 year olds
- **Septic conditions:** usually younger age groups, rare in adolescents
- **Perthes' disease:** 4–10 year olds
- **Slipped upper femoral epiphysis:** 10–15 year olds

Trauma

Older children can usually give a history of trauma, unless they have something to hide. A child who has sustained an injury while engaged in an activity forbidden to them may not tell, for fear of getting into trouble. A child who has been abused may also be frightened to tell. Younger children may not have the means to say what has happened. They may not complain of pain; instead they refuse to weight bear and return to crawling to get around. Upper femoral or pelvic fractures in children are rare and usually the result of major trauma.

Involvement of other joints

Perthes' disease and SUFE may be bilateral in up to 25 per cent of cases.

Fever and systemic upset

A child with an acute febrile illness and a tender joint or limb must have septic arthritis or osteomyelitis excluded, because prompt treatment is necessary to prevent bone destruction (Figure 33.2).

Subacute osteomyelitis may have more insidious features, but radiographic changes are usually present at the presentation, although the latter may be confused with neoplasia of the bone. Children with transient synovitis may have a mild fever.

Pain

The pain and degree of severity may give diagnostic clues. Osteomyelitis and septic arthritis are acutely painful, and the former has sharply localized tenderness on palpation. Osteoid osteoma, a benign tumour of adolescents, is much more painful at night and there may be some localized tenderness. The pain in transient synovitis is present on movement of the joint.

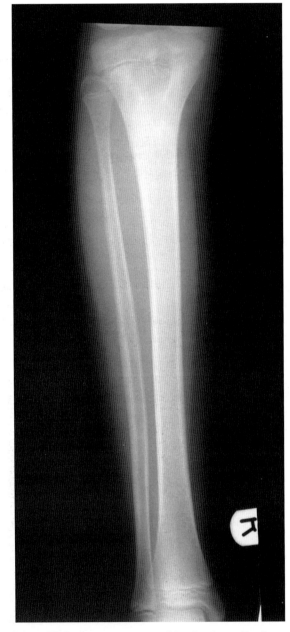

Figure 33.2 Chronic osteomyelitis showing a Brodie abscess of the proximal end of the tibia. (With thanks to Dr L Abernethy for providing the radiograph.)

Emotional problems

In older children, limb pain may be related to psychological stress or result from over-protection of the limb following minor injury. It may be important to observe the child when he or she isn't aware of being watched.

Systemic juvenile chronic arthritis (JCA), rheumatic fever and Henoch–Schoenlein purpura (HSP) are unlikely to cause diagnostic confusion in a child presenting solely with pain in the hip. HSP (with its typical rash, see Chapter 23) and rheumatic fever usually present with involvement of more than one joint. JCA usually involves several joints, although the pauciarticular or oligoarticular type may involve four joints or fewer, more usually the knee, wrist or ankle.

Meaning of the history in Patrick

Patrick's pain is present on movement and is relieved by rest. He denies any trauma and his demeanour gives no reason to suggest that he might be covering anything up. Trauma sustained at football would occur more acutely, not 3 days later. Patrick hasn't complained of systemic upset or rash, which makes a systemic condition less likely. There isn't anything in the history to suggest that Patrick has an emotional cause for the hip pain – he is an active outgoing boy who likes school.

Self-test 3: A 3-year-old girl presents with pain in both legs that wakes her at night. She doesn't have any pain during the day and is lively. The examination is normal. What is the likely diagnosis?

Answer: Growing pains. The term 'growing pains' is a misnomer, because they don't appear to have anything to do with growth. They are common in preschool and primary school-age children. They are mainly confined to the lower limbs and to the calf and thigh muscles, and are non-articular. They are more common after fatigue and exertion. They usually occur at night and wake the child from sleep. The pain usually settles with massage or comforting. They more rarely occur during the day and are not associated with organic disease.

Examination

- Growth: height and weight both on the 25th centile
- Temperature: 37.2°C
- Looks well
- Mildly inflamed throat
- Right hip: hip held flexed and externally rotated with limited abduction, internal and external rotation; pain on movement of joint, no increased heat
- Right knee: full movements, non-tender
- No other joint or bone pain
- No rashes

Interpretation of the examination

Patrick is well, there is no fever or evidence of systemic illness or infection, and he has isolated pain in his right hip. He is likely to have transient synovitis, which is the most common cause of acute hip pain in children, although Perthes' disease and SUFE are also possible.

Self-test 4: Which investigation will differentiate transient synovitis, Perthes' disease and slipped upper femoral epiphysis?

Answer: Radiograph of the hips in two planes.

Investigations

- Neutrophil count normal
- C-reactive protein slightly raised
- Erythrocyte sedimentation rate (ESR) normal
- Blood cultures negative
- Radiograph of hips normal
- Ultrasonography of hips – small joint effusion on right

Radiograph of the hips will be abnormal in SUFE and Perthes' disease, although in the latter it may be normal in the early stages, when transient synovitis may be diagnosed. Follow-up radiographs would be required if symptoms persisted (Figures 33.3 and 33.4).

Diagnosis

Transient synovitis.

Treatment and follow-up plan

The management of transient synovitis is bed rest and analgesia. Mild cases can be managed at home, but patients with more severe symptoms require admission. Traction is no longer recommended because it may increase the intra-articular pressure

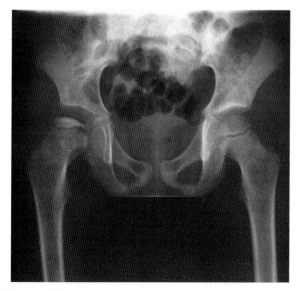

Figure 33.3 Perthes' disease of the right hip. (With thanks to Dr L Abernethy for providing the radiograph.)

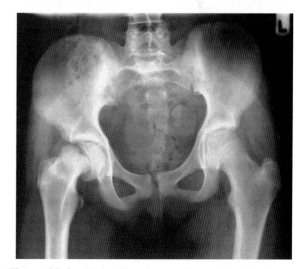

Figure 33.4 Right slipped upper femoral epiphysis (SUFE). (With thanks to Dr L Abernethy for providing the radiograph.)

In view of the severity of Patrick's symptoms, the A&E doctor refers him to the orthopaedic team. The orthopaedic surgeon considers that Patrick's mother will be able to manage him at home. He is discharged with instructions to rest in bed and a non-steroidal anti-inflammatory agent is prescribed, to be taken regularly.

Patrick is reviewed 2 days later and his symptoms have started to improve. He is advised to continue with bed rest and his symptoms resolve over the next few days. He is discharged and makes a full recovery.

How to manage acute pain

Who feels pain?

All children, including neonates, feel pain. Pre-verbal children cannot tell us about their pain and verbal children up to the age of 7 years are unable to describe their pain.

How can pain be assessed?

Listening to parents is important – they know their children better than anyone.

There are validated, reliable instruments to measure and assess pain in children over the age of 3 years, and they may be useful particularly in children with chronic pain. Such self-report measures make use of pictures or word descriptions to describe pain, e.g. Wong's 'smiley' face scale has a smiling face at one end and a distraught crying face at the other, with several gradations in between.

Pain can be assessed in infants by measuring physiological responses to painful stimuli such as blood pressure or heart rate.

General principles

- Select the most appropriate analgesic agent to match the degree of pain that is expected
- Prescribe regular analgesia, to prevent suffering while waiting for an 'as-required' prescribed dose to work
- Titrate dose according to need
- Avoid intramuscular administration – why inflict pain to relieve pain

Medication

- **Paracetamol:**
  - indication: first-line management of mild-to-moderate general pain; antipyretic
  - preparations: suspension, tablets, soluble tablets, suppositories
  - duration of effect: 4–8 hours
  - side effects: none
  - cautions: liver and renal impairment
  - if pain control is inadequate with regular administration, consider adding ibuprofen, diclofenac or codeine
- **Non-steroidal anti-inflammatory agents:**
  - indication: ibuprofen for mild-to-moderate pain, an antipyretic; diclofenac for moderate pain and inflammation, musculoskeletal, bone pain, and as an adjunct to morphine in severe pain to reduce morphine requirements
  - preparations: suspension, tablets, suppositories, injection (diclofenac)
  - duration of effect: depends on individual drug
  - side effects: gastrointestinal irritation
  - cautions: do not use if patient has a bleeding disorder, active peptic ulceration, poor renal function or severe asthma
- **Opiates:**
  - indication: codeine for moderate pain – visceral, oncology, dental, postoperative; morphine for moderate-to-severe pain – postoperative, orthopaedic, visceral, terminal care, burns, trauma, oncology; fentanyl for severe pain – favoured for short procedures because of rapid onset and short action, e.g. fracture reductions
  - preparations: syrup, tablets, suppositories, injection (varies with drug)
  - duration of effect: fentanyl 1 hour, others 4–8 hours
  - side effects: constipation (consider routine use of laxatives), sedation, respiratory depression, nausea, vomiting
  - cautions: use only one opiate at a time

Complex pain
Many specialist paediatric units have a dedicated pain team and/or a palliative care team to deal with complex cases.

Background information

Transient synovitis (irritable hip)

'Irritable hip' is the most common cause of acute pain in the hip or limp in children, with an incidence of 1–4 per 1000. The most commonly affected age group is 3–8 years with a male:female ratio of 2:1. It is a transient mild synovitis resulting in an effusion in the hip joint. Both hips can be affected in 5 per cent of cases, but not usually simultaneously. It often follows or occurs with a mild viral infection, but the exact aetiology is unclear.

- **Presentation:** sudden onset of pain in the hip or a limp, as a result of intra-articular pressure caused by the effusion
- **Examination:** reduced range of movements of the hip; child holds the hip flexed and externally rotated to relieve pain. The child may have a mild fever, but is otherwise well
- **Investigations:** blood cultures are negative, the neutrophil count and acute phase reactants are usually normal, but may be slightly raised. Radiographs of the hips are normal. Ultrasonography of the hip joint may detect a small effusion
- **Management:** simple analgesia and bed rest; transient synovitis seldom lasts longer than a few days or weeks
- Prognosis is good, but recurrence rates of up to 10 per cent have been reported

Perthes' disease

The aetiology is unknown but results in segmental avascular necrosis of the femoral head. It affects mainly boys (male:female ratio 4:1) aged 4–10 years. It is bilateral in 10 per cent of cases.

Pathological process

There is infarction of the capital femoral epiphysis to a varying degree. In some cases the epiphysis revascularizes within weeks without any long-term problems. In established disease, four stages are recognized (based on the radiological features) that may last up to 4 years:

1. Avascular necrosis
2. Fragmentation
3. Healing
4. Remodelling

Presentation

Limp with or without pain in the hip or knee joint, hip mobility, especially abduction and internal rotation, is limited.

Diagnosis

Based on clinical findings and radiological features.

Prognosis

Good, particularly in those under 6 years of age with involvement of less than half the femoral epiphysis. When over half the epiphysis is affected and the child is older, deformity of the femoral head and metaphyseal damage are more likely, resulting in subsequent degenerative arthritis in later life.

Management

Controversial – if less than half of the femoral epiphysis is affected, activity should be encouraged; however, reduced activity and partial weight bearing may be required if symptoms worsen. In more severe disease, the femoral head needs to be covered by the acetabulum to act as a mould for the reossifying epiphysis. This is done by maintaining the hip in abduction with plaster or callipers, or by femoral or pelvic osteotomy.

Slipped upper femoral epiphysis

This is a common cause of hip pain in adolescents in which there is gradual displacement of the femoral head downwards and posteriorly. It is most common during the adolescent growth spurt (girls at 10–14 years and boys at 12–16 years), particularly in obese boys. Males are affected more frequently than girls in a ratio of 3:1. It is bilateral in 25 per cent of cases.

Presentation may be:

- **Acute:** sudden onset of severe pain and weight bearing may be impossible. May be a history of minor trauma
- **Acute on chronic:** similar to acute but also a previous history of chronic pain or limp
- **Chronic:** gradual onset of pain or limp, which may have been present for several weeks or months. Pain in the region of the hip, but often referred to the thigh or knee, which may delay the diagnosis

In all cases the hip joint is often irritable with restricted range of movements, and in advanced cases the affected leg may appear shorter and externally rotated.

The diagnosis is confirmed on radiograph, but early signs may be missed unless a lateral view is taken. Management is by internal fixation.

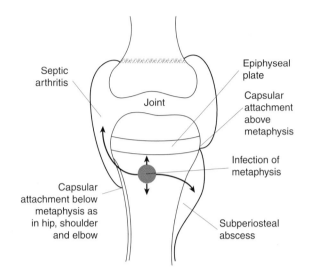

Figure 33.5 Osteomyelitis showing possible spread of infection.

Further sources of information

Articles

Beyer JE. Key issues surrounding the assessment of pain in children. *Paediatric and Perinatal Drug Therapy* 1998; **2**: 3–13

Hill H, Gill A. Analgesic guidelines in children. *Paediatric and Perinatal Drug Therapy* 1997; **1**: 15–19

Zadeh HG, Monsell F. The painful hip. *Current Paediatrics* 1998; **8**: 11–18

Self-test 5: Eighteen-month-old Patricia presents at A&E with a history of becoming acutely unwell with a high fever. She is refusing to weight bear and she screams when her left leg is moved.

A What are the two most likely diagnoses?
B What is the cause of these conditions?
C How are they spread?
D How are they diagnosed?
E What is the treatment?

Answer:

A Septic arthritis or osteomyelitis. The former is a serious infection of the joint space. In the latter, the metaphysis of long bones is infected. Common sites are the distal femur and proximal tibia

B Infection is usually caused by *Staphylococcus aureus* in older children and *Haemophilus influenzae* in children under 2, although this has lessened with the introduction of the Hib immunization. TB may present as septic arthritis, osteomyelitis or in combination. It usually presents with a low-grade fever, weight loss and localized pain

C Both usually result from haematogenous spread, but can also arise directly from an infected wound. In younger children septic arthritis can result from spread from adjacent osteomyelitis into joints where the capsule inserts below the epiphyseal growth plate. In osteomyelitis, the growth plate limits the spread of infection but, in infants, infection can spread directly through the immature growth plate to cause joint destruction (Figure 33.5)

D For both, diagnosis is made on history and clinical findings, elevated acute phase reactants, plus:
Septic arthritis – ultrasound-guided joint aspiration with Gram staining and culture may be helpful
Osteomyelitis – radiological changes are absent in the first 2–3 weeks. Bone scintigraphy and magnetic resonance imaging are usually positive early on

E Septic arthritis: intravenous antibiotics and surgical drainage and lavage of the joint. Osteomyelitis: antibiotics, usually a 6-week course and rest. Surgical drainage of abscesses and necrotic tissue

Weight loss and passing lots of urine

Age: 12 years

LEENA PATEL

Presentation

Joseph is 12 years old. His parents are quite worried because he has been passing urine frequently, and even having to get up at night to go, for the past 2 weeks. He has been drinking a lot and his clothes are rather loose. They telephoned their general practice and their GP saw Joseph later that day.

Self-test 1: The GP sees Joseph the same day because the condition he suspects from Joseph's symptoms is worrisome and can lead to an acute life-threatening complication if untreated. What is this complication and what causes death?

Answer: Diabetic ketoacidosis. Children can die from diabetic ketoacidosis as a result of:
- Hypokalaemia
- Cerebral oedema

Initial considerations and action

The symptom of passing urine frequently and even having to get up at night suggests polyuria associated with increased urine volume. It needs to be differentiated from increased frequency caused by bladder inflammation or irritation. Type 1 diabetes mellitus (insulin-dependent diabetes mellitus or IDDM, or juvenile diabetes) should be considered (Table 34.1) in children with:

- The classic symptoms and
- Duration of symptoms of a few days to a few weeks

Table 34.1   When to consider type 1 diabetes mellitus

Classic symptoms
- Polyuria (excessive urination), especially at night (nocturia) or bedwetting in a previously bladder-trained child (secondary nocturnal enuresis)
- Increased thirst
- Weight loss
- Polyphagia

Recent unexplained weight loss

Acute dehydration without a gastrointestinal disorder

Joseph's urine examined with a dip stick shows glucose 4+. This supports the diagnosis of diabetes mellitus. The GP tells Joseph and his parents about this. He telephones the local hospital and asks the paediatric doctor on call to see Joseph urgently.

Self-test 2: What conditions will you think of if a child:

A Has an acute history of passing small amounts of urine frequently?

B Drinks a lot of fluids but refuses water?

C Has polyuria, excessive thirst and weight loss but no glycosuria?

Answers:

A Bladder inflammation or irritation associated with urinary tract infection (more common) or a stone (less common)

B Primary polydipsia (habit drinking or behavioural problem)

C Diabetes insipidus

Immediate assessment in A&E

Diabetic ketoacidosis is common in children who first present with type 1 diabetes mellitus. The child may have vomiting, severe dehydration, hypovolaemic shock and altered consciousness, and therefore requires immediate assessment and attention to:

- **A**irway
- **B**reathing
- **C**irculation
- **D**egree of dehydration

A Joseph talks in sentences and clearly his **a**irway is patent. As he is not vomiting, a nasogastric tube is not inserted

B His **b**reathing is rapid and deep. This is called Kussmaul's breathing and is a compensatory hyperventilation, in order to excrete excess CO_2, associated with metabolic acidosis. Joseph's breath has a fruity smell like nail polish remover and this is caused by acetone (derived from the ketone acetoacetate)

C Oxygen saturation in air is 98 per cent and assessment of **c**irculation reveals tachycardia, pulse volume in radial and carotid arteries normal and symmetrical (suggesting normal stroke volume), normal blood pressure (BP), warm hands and normal capillary refill. These suggest no significant impairment in circulation and perfusion to the brain has not been compromised because Joseph is alert and not agitated or confused

D The **d**egree of dehydration is estimated to be moderate because Joseph is very thirsty, has dry mucous membranes, reduced skin turgor and tachycardia, although his eyeballs are not sunken and his BP is normal (see Chapter 4, Table 4.3 for how to assess the degree of dehydration clinically)

Had Joseph been shocked (very poor capillary refill, markedly reduced pulse volume, hypotension, cold mottled skin, altered mental state), he would have been given 100 per cent oxygen and fluid resuscitation (0.9 per cent sodium chloride 10 ml/kg as quickly as possible, repeated as necessary to 30 ml/kg).

A peripheral venous cannula is inserted and blood samples are taken (see 'Investigations and results').

A urine sample is also obtained and Joseph's weight and height are measured.

Quick tests in A&E reveal hyperglycaemia (BM stick reading 44 mmol/L), glycosuria (urine glucose 4+) and ketonuria (urine ketones 3+).

These, along with the clinical assessment, indicate that Joseph has diabetic ketoacidosis with 5–10 per cent dehydration. The hospital's 'Guidelines for the Management of Diabetic Ketoacidosis' are followed (Table 34.2).

Table 34.2 Categorizing patients for management of diabetic ketoacidosis

Clinical assessment	Not clinically unwell	Unwell child
	≤5 per cent dehydration	>5 per cent dehydration
		With or without drowsiness, vomiting, Kussmaul's breathing
	↓	↓
Management	Oral rehydration	Consult hospital guidelines and inform senior doctor – consultant
	Subcutaneous insulin	Admit to intensive care unit if >10 per cent dehydrated with shock or altered consciousness

Self-test 3: What is orthostatic hypotension and how will you identify it?

Answer: It is low BP in the upright position. It indicates volume depletion and is identified by increase in pulse and decrease in BP in the standing position for at least 5 minutes, compared with sitting or prone positions.

Self-test 4: Why is Joseph so thirsty? From your understanding of the physiological actions of insulin, explain how insulin deficiency results in the clinical features that Joseph has. Are any other hormones involved in the pathophysiology of ketoacidosis?

Answer: The pathophysiological effects of insulin deficiency on carbohydrate, fat and protein metabolism are shown in Figure 34.1. The classic features of type 1 diabetes mellitus are shown in green and of ketoacidosis

in pink. Ketoacidosis results from a combination of:

- Insulin deficiency and
- Excess of the counter-regulatory stress hormones – adrenaline (epinephrine), cortisol, glucagon and growth hormone (Figure 34.2)

History (see Table 34.3)

After the immediate assessment in A&E, the hospital doctor obtains the following history from Joseph's parents:

Until 2 weeks ago, Joseph had been perfectly fit apart from the odd cold. Then he gradually began drinking a lot and, at first, his parents put it down to the hot weather. He drinks whatever he can get hold of: juice, pop and even water. It was only when they heard him passing urine in the middle of the night three nights in a row that they became concerned.

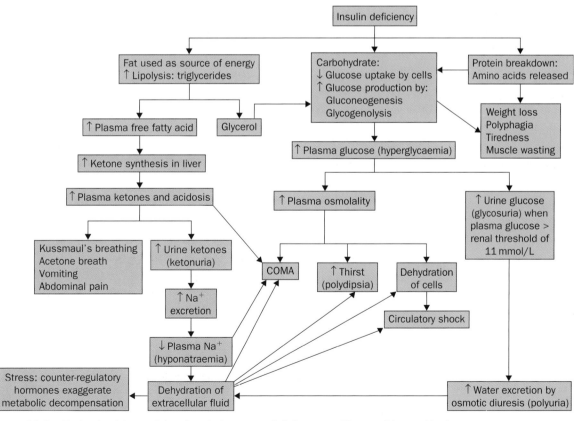

Figure 34.1 Pathophysiology of the classic features of diabetes mellitus and ketoacidosis.

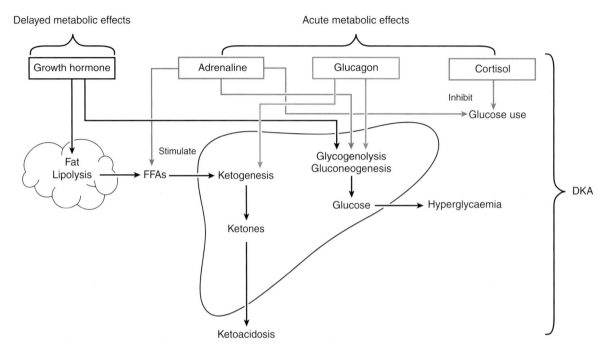

Delayed metabolic effects

Acute metabolic effects

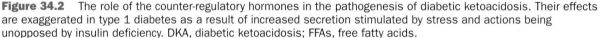

Figure 34.2 The role of the counter-regulatory hormones in the pathogenesis of diabetic ketoacidosis. Their effects are exaggerated in type 1 diabetes as a result of increased secretion stimulated by stress and actions being unopposed by insulin deficiency. DKA, diabetic ketoacidosis; FFAs, free fatty acids.

He has needed the toilet quite frequently during the day time as well. They had to find a belt because his trousers are so loose. His mum could not understand this because Joseph has been eating well. He complained of tummy ache this morning but has not vomited. Generally a lazy child, he has been more so this past week. The sore throat that he picked up from his sister 2 days ago has knocked him out completely. The pregnancy with Joseph and his birth were uneventful. There is no family history of diabetes mellitus.

Interpretation of the history

In addition to eliciting the classic symptoms of diabetes mellitus, the history is helpful in exploring whether there is:

- Any intercurrent infection triggering ketoacidosis
- Clues about the aetiology; Joseph has been worse since a recent upper respiratory tract infection

Previous good health and normal growth exclude any undiagnosed chronic autoimmune disease such as coeliac disease, thyroid disease or adrenal insufficiency.

He has not been on any medication that causes hyperglycaemia. A family history is common for type 2 diabetes but not for type 1.

Examination

Joseph's vital signs and neurological state are re-examined:

He has not deteriorated since the initial assessment but will continue to be closely observed, especially for warning signs of cerebral oedema (see Self-test 5). Cerebral oedema may become apparent only several hours after treatment has started, when the hyperglycaemia, dehydration and acidosis are improving.

Examination of the chest does not reveal any signs of a lower respiratory tract infection.

His abdomen is carefully examined and there is no abdominal distension, tenderness or guarding, and normal bowel sounds are heard. Although abdominal pain and vomiting are features of diabetic ketoacidosis, a surgical cause such as

Table 34.3 Important points in the history and examination of a child with suspected diabetes mellitus (DM)

History	Examination
Classic symptoms of DM:	*For diabetic ketoacidosis*:
• Polyuria, nocturia, secondary nocturnal enuresis (dysuria suggests a urinary tract infection)	• Vital signs and A, B, C
	• Signs of dehydration and intravascular volume depletion
	• Signs of ketoacidosis: rapid deep Kussmaul's breathing and smell of ketones on breath
• Excessive thirst (polydipsia)	• Neurological status
• Weight loss	• Pupils and fundi
• Excessive eating (polyphagia)	• Abdomen for medical (acute gastric dilatation, paralytic ileus) and surgical causes of abdominal pain (e.g. appendicitis)
Symptoms suggestive of diabetic ketoacidosis:	• Triggering infection, e.g. lower or upper respiratory tract infection
• Abdominal pain	*Associated infection*:
• Vomiting	• Candida vulvovaginitis
• Difficulty breathing	*Weight, height and stage of puberty, and previous measurements for comparison*:
Factors precipitating diabetic ketoacidosis:	• Weight loss in type 1 diabetes mellitus, obesity in type 2 diabetes
• Infection	• Deceleration in height velocity and delayed puberty indicates prolonged uncontrolled hyperglycaemia
• Injury	
Clues to associated aetiology:	*Signs of autoimmune disease*:
• Autoimmune disorders, e.g. coeliac disease, thyroiditis, Addison's disease	• Coeliac disease
	• Thyroid: goitre, hypo- or hyperthyroidism, exophthalmos
	• Adrenal: hyperpigmentation associated with primary adrenal insufficiency
• Medications, e.g. glucocorticoids	• Pernicious anaemia
• Family history of diabetes mellitus for type 2 diabetes mellitus	*Skin changes in type 2 diabetes mellitus*
	• Acanthosis nigricans at the back of the neck or axillae

acute appendicitis needs to be excluded in an unwell child (see Chapter 24). Paralytic ileus (when the abdomen would be distended and silent) is associated with metabolic acidosis, reduced splanchnic blood flow and potassium depletion.

- Small pupils
- Papilloedema
- Respiratory impairment, decreased oxygen saturation
- Incontinence

Self-test 5: What are the warning features of cerebral oedema?

Answer:
- Severe headache
- Persistent vomiting
- Confusion, irritability, reduced conscious level
- Fits
- Slowing pulse, increasing BP

Interpretation of the examination

The diagnosis of type 1 diabetes mellitus is straightforward with recent onset of classic symptoms. With increased public awareness, it is not uncommon for parents to have suspected the diagnosis. At first presentation and in children known to have type 1 diabetes, ketoacidosis should be considered when there is vomiting with or without abdominal pain. The important points in the history and examination, and the differential diagnosis in the absence of glycosuria, are shown in Tables 34.3 and 34.4.

Investigations and results

Blood and urine samples are obtained from Joseph for a number of urgent and non-urgent investigations, which help with the diagnosis and acute management (Table 34.5).

Diagnosis

Joseph has type 1 diabetes mellitus and ketoacidosis with moderate dehydration triggered by an upper respiratory tract infection (Table 34.6).

Management and follow-up

The management of a child such as Joseph presenting with diabetic ketoacidosis needs to be supervised by a senior doctor and includes:

- Resuscitation to establish A, B, C
- Management of the acute problem – correction of diabetic ketoacidosis and dehydration
- Management of the primary diagnosis – type 1 diabetes mellitus
- Long-term management of the life-long condition

Immediate assessment in A&E revealed that Joseph did not require any resuscitation. The other aspects of management are discussed below.

Management of diabetic ketoacidosis and dehydration

Aims of management of ketoacidosis and dehydration are to:

- Expand intravascular volume
- Correct deficits in fluid, sodium, potassium and acid–base status
- Normalize blood glucose with insulin infusion
- Observe and monitor very closely

Table 34.4 Differential diagnosis of the clinical features seen with diabetes mellitus and diabetic ketoacidosis

Clinical feature	Differential diagnosis	Supporting clues in addition to no glycosuria
Polyuria, nocturia	Urinary tract infection	Dysuria, urine culture diagnostic
	Diabetes insipidus	Low urine osmolality, plasma Na^+ normal or high
	Primary polydipsia	Fussy about type of fluid and may refuse water, no weight loss, urine osmolality normal from first morning sample or after water deprivation
Polydipsia	Diabetes insipidus	as above
	Primary polydipsia	
Weight loss	Anorexia nervosa	History and behaviour characteristic
	Gastrointestinal tract or other systemic disease	Specific features in history and examination
Hyperglycaemia	Drug induced	History of medication
Glycosuria	Benign glycosuria	Plasma glucose <normal renal threshold
Kussmaul's breathing, ketoacidosis	Salicylate overdose	Specific features in history and examination
	Renal failure	
	Lactic acidosis	
	Reye's syndrome	

Table 34.5 Investigations in a child presenting with diabetic ketoacidosis: Joseph's results and what they indicate

Urgent investigations	Joseph's results
Urine	
Glucose	4 +glycosuria
Ketones	3 +ketonuria
Microscopy and culture	Normal microscopy, no growth on culture – excludes UTI
Blood	
Glucose	40 mmol/L – hyperglycaemia
Urea and electrolytes:	Urea 6.9 mmol/L, creatinine 88 μmol/L – dehydration Na^+ 127 mmol/L, K^+ 3.2 mmol/L – electrolyte imbalance
Calcium, albumin:	Ca^{2+} 2.45 mmol/L, albumin 29 g/L – normal
Gases, bicarbonate:	pH 7.27, P_{CO_2} 3.1 kPa (23 mmHg), P_{O_2} 12 kPa (90 mmHg), HCO_3^- 10 mmol/L, base deficit −15 – metabolic acidosis
Full blood count:	Hb 15.1 g/dL, WBC $\times 10^9$/L, 7.6, neutrophils 66%, lymphocytes 25%, platelets 268 $\times 10^9$/L – Hb concentrated as a result of dehydration, leucocytosis common in uncomplicated diabetic ketoacidosis

Other urgent investigations (not indicated for Joseph)

- Blood culture if septicaemia suspected
- Chest radiograph if lower respiratory tract infection suspected
- Abdominal radiograph and ultrasonography if suspicion of a surgical cause for abdominal pain (see Chapter 24)

Non-urgent blood tests (Joseph has blood samples taken for these)

- HbA_{1c}: reflects blood glucose level over past 2–3 months
- Fructosamine: reflects blood glucose level over past 2–3 weeks
- Insulin and C-peptide: low in type 1 diabetes (usually high in type 2)
- Islet cell antibodies: may be present in type 1 diabetes
- Thyroid function and thyroid antibodies: for associated autoimmune thyroiditis
- Anti-endomysial and anti-gliadin antibodies: for associated coeliac disease (see Chapter 6)

UTI, urinary tract infection; WBC, white blood cell count.

Table 34.6 Clinical definition of diabetic ketoacidosis

- Classic features of diabetes mellitus: polyuria, polydipsia, weight loss
- Dehydration
- Vomiting, abdominal pain
- Hyperglycaemia: blood glucose > 11 mmol/L
- Ketonaemia: acetone breath
- Metabolic acidosis: Kussmaul's breathing, blood pH < 7.30 and bicarbonate < 15 mmol/L
- Glycosuria: urine glucose > 55 mmol/L
- Ketonuria

Fluid and electrolytes

Joseph is dehydrated but not shocked and does not require any fluid to expand his intravascular volume. The total fluid requirement (sum of deficit +maintenance) is replaced slowly and evenly over 48 hours because it is crucial to correct the hyperosmolality gradually (see Self-tests 6 and 7). Intravenous 0.9 per cent sodium chloride is given initially and changed to 0.45 per cent sodium chloride with 5 per cent dextrose when blood glucose has fallen to 12–15 mmol/L. Potassium chloride is replaced by adding 20 mmol to every 500-mL bag of fluid, provided that there is no anuria and no tented T waves on the ECG.

Oral fluids should be offered only after substantial clinical improvement and provided that there is no vomiting. The volume of oral fluid has to be subtracted from the total fluid requirement and intravenous fluids reduced accordingly. Although Joseph is very thirsty and asks for drinks, he is initially allowed only sips of oral rehydration solution.

Resuscitation, fluid therapy and administration of insulin facilitate correction of the metabolic acidosis, and bicarbonate infusion is not recommended.

Self-test 6: Joseph's weight is 38.6 kg and he has moderate (7.5 per cent of body weight) dehydration. Calculate his total fluid requirement.

Answer: Joseph's 48-h total fluid requirement is 6755 mL and this is given at a rate of 140 mL/h:

48-h total fluid requirement =
 Maintenance (Table 34.7) + Deficit

50 mL/kg per 24 h × 2 + 7.5 per cent of body weight in g

i.e. 50 × 38.6 × 2   + 0.075 × (38.6 × 1000)
i.e. 3860 mL   + 2895 mL

Self-test 7: Why is it important to correct the fluid deficit slowly over 48 hours?

Answer: Cerebral oedema is an unpredictable and frequently fatal complication of diabetic ketoacidosis. It becomes clinically apparent several hours after treatment

Table 34.7 Maintenance fluid requirement at different ages

Approximate age (years)	Weight (kg)	Maintenance fluid (ml/kg per 24 h)
<1	3–9	80
1–5	10–19	70
6–9	20–29	60
10–14	30–50	50
>15	>50	35

has begun. The pathophysiology of cerebral oedema is not known but risk factors associated with it include:

- At presentation:
  - high plasma sodium
  - low arterial P_{CO_2}
  - high plasma urea (in turn associated with longer duration of symptoms)
- During fluid therapy:
  - rapid decline in plasma osmolality – plasma osmolality can be measured in the laboratory or calculated:

    Plasma osmolality = 2(Na$^+$ + K$^+$) + Blood glucose (mosmol)

  - too much insulin and rapid fall in blood glucose by >5 mmol/L per hour
  - failure of plasma sodium to rise as plasma glucose declines
  - too rapid fluid replacement (e.g. wrong calculation, oral fluid intake not subtracted from total fluid requirement)
  - bicarbonate therapy

Insulin

After any shock has been corrected and replacement fluid started, insulin is commenced as an intravenous infusion at 0.1 unit/kg per hour. The infusion rate may have to be reduced to ensure that blood glucose does not fall more rapidly than 4–5 mmol/L per hour.

Insulin by subcutaneous injection is started when oral intake is tolerated. To prevent rebound hyperglycaemia, the intravenous insulin infusion should be continued until 60 minutes after the first subcutaneous injection of insulin.

Monitoring

Joseph requires close monitoring (Table 34.8) and vigilance for warning features of the two most serious complications: cerebral oedema (see Self-test 5) and hypokalaemia (Table 34.9).

In the presence of hyperglycaemia and hyperosmolality, plasma sodium is diluted as water is drawn out of cells and into extracellular space. Thus, measured plasma sodium is 2 mmol/L lower than true plasma sodium for a blood glucose that is 5.5 mmol/L higher.

Although Joseph's plasma sodium and blood glucose are 127 mmol/L and 40 mmol/L, respectively, his true plasma sodium is likely to be 138 mmol/L (127 + [2(40–10)/5.5]).

During fluid management:

- Measured plasma sodium should rise by 2 mmol/L for every 5.5 mmol/L fall in blood glucose
- Blood glucose should fall by 4–5 mmol/L every hour

At 8 am the following morning, 10 hours after he presented to hospital, Joseph is sitting up in bed watching television, has tolerated oral rehydration fluid and is keen to have some breakfast. His blood results show that the blood glucose has come down gradually, the electrolytes are normal and the acidosis is improving (glucose 10.5 mmol/L, Na^+ 135 mmol/L, K^+ 3.8 mmol/L, urea 4.9 mmol/L, creatinine 66 nmol/L, pH 7.32, bicarbonate 16 mmol/L, base deficit −8). He is given subcutaneous short-acting insulin, has breakfast cereal 30 minutes later, and the intravenous fluids and insulin infusion are stopped thereafter.

Table 34.8 Observations in a child with diabetic ketoacidosis

- Continuous ECG – watch changes in T wave, appearance of U waves and rhythm
- Intravenous and oral fluid input
- Urine output and other losses
- Hourly pulse rate, respiratory rate, BP
- Hourly neurological observations
- Hourly finger-prick blood glucose with BM stick
- Hourly capillary blood gas
- Urine glucose and ketones from every sample
- Blood glucose and electrolytes 2 hours after start of intravenous therapy and then 4 hourly
- Weigh once or twice a day

Table 34.9 Warning features of hypokalaemia

ECG shows:
- Broad flat T waves
- ST segment depression
- QT interval prolonged
- Ventricular arrhythmia

Self-test 8: The following contribute to the life-threatening hypokalaemia in diabetic ketoacidosis:

A Impaired renal function
B Metabolic acidosis
C Administration of insulin
D Administration of sodium bicarbonate
E Hypocalcaemia

Answers: C and D are true. Impaired renal function, metabolic acidosis and hypocalcaemia are associated with hyperkalaemia.

Management of type 1 diabetes mellitus

Joseph and his parents have been informed about the diagnosis and the management so far. It is hard for any family to take all this in, and they are supported and helped by the diabetes care team, which includes doctors, specialist nurses, dieticians, family counsellors and clinical psychologists. With time, Joseph and his family need to become experts in order to manage well with his diabetes. They are informed and involved with various aspects of management while Joseph is in hospital to stabilize his blood glucose, and thus a gradual process of education is initiated (Table 34.10).

Goals of treatment

- Control blood glucose and aim for glycated haemoglobin (HbA_{1c}) in the normal range, which varies according to the assay used
- No symptoms of high or low blood glucose day to day
- Prevent ketoacidosis
- Overall good health
- Normal growth and puberty
- Normal development, schooling and family life
- Prevent long-term complications

Subcutaneous insulin injections

There are many insulin preparations that can be administered with a syringe or different pen injection devices. There are three main types according to the onset and

Table 34.10 Various aspects of management of a child with type 1 diabetes mellitus, which the child and family need to be informed about

Subcutaneous insulin injections

- Types of insulin, dose and timing, injection technique, changing sides and rotating sites, storing
- Altering dose for specific situations: birthdays, parties, holidays, acute illness, gastroenteritis, operation, intense exercise

Diet

General principles:
- Nutritional requirements similar to those of a healthy non-diabetic child
- Carbohydrate intake and insulin need to be carefully matched
- Carbohydrate as starch rather than sugar, low fat, high fibre
- Meals and snacks distributed throughout the day

Monitoring

Self-monitoring:
- Normal blood glucose levels, finger-prick technique, frequency of testing, recording results
- Urine testing for ketones
- HbA$_{1c}$
- Urine for microalbuminuria

Problems with glucose control

Hypoglycaemia:
- Causes, symptoms and signs, treatment, prevention

Hyperglycaemia and ketoacidosis:
- Causes, symptoms and signs, treatment, prevention

Intermediate-term complications:
- Impaired growth
- Delayed puberty

Long-term complications:
- Small blood vessels: eyes – retinopathy; kidneys – nephropathy; nerves – neuropathy
- Large blood vessels: accelerated atherosclerosis, peripheral vascular disease (gangrene), cardiovascular disease

Sources of parent support and information outside the hospital

- Local parents' group
- Charities such as Diabetes UK

duration of action:

1 Short acting – rapid onset (15–30 min) and short duration (3–4 hours): soluble insulin such as Human Actrapid, insulin lispro
2 Intermediate acting (12–18 hours), e.g. isophane insulin, insulin zinc suspension
3 Long acting (12–24 hours), e.g. Human Ultratard

The type of insulin, dose and frequency of administration need to be tailored to the individual child.

For a brief period after diagnosis (several weeks to months), insulin requirement may be reduced (from 1 unit/kg per day to <0.5 unit/kg per day) as a result of some residual insulin secretion from β cells. This is called the honeymoon or remission phase. Higher doses are usually required during puberty.

The insulin regimen can vary from twice-daily injections before meals of a short-acting insulin mixed with intermediate-acting insulin to multiple injections of short-acting insulin before meals and intermediate-acting insulin at bedtime.

Short-acting insulin is recommended for acute illness, surgery or other stress.

Absorption of insulin varies from different subcutaneous sites, being relatively rapid from the stomach compared with the thigh. It is therefore advisable to keep a consistent site for each time of the day. However, to prevent lipodystrophy and erratic absorption of insulin, Joseph is told to change sides and rotate within sites (Figure 34.3).

Self-test 9: For certain situations, Joseph is most likely to require the following alterations:

A Reduce the dose of insulin with an acute febrile illness

B Reduce the dose of insulin with acute gastroenteritis

C Omit insulin with intense physical activity

Answers:

A False: an acute febrile illness increases blood glucose as a result of insulin resistance and increased secretion of stress hormones. It may even be the trigger for ketoacidosis. Joseph will certainly need to take insulin and may need a higher dose

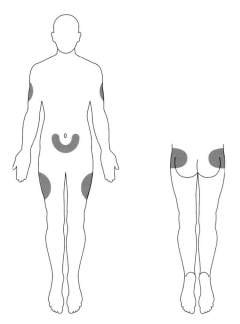

Figure 34.3 Sites suitable for injecting insulin subcutaneously in children and teenagers.

depending on his blood glucose reading, how unwell he is and his appetite

B True: as a result of rapid intestinal transit and impaired digestion and absorption, blood glucose may fall during acute gastroenteritis. Therefore, the dose of insulin may have to be reduced

C False: the need for insulin is lower with exercise but not zero. Insulin is required to transport glucose into cells. Even more glucose is transported into cells during intense physical activity and hypoglycaemia may occur. If insulin is omitted, intracellular glucose deficiency results in excess secretion of counter-regulatory hormones and consequently hyperglycaemia. Therefore, the dose of insulin may have to be reduced but it should not be omitted

Hypoglycaemia

Causes
- Not enough food, e.g. skipped or delayed meal
- Too much insulin, new site, e.g. abdomen instead of thigh
- Unusually heavy exercise
- Alcohol

Clinical features
See Table 34.11.

Management
An unconscious child requires a subcutaneous or intramuscular glucagon injection.

When symptomatic and conscious, immediate treatment is ingestion of roughly 10 g glucose which is available from three glucose tablets (each contains 3 g glucose), two to three teaspoons of sugar or jam, or a glass of fruit juice. These may need to be repeated in 5 minutes if there is no improvement.

To maintain the blood glucose level, a longer-acting carbohydrate (such as a few biscuits, a sandwich, a packet of crisps or yoghurt) should be taken 15 minutes later.

Blood glucose should be measured at the time of hypoglycaemia and every 30 minutes for 90 minutes.

Hyperglycaemia

Causes
- Not enough insulin
- Too much carbohydrate
- Less exercise than usual
- Excitement or emotional stress
- Intercurrent illness, fever

Clinical features
- Polyuria
- Increased thirst

These symptoms at a particular time of the day (e.g. afternoon) indicate when blood glucose control is poor.

Hyperglycaemic phenomenon
Rebound phenomenon (or posthypoglycaemic hyperglycaemia)
- Hyperglycaemia following hypoglycaemia
- Associated with a counter-regulatory hormone response to low blood glucose when insulin levels are also low (high levels of insulin reduce secretion of counter-regulatory hormones), e.g. after hypoglycaemia caused by exercise or not eating enough

Table 34.11 Clinical features of hyperglycaemia

As a result of adrenaline release and autonomic nervous system activity (adrenergic)	As a result of reduced cerebral glucose and oxygen use (neuroglycopenic)
Sweating	Headache
Tremors, shakiness, jitteriness	Weakness, tiredness
Anxiety, nervousness	Poor concentration, short-term memory and judgement
Tachycardia, palpitations	Double or blurred vision, disturbed colour vision (especially red–green colours)
Hunger	
Nausea	Slurred speech
Pallor	Unsteadiness, poor coordination
	Behavioural and personality changes – irritability, temper tantrums, bizarre behaviour
	Nightmares
	Confusion, drowsiness, impaired consciousness
	Convulsions

Somogyi phenomenon

- Rebound hyperglycaemia on waking in the morning caused by low blood glucose at night
- Associated with pre-bedtime dose of insulin being too high

Dawn phenomenon

- Rise in blood glucose early in the morning not preceded by hypoglycaemia
- Associated with physiological increased secretion of growth hormone
- More pronounced during the pubertal growth spurt

Self-test 10: In hospital, Joseph has finger-pricks before every meal and also before bedtime. He resents them because his fingers are sore. His parents ask whether they can test Joseph's urine for glucose instead of doing finger-prick blood glucose. Is this appropriate?

Answer: No. The risks of complications can be reduced by good metabolic control. Treatment is aimed at keeping pre-meal blood glucose within the range 4–9 mmol/L. This information is provided by finger-prick blood glucose testing, but not by urine glucose testing

because the latter will be positive only when the blood glucose is greater than the normal renal threshold (>11 mmol/L).

Routinely, it is not necessary to check blood glucose more than once or twice a day. However, the time should be altered each day so that by the end of the week there is a profile of readings for before breakfast, lunch, dinner and bedtime. Home urine testing for ketones is recommended:

- If blood glucose is >11 mmol/L for more than 6 hours
- With acute illness and
- If there is any vomiting or abdominal pain

Follow-up for a child with type 1 diabetes mellitus

Four days after he presented to hospital, Joseph is ready to be discharged and the GP is informed.

Joseph has been established on a twice-daily insulin regimen. His father is competent in giving insulin, his mother intends to learn over the next few days, but Joseph is still hesitant. He has, however, learnt to do his own finger-pricks and blood glucose tests.

The diabetes specialist nurse arranges a home visit for the following day and will maintain regular contact over the coming weeks, when the family will be adjusting to Joseph's diagnosis and its management.

He requires life-long follow-up by the multidisciplinary team. During childhood, he will be reviewed every 3 months in the outpatient clinic (Table 34.12) and will also have detailed annual assessments (Table 34.13).

Background information

Differentiating type 1 from type 2 diabetes mellitus

See Table 34.14.

Diagnostic algorithm for diabetes mellitus

Figure 34.4 (p. 367) is adapted from the guidelines of the World Health Organization and International Diabetes Federation guidelines.

WHO classification of diabetes mellitus

- Type 1: β-cell destruction, insulin deficiency – ketosis prone:
  - type 1A: autoimmune aetiology
  - type 1B: no demonstrable autoimmunity
- Type 2: variable degree of insulin resistance and deficiency – not ketosis prone
- Other specific types:
  - genetic causes of impaired β-cell function: maturity-onset diabetes of youth (MODY)
  - defects in insulin action: type A insulin resistance, congenital lipoatrophy
  - secondary to pancreatic disease: cystic fibrosis, thalassaemia, haemochromatosis
  - secondary to other endocrine disease: Cushing's disease, pituitary gigantism
  - drugs/toxins: glucocorticoids, thiazides, asparaginase
  - infection: congenital rubella

Source: www.nzgg.org.nz/library/gl_complete/ diabetes/who_report_diabetes_diagnosis.pdf

Table 34.12 What to assess at each outpatient clinic visit

- Any hyper- or hypoglycaemic symptoms, explore contributing factors
- Height, weight and stage of puberty and compare with previous assessments
- Blood pressure
- Blood glucose control: home testing and HbA_{1c}
- Self-monitoring of blood glucose and urine for ketones, insulin dose, injection technique, injection sites, diet, physical activity
- Family and school life
- Discuss any concerns
- Discuss general and specific knowledge, enhance understanding
- Discuss realistic targets

Table 34.13 What to check at each annual assessment

- Blood pressure
- Eyes: visual acuity, lens for cataract, fundus examination
- Hands, feet: pulses, neurology
- Biochemical tests of metabolic control: HbA_{1c}
- Screening tests for complications: urine for microalbuminuria, plasma lipids
- Tests for autoimmune disorders: thyroid antibodies, thyroid function, anti-endomysial and anti-gliadin antibodies

  - genetic disorders: syndromes – Down's, Klinefelter's, Prader–Willi, Turner's

Further sources of information

Book

Hanas R. *Insulin-dependent Diabetes in Children, Adolescents and Adults. How to become an expert on your own diabetes.* Uddevalla, Sweden: Piara HB, 1998

Table 34.14 Differentiating type 1 from type 2 diabetes mellitus

	Type 1 diabetes mellitus	Type 2 diabetes mellitus
Also called	Insulin-dependent diabetes mellitus (IDDM) Juvenile diabetes mellitus	Non-insulin-dependent diabetes mellitus (NIDDM)
Age of onset	Usually before age 35 years	Usually after age 35–40 years
Peak age	5–7 years, at time of puberty	Mid to late puberty
Prevalence	<5 years age: 1 in 1500 5–18 years age: 1 in 400	Increasing as a result of escalating trend in childhood obesity
Gender	Occurs equally in boys and girls	More common in girls
Ethnic origin	White people of northern European descent living in temperate climates Most common in Scandinavia	Any but most common in African–Caribbean and Indo-Asian communities
Basic defect	Destruction of β cells and insulin deficiency	Increased insulin secretion and down-regulation of insulin receptors leading to insulin resistance
Associations	Certain MHC loci on chromosome 6 Islet cell antibodies Other autoimmune manifestations Viral infections, e.g. congenital rubella, mumps, Coxsackie virus	Obesity Sedentary lifestyle Gestational diabetes
Presentation	Obvious symptoms for a few days to few weeks	Symptoms may be mild and go unnoticed for months to years
Ketoacidosis	Always a possibility	Unlikely to occur
Treatment	Insulin required from the onset	Drugs that increase insulin sensitivity or increase release of insulin from the pancreas

MHC, major histocompatibility complex.

Articles

Epstein FH. Protection of acid–base balance by pH regulation of acid production. Mechanisms of disease. *New England Journal of Medicine* 1998; **339**: 819–26

Inward CD, Chambers TL. Fluid management in diabetic ketoacidosis. Have we got it right yet? *Archives of Disease in Childhood* 2002; **86**: 443–5

Glaser N, Barnett P, McCaslin I et al. Risk factors for cerebral oedema in children with diabetic ketoacidosis. *New England Journal of Medicine* 2001; **344**: 264–9

Self-test 11: Are there any similarities between prolonged starvation (such as in someone with anorexia nervosa) and diabetic ketoacidosis?

Answer: In both there is intracellular glucose deficiency in the presence of low insulin activity. This results in ketone production because fat rather than glucose is used as an energy source. The intracellular glucose deficiency is the result of:

- Low extracellular glucose concentrations in starvation but
- Insulin deficiency in type 1 diabetes mellitus

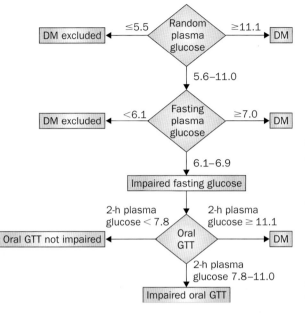

Figure 34.4 Algorithm for diagnosis of diabetes mellitus (DM) from guidelines of the World Health Organization and the International Federation of Diabetes. Plasma glucose concentrations are in millimoles per litre. GTT, glucose tolerance test. Redrawn from Lamb EJ, Day AP, New diagnostic criteria for diabetes mellitus; are we any further forward? *Annals of Clinical Biochemistry* 2000; **37**: 588–92, with permission from Blackwell Publishing.

In both starvation and ketoacidosis, increased gluconeogenesis results in increased glucose being released into the extracellular fluid. This is appropriate in starvation but aggravates the hyperglycaemia in type 1 diabetes mellitus (Figure 34.5).

Self-test 12: What measures help prevent diabetic ketoacidosis in a child known to have type 1 diabetes mellitus?

Answers:
- Patient and family education so that the dose of insulin is not reduced or withheld during an acute illness when there is actually a greater insulin requirement
- Improved patient compliance with management

Self-test 13: Macy has cystic fibrosis and both α and β cells in the islets of Langerhans are damaged. This results in diabetes mellitus but ketoacidosis is less likely to occur. Why?

Answer: Because Macy has a deficiency of glucagon, secreted by the α cells, as well as a deficiency of insulin. Ketoacidosis develops when there is insulin deficiency along with exaggerated effects of the counter-regulatory hormones (see Figure 34.2, p. 356). Glucagon is a major counter-regulatory hormone and its deficiency reduces the likelihood of ketoacidosis developing.

Self-test 14: Polyuria, dehydration and thirst are common after a few alcoholic drinks. Does this sound familiar? Can you explain why, considering that alcohol reduces blood sugar?

Answer: Alcohol inhibits antidiuretic hormone (ADH) secretion from the posterior pituitary and this results in polyuria (dehydration). Initially alcohol blocks gluconeogenesis, and the slight fall in blood glucose stimulates appetite. It also suppresses secretion of cortisol and growth hormone. These, along with depletion of glycogen stores, lead to hypoglycaemia (headache) for several hours after drinking large amounts of alcohol.

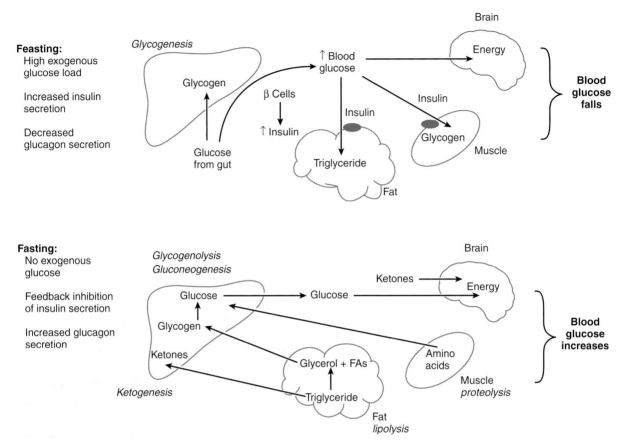

Figure 34.5 Regulation of blood glucose with feasting and fasting. There is a feedback relation between blood glucose and secretion of insulin and glucagon. FAs, fatty acids.

Bad asthma attack

Age: 13 years

LEENA PATEL

Presentation

It is 6 pm on Friday evening and Tomayo (13 years old), accompanied by his mother, is brought to the accident and emergency department (A&E) by ambulance with a 'severe asthma attack'. He has had high-flow oxygen and two doses of salbutamol 10 mg nebulized on the way to hospital. The asthma attack started that morning; the cough worsened very quickly in the evening and Tomayo collapsed, unable to breathe. His older sister gave mouth-to-mouth breathing while mother called the ambulance.

Self-test 1: What might you do first if you were the doctor in A&E?

Answer: Primary assessment of A, B, C.

Initial considerations and action

The priority in managing Tomayo is primary assessment of vital functions – ABCD and resuscitation (see Chapter 22). Secondary assessment of his 'asthma attack' will be undertaken thereafter to provide specific emergency treatment.

Primary assessment, which takes no longer than a minute, reveals the following:

- **Airway:** patent – Tomaya is not talking but is breathing spontaneously
- **Breathing:** difficulty – suprasternal and intercostal recessions, use of accessory muscles, tachypnoea (respiratory rate 45/minute), no wheeze, poor air entry, arterial oxygen saturation (Sao$_2$) 92 per cent in 15 L O$_2$

- **Circulation:** adequate – pulse 135/minute regular and normal volume, capillary refill <2 seconds, blood pressure (BP) 106/66 mmHg
- **Disability:** responds to voice – pupils equal and reactive, no convulsions

The anaesthetic registrar arrived in A&E immediately. Tomayo has significant respiratory distress and hypoxia but does not require ventilatory support at this stage. As a result of the possibility of a 'severe asthma attack', he is given another dose of nebulized salbutamol 10 mg with oxygen.

A peripheral venous cannula is inserted for intravenous access. Whether he has indeed had a severe asthma attack or another acute problem will now be considered from the history and examination (secondary assessment) so that appropriate emergency treatment can be given.

Self-test 2: What other acute problem could Tomayo have?

Answer: A pneumothorax.

History

For the purpose of secondary assessment, a concise history is obtained from the mother as well as the paramedics focusing on:

- The duration and progress of symptoms
- Peak expiratory flow rate (PEFR) if measured at home
- Treatment already given and response
- Course of previous attacks

Tomayo's mother reveals that Tomayo has had asthma since he was 7 years old and is under a specialist at the hospital. He had mild attacks of asthma until a few years ago, but has not had any admissions.

Tomayo had a runny nose and dry cough this morning. He was a little wheezy at school but could not take any inhalers because he has not been carrying them around for some time. He managed to catch the bus but felt tight and out of breath by the time he got home. He took two puffs of his salmeterol Accuhaler because his salbutamol had run out. Nothing happened so his mother made him take 10 puffs of his sister's salbutamol spray. The cough got worse and Tomayo complained that he could not breathe. Just as mother was getting ready to bring him to hospital he slumped and passed out on the settee. The ambulance men found him unconscious, breathing spontaneously and cyanosed.

Interpretation of the history

The history reveals acute asthma symptoms triggered by a cold (see Chapter 26) and rapid worsening of symptoms in a teenager known to have asthma. The symptoms of acute asthma are:

- Dry cough
- Wheeze
- Chest tightness
- Difficulty breathing

The symptoms of worsening asthma are:

- Worsening cough, wheeze and breathlessness
- Difficulty in sleeping, walking, talking and eating
- Increasing need for reliever bronchodilator (indicates response is not prompt and not sustained for at least 3 hours)

Chest tightness may be described as a pain over the sternum and it is important to differentiate this from the pain associated with a pneumothorax. The symptoms of a pneumothorax are sudden onset of breathlessness and unilateral chest pain.

Tomayo's symptoms rapidly worsened, probably as a result of:

- A delay in taking any treatment
- Inappropriate treatment and
- The physical exertion in getting home from school

Salmeterol does not relieve acute symptoms because it is a long-acting β_2 agonist with slow onset of action, compared with short-acting β_2 agonists such as salbutamol or terbutaline (see Figure 35.4). His sister's 'spray' is an aerosol delivered with a metered dose inhaler (MDI). Using an MDI is difficult because inhalation has to be synchronized with inspiration (see Chapter 26). Thus, drug delivery to the airway is poor, and more so during an acute attack when the inspiratory flow rate is low. It is not surprising that the MDI had no effect despite 10 puffs of salbutamol. This dose, inhaled with a large-volume spacer might have been effective early on in the attack because a β_2 agonist administered with a large-volume spacer is as effective as a nebulizer for a moderately severe acute attack. However, during a severe attack, even a spacer is used less effectively because of distress and panic.

Examination

The purpose of the examination is to assess the severity of the asthma attack and confirm that there are no signs of a pneumothorax.

In addition to the observations made during the primary assessment, Tomayo's chest movements are symmetrical and regular. He is working hard to breathe, using his accessory muscles, and is unable to blow into a peak flowmeter. He is restless and too breathless to talk but responds to questions by moving his hand. Air entry is reduced bilaterally. The trachea is central, the apex beat is not displaced and the percussion note is resonant.

Meaning of the examination

In an acute asthma attack, wheeze (may be absent if the airflow is very low as in Tomayo, or loud) and respiratory rate (may be fast like Tomayo's or slow) are poor indicators of severity.

Recessions during inspiration suggest that high negative intrathoracic pressure is generated by airway obstruction. Use of accessory muscles reflects the increased work of breathing and significant respiratory distress.

In a patient with respiratory distress, the ability to walk, talk, eat and drink indicates the degree of

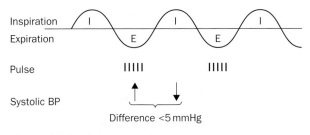

Figure 35.1 Pulsus paradoxus.

breathlessness. Inability to blow into a peak flowmeter implies poor respiratory effort.

Pulsus paradoxus is a sign of severe airway obstruction. It is assessed from disappearance of the pulse during inspiration and a difference of $\geq 20\,\mathrm{mmHg}$ between the systolic pressure on inspiration and that on expiration (Figure 35.1). However, it may be difficult to measure in children like Tomayo who are tachypnoeic. Prolonged expiration is a feature of intrathoracic airway obstruction, but it may also be difficult to appreciate in a tachypnoeic child.

Air entry is reduced bilaterally in severe diffuse airway obstruction. Unilateral reduced air entry indicates localized airway narrowing (e.g. foreign body or tumour), collapse of a segment or lobe, pneumothorax or pleural effusion. A significant pneumothorax would displace the mediastinum and result in displacement of the trachea and apex beat.

Self-test 3: Explain why expiration is prolonged in intrathoracic airway obstruction.

Answer: Normally, the intrathoracic airways collapse slightly during expiration because pressure in the airways is lower than in the alveoli. When there is intrathoracic airway obstruction, there is greater resistance to airflow and it takes longer to move air out of the alveoli (see Chapter 9).

Interpretation of the examination

Tomayo had rapidly worsening acute asthma symptoms and was brought to A&E by ambulance after collapsing at home. The collapse may have been the result of hypoxia and exhaustion. He has had high-flow oxygen, two doses of nebulized salbutamol in the ambulance and a further dose in A&E, does not appear to have deteriorated since, and is not unconscious in A&E. Examination suggests a severe asthma attack and the major concern is that Tomayo may soon get exhausted from the sheer effort of working so hard to breathe (Table 35.1).

Investigations and results

Serial arterial blood gas monitoring is indicated in view of the severe asthma attack and concerns about exhaustion. A sample is obtained from the left radial artery soon after starting emergency treatment, approximately 20 minutes after Tomayo was brought to A&E. A chart of the investigations and treatment given is shown in Table 35.2.

During an acute attack of asthma resistance varies throughout the lower airway, resulting in both over-ventilated and under-ventilated lung units. This diffuse ventilation–perfusion mismatch results in varying degrees of hypoxia. Early in an asthma attack patients have respiratory alkalosis (low $P\mathrm{CO_2}$) from hyperventilation. As airway obstruction progresses, alveolar hypoventilation and respiratory muscle fatigue lead to hypercapnia and respiratory acidosis ($Pa\mathrm{CO_2} \geq 6\,\mathrm{kPa}$ or $45\,\mathrm{mmHg}$) (for 'How to read a blood gas report' see Figure 3.5 in Chapter 3).

A chest radiograph does not alter management and is indicated if pneumothorax is suspected. It may show free air (pneumothorax or pneumomediastinum), infiltrates or atelectasis.

Self-test 4: Interpret the chest radiographs in Figure 35.2 from children who presented acutely with difficulty breathing. What might be the other distinguishing features in the history? (See Chapter 9 for 'How to interpret a chest radiograph'.)

Answer:
A Hyperlucency of both lungs and hyperinflation with flattening of the diaphragm and narrow heart shadow (from air trapping) in severe asthma. A bell-shaped thoracic cage suggests long-standing asthma.

Table 35.1 Clinical features helpful in assessing the severity of an asthma attack

Examination	Mild	Moderate	Severe	Respiratory arrest imminent
Breathlessness	On walking	On talking	At rest, respiratory rate >50/min if <5 years of age and >40/min if >5 years age	Exhaustion; respiratory effort poor, feeble, irregular
Talking	In sentences	Single words	Too breathless to talk or feed	Cannot talk
Posture	Can lie flat	Prefers sitting	Hunched forward	Supine
Alertness	May be agitated	Usually agitated	Agitated	Confused, drowsy, unconscious
Sao_2 in air (%)	>95	92–95	<92	<85, cyanosis
PEFR (% of expected or best)	>80	50–80	30–50	<30
Other signs			Breath sounds reduced in intensity, pulse >140/min if age <5 years and >120/min if age >5 years	Bradycardia, hypotension, silent chest
			Transfer to paediatric intensive care unit Mechanical ventilation if: • Persistent hypoxia, $Pao_2 < 8\,kPa$ • $Paco_2 > 8\,kPa$ • Increasing exhaustion	

Table 35.2 Results of Tomayo's investigations

	Time			
	6.20 pm	7 pm	7.30 pm	9 pm
Arterial blood gas				
pH	7.05	7.24	7.33	7.36
Pco_2 (mmHg)	101	60	42	42
Po_2 (mmHg)	210	207	191	202
HCO_3 (mmol/L)	25	25	23	24
Base excess	−8	−3	−2	−1
Plasma urea and electrolytes				
Na^+ (mmol/L)	137			138
K^+ (mmol/L)	3.9			3.6
Urea (mmol/L)	3.4			
Creatinine (μmol/L)	82			
Time	6.05 pm	6.15 pm	6.30 pm	
Treatment	Oxygen Salbutamol neb	Oxygen Salbutamol neb Hydrocortisone i.v.	Oxygen Salbutamol neb Aminophylline infusion	

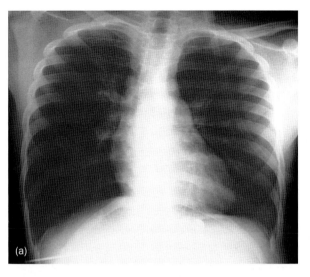

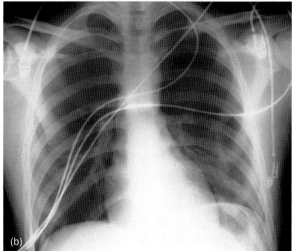

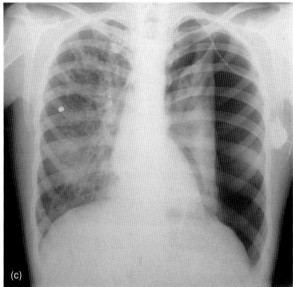

Figure 35.2 Radiographs for (a) person A, (b) person B and (c) person C in Self-test 4.

Presentation with acute cough, wheeze, chest tightness and shortness of breath in a child known to have asthma

B Left pneumothorax, right lung normal, no central venous lines, no rib fractures. Presentation is with sudden onset of breathlessness and 'sharp' pain in the left side of the chest. May be spontaneous or caused by blunt chest injury. Spontaneous pneumothorax typically occurs in tall thin boys

C Left pneumothorax and lungs are abnormal throughout: linear parallel shadows and ring shadows indicate bronchial wall thickening and inflammation. Diffuse ill-defined shadows are caused by distended airways filled with mucus, areas of collapse, lung damage and fibrosis. Presentation as for B and associated with an exacerbation of respiratory symptoms in a girl known to have cystic fibrosis and severe lung disease

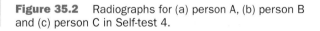

Causes of pneumothorax

- Spontaneous in previously healthy person
- Secondary to lung disease, e.g. asthma, cystic fibrosis

- Chest injury: penetrating or blunt
- Iatrogenic, e.g. insertion of central venous catheter

Diagnosis

The secondary assessment reveals that Tomayo has had a severe asthma attack triggered by a cold. An acute asthma attack is the most common cause of hospital admissions in the UK. The mortality from asthma in children under 10 years of age is low and has declined in the past decade. However, asthma in adolescents is associated with higher mortality rates (5 per million for those aged 10–14 years) than in younger children (4 per million for children aged 0–4 years; fewer than 2 per million for children aged 5–9 years). Morbidity is also high in adolescents and asthma symptoms can interfere with school and physical activity. An acute attack must always be considered a failure of preventive treatment. Tomayo's preventive treatment will need to be reviewed once this acute attack is controlled and before discharge.

Factors associated with a high risk of asthma-related death

- Non-adherence with treatment, poor supervision
- Denial of asthma or its severity, inappropriate perception of severity
- Recent discontinuation of oral prednisolone or high-dose inhaled corticosteroid treatment
- Previous severe attack of asthma requiring mechanical ventilation or intensive care
- More than two admissions to hospital in the past year with asthma attacks
- Acute attack of asthma requiring hospital management in the previous month
- Major psychosocial problems

Management and follow-up

Emergency treatment

For Tomayo, emergency management includes:

- Continuing high-flow oxygen to maintain $SaO_2 > 95$ per cent

Table 35.3 Drugs used for emergency management of acute severe asthma

- High-flow oxygen
- Salbutamol 2.5–10 mg or terbutaline 2.5–10 mg nebulized continuously or every 30 min according to severity
- Ipratropium bromide 250 µg nebulized every 6 hours
- Prednisolone (1–2 mg/kg, maximum 40 mg) orally

If life-threatening features:

- Hydrocortisone 1 mg/kg per h of infusion
- Aminophylline 5 mg/kg infusion over 20 minutes of loading dose (omit this if child already on oral theophylline) followed by 1 mg/kg per h of infusion
- Salbutamol 4–6 µg/kg i.v over 10 min followed by 0.1–1.0 µg/kg per min of infusion

- Short-acting β_2 agonist (salbutamol 10 mg or terbutaline 10 mg) nebulized with oxygen immediately and repeated in order to deliver continuously
- Hydrocortisone 100 mg i.v. as a bolus (Table 35.3)

How to reassess and review a child admitted with an acute asthma attack

- Compare with earlier assessments

From nurses' observation chart
- Oxygen saturation, oxygen requirement
- Respiratory rate and heart rate
- Peak flow readings
- Temperature

History from child, parents and nurses
- Change in symptoms
- Oral intake

Examination
- Posture
- Pallor, cyanosis
- Ability to talk
- Signs of respiratory distress
- Chest auscultation

Results of any investigations undertaken

- Blood gases
- Plasma electrolytes
- Chest radiograph

Treatment

- Frequency, dose and mode of delivery of inhaled bronchodilator
- Other treatment

Tomayo's progress

Reassessment reveals that Tomayo now has a bilateral wheeze and there is some improvement in air entry. However, he is still too breathless to talk and the arterial blood gas taken soon after starting this treatment shows respiratory acidosis (at 6.20 pm – see Table 35.1). He continues to have high-flow oxygen and nebulized salbutamol and is also given treatment with:

- Aminophylline 5 mg/kg i.v. over 15 minutes as a loading dose followed by infusion at 1 ml/kg per hour
- Hydrocortisone 1 mg/kg per hour of infusion
- Intravenous fluids at 75 per cent of maintenance requirement

A severe acute asthma attack may progress very rapidly to respiratory failure. Tomayo is therefore admitted to the paediatric intensive care unit for close monitoring and may require mechanical ventilation if he deteriorates.

Tomayo continues to improve over the next few hours. By 9 pm, he is able to sit up and talk, has bilateral expiratory wheeze, prolonged expiration and peak flow 200 L/min (50 per cent of his personal best reading of 400).

He is still tachypnoeic (respiratory rate 35/min), has tachycardia (heart rate 120/min) and requires oxygen to maintain SaO_2 >95 per cent.

Improved ventilation is associated with correction of the respiratory acidosis (Table 35.2 shows the results of serial arterial blood gas monitoring).

Overnight, treatment is continued with oxygen, salbutamol nebulizer every 2 hours, aminophylline and hydrocortisone infusion.

Tomayo is able to have breakfast the following morning and talks about how his asthma attack started. He is no longer breathless, and his respiratory rate and heart rate are coming down towards normal (30/min and 100/min, respectively).

During the day, the following changes are made to his treatment:

- Oxygen is discontinued
- The interval between doses of nebulized salbutamol is increased to 4 hours
- Aminophylline and hydrocortisone infusion rate is halved and later discontinued
- Prednisolone 40 mg daily is started

Tomayo is then transferred to the paediatric ward.

Three days after admission, Tomayo has no respiratory distress and his peak flow readings are 320–340 L/min (his personal best is 400). His lung function is assessed with a spirometer so that future measurements can be compared (Figure 35.3 and Table 35.4).

Self-test 5: Explain and interpret Tomayo's spirometer measurements (Figure 35.3, Table 35.4).

Answer: Spirometry measures the volume of air exhaled during forced expiration. Forced expiration begins at TLC (total lung capacity), after a full inspiration, and ends at RV (residual volume). It normally takes less than 3 seconds and can be longer in patients with airway obstruction. FVC (forced vital capacity) is the total volume of air that can be exhaled. Tomayo's FVC is reduced as a result of air trapping. The FEV_1 (forced expiratory volume in 1 second) is the volume of air exhaled in the first second. PEFR is the rate at which air is exhaled. PEFR and FEV_1 indicate what happens in early expiration and are influenced by large airway resistance and effort. They are reduced in keeping with airway narrowing and the FEV_1/FVC ratio of less than 75 per cent reflects obstructive lung disease. The midexpiratory flow between 25 and 75 per cent of expired vital capacity (MEF_{25-75}) gives a measure of flow at lower lung volumes and is influenced by resistance in the smaller airways. Tomayo's curve is concave on the right. This and the reduced MEF_{25-75} indicate reduced airflow through smaller airways. (See Chapter 36 for differences in lung function between obstructive and restrictive lung disease.)

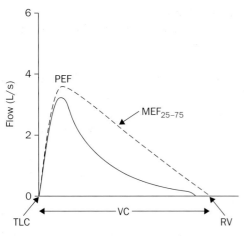

Figure 35.3 Tomayo's lung function assessed with a spirometer 3 days after he presented with a severe asthma attack. — Patient's curve; ---- predicted curve. MEF$_{25-75}$, midexpiratory flow between 25 and 75 per cent of expired vital capacity (VC); PEF, peak expiratory flow; RV, residual volume; TLC, total lung capacity.

Table 35.4 Measurements shown in Figure 35.3

Measure	Actual value	Percentage of predicted
PEFR	340 L/min	94
FEV$_1$	1.68 L	70
FVC	2.31 L	80
FEV$_1$/FVC	73%	
MEF$_{25-75}$	1.46 L	50

FEV$_1$, forced expiratory volume in 1 second; FVC, forced vital capacity; MEF$_{25-75}$, midexpiratory flow between 25 and 75 per cent of expired vital capacity; PEFR, peak expiratory flow rate.

Self-test 6: (A) What electrolyte abnormality will you look out for during treatment of acute severe asthma and (B) what contributes to it?

Answer:

A Hypokalaemia

B Alkalosis and the treatments – corticosteroids, aminophylline and salbutamol – contribute to it

Tomayo's detailed past history

The day after admission, a detailed history is obtained from Tomayo and his mother to identify factors that might have contributed to the severe attack and poor asthma control.

Tomayo was diagnosed to have asthma at 7 years of age. He had then had an intermittent dry cough and wheeze, which occurred at night, in the mornings and with physical activity. Various puffers from the GP did not help. He was referred to the hospital when he was 9 and was seen by the specialist and the asthma nurse. He was given an 'orange Accuhaler 125' twice a day as a preventer, a 'blue Accuhaler' to carry around as a reliever, and told to check his blows regularly (Accuhalers are dry powder inhalers). These inhalers helped but Tomayo did not take them regularly after some time. His mother is not sure whether he has been taking any treatment recently other than the green inhaler he had today.

Tomayo's mother lives on her own with the five children: two girls older than Tomayo also have asthma and the 3 year old has eczema. His mother has hayfever. No one smokes and there are no pets.

The medical records reveal that Tomayo was seen regularly in clinic from age 9 to 10.8 years. There is a note at 10.5 years that he 'forgets to take fluticasone regularly' and his peak flow reading was 250 L/min. Thereafter he stopped treatment and had troublesome symptoms. The asthma nurses saw him regularly. On salmeterol 50 µg and fluticasone 125 µg twice a day with an Accuhaler, his symptoms were controlled and the peak flow readings were 370–400 L/min. However, he did not return for follow-up despite three clinic appointments.

Meaning of the past history

Tomayo's history suggests recurrent asthma symptoms since he was 7 years old, which were troublesome enough to warrant regular preventive treatment with inhaled long-acting bronchodilator and corticosteroid. As he has been managed by a hospital specialist and seen repeatedly by asthma specialist nurses, he and his mother are expected to:

- Have received information about asthma and its management

- Understand the importance of taking the inhalers regularly as recommended
- Have had his inhaler technique checked and optimized
- Know the advantages of home peak flow monitoring
- Know what to do during an acute attack

Whether Tomayo and his mother appreciate all this is questionable because his adherence with treatment is poor and he has failed to attend follow-up. Poor adherence is complex, not simply caused by a lack of information and understanding (unintentional non-adherence) and may be a result of a patient's/parents' conscious decision (intentional non-non-adherence) (see Chapter 36). Adherence to treatment is not static, often declines as a child gets older and is lowest during adolescence. Possible explanations for this might be the adolescent's transition to greater self-care, rebellious assertion of autonomy, desire to conform to peer pressure and be like everyone else, or denial (Table 35.5). Adherence may be improved by giving patients such as Tomayo the opportunity to talk about concerns, difficulties, fears and expectations related to asthma and its treatment.

Asthma management plan before discharge

For successful management, Tomayo and his mother require ongoing education about the following:

- Preventive steps:
  - daily medication and ways of remembering (e.g. calendar)
  - triggers to avoid
- Self-monitoring with symptom diary and PEFR
- How to recognize worsening asthma
- How to treat worsening asthma
- How and when to seek medical attention

Background information

Acute respiratory failure

Acute respiratory failure is a state of inadequate ventilation, oxygenation or both, and intervention is required to prevent respiratory or cardiac arrest.

Some important causes of acute respiratory failure

In any child:

- **Upper airway obstruction:** foreign body inhalation, laryngeal oedema with acute allergic reaction, epiglottitis, bacterial tracheitis
- **Lower airway obstruction:** severe asthma attack
- **Lower respiratory infection:** bronchiolitis, pneumonia
- **Pleural abnormalities:** large pneumothorax, pleural effusion

Table 35.5 Factors contributing to poor adherence with treatment

	Treatment-related factors	Other factors
Unintentional	Not understanding the reasons for preventive and reliever treatment	Lack of supervision
		Inappropriate expectations
		Forgetfulness
		Busy life style
Intentional	Impractical regimen: too many medicines, too many doses	Denial of symptoms or attacks
	Dissatisfaction or difficulty with inhaler device	Dissatisfaction with health-care professionals
	Fear of side effects	Social and peer pressure
	Disliking treatment	Rebellion
	Difficulty in obtaining prescriptions	Cultural issues: traditions, beliefs
	Feeling better	

Table 35.6 How to interpret blood gas results

Pco_2	pH Low	Normal	High
Low		**Compensated metabolic acidosis** Bicarbonate low and compensated by low Pco_2, e.g. renal tubular acidosis Compensated respiratory alkalosis, e.g. later in an uncontrolled asthma attack	**Uncompensated respiratory alkalosis** Bicarbonate normal, e.g. early in an asthma attack, hysterical hyperventilation
Normal	**Acute metabolic acidosis** Bicarbonate low, e.g. hypotension and shock, diabetic ketoacidosis		**Uncompensated metabolic alkalosis** Bicarbonate high, e.g. pyloric stenosis
High	**Acute respiratory acidosis** Acute respiratory failure: bicarbonate normal or slightly raised, e.g. acute asthma, bronchiolitis	**Chronic respiratory acidosis** Chronic respiratory failure: compensated by high bicarbonate, e.g. chronic lung disease **Compensated metabolic alkalosis**	

- **Respiratory muscle weakness:** Guillain–Barré syndrome
- **Depression of respiratory centre:** acute central nervous system (CNS) disease, e.g. viral encephalitis, or overdose, e.g. barbiturates
- **Accidents:** smoke inhalation, near drowning

Any acute respiratory problem in children who are more prone because of:

- **Chronic lung disease:** chronic lung disease of prematurity, cystic fibrosis
- **Congenital heart defect:** moderate-to-large, left-to-right shunts
- **Immunodeficiency:** congenital or acquired
- **Immunosuppression:** leukaemia, drug induced
- **Neuromuscular weakness:** spinal muscular atrophy, cerebral palsy

How to interpret arterial blood gas results

For explanations refer to Chapter 3 and see Table 35.6.

Effects of stimulation of α- and β-adrenoceptors

These effects are shown in Table 35.7.

Pharmacodynamics of β_2 agonists

The β_2 agonists can be differentiated by their onset and duration of action (Figure 35.4). These are influenced by their biophysical properties and receptor interactions (Figure 35.5). β_2-Adrenoceptors are located in airway smooth muscle cells and the receptor density is greater in smaller airways. Salbutamol and terbutaline are hydrophilic and interact directly with the receptor. They have a fast onset and short duration of action, and are used as 'relievers'. Salmeterol is highly lipophilic, partitions into the cell membrane and then diffuses through the cell membrane to the receptor. This results in a slow onset of action. Formoterol is moderately lipophilic, partitions reversibly into the cell membrane as a depot and is released to interact with the receptor.

Table 35.7 Effects of stimulation of α- and β- adrenoceptors

| α-Receptor | β-Receptor | |
	β₁	β₂
Vasoconstriction	Increased heart rate	Bronchodilatation
Pupil dilation	Increased myocardial strength	Vasodilatation
Reduced intestinal motility and sphincter contraction		Reduced intestinal motility
Bladder sphincter contraction		Bladder wall relaxation
Uterus contraction		Uterus relaxation
		Insulin release from pancreas
		Glycogenolysis

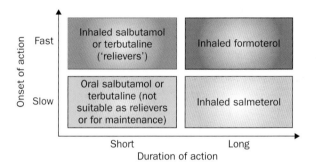
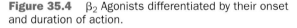

Figure 35.4 β₂ Agonists differentiated by their onset and duration of action.

Its onset of action is rapid. Salmeterol and formoterol have sustained effects and are suitable for maintenance treatment of asthma.

Further sources of information

Articles

British Thoracic Society, Scottish Intercollegiate Guidelines Network. British guidelines on the management of asthma. *Thorax* 2003; **58**(suppl 1): i1–94 (also available on BTS website)

FitzGerald M. Acute asthma. Extracts from 'Clinical Evidence'. *British Medical Journal* 2001; **323**: 841–5

Peek GJ, Morcos S, Cooper G. The pleural cavity. *British Medical Journal* 2000; **320**: 1318–21

Websites

www.brit-thoracic.org.uk

British Thoracic Society's website.

www.sign.ac.uk/guidelines/published/

Scottish Intercollegiate Guidelines Network (SIGN) Clinical Guidelines' website.

Self-test 7: Interpret the arterial blood gas from a teenage girl who has presented to A&E and has a rapid respiratory rate (normal values are shown in Table 35.8): pH 7.49; $P\text{co}_2$ 3.3 kPa or 25 mmHg; $P\text{o}_2$ 11.7 kPa or 88 mmHg; bicarbonate 22 mmol/L.

Answer: The pH is high, $P\text{co}_2$ low, and $P\text{o}_2$ and bicarbonate normal, suggesting respiratory alkalosis. The rapid respiratory rate may be caused by hysterical hyperventilation.

Self-test 8: The following are known side effects of β₂ agonists:

A Bronchoconstriction

B Hypoglycaemia

C Tremor

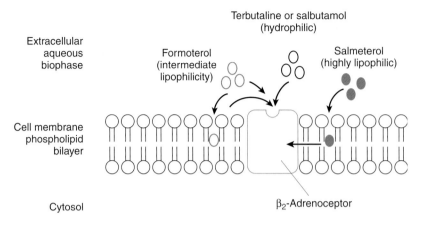

Figure 35.5 Proposed interactions of β_2 agonists, the β_2-adrenoceptor and the cell membrane. Redrawn from Johnson M, Beta$_2$-adrenoceptors: mechanisms of action of beta$_2$-agonists, *Paediatric Respiratory Reviews*, 2001; **2**: 57–62, with permission from Elsevier.

Table 35.8 Normal values for arterial blood gases

pH	$P\text{co}_2$ (kPa)[a]	$P\text{o}_2$ (kPa)[a]	Base excess (mml/L)	Bicarbonate (mmol/L)
7.36–7.44	4.7–6.0 (35–45)	10.6 (>80)	>0–2	20–26

[a]Values in parentheses are millimetres of mercury.

D Palpitations

E Headache

Answer: A, C, D and E are true. Bronchoconstriction is a paradoxical effect of inhaled β_2 agonists and may be caused by the propellants.

Self-test 9: The old-fashioned treatment of asthma included adrenaline (epinephrine) and isoprenaline. Why have these been superseded by newer drugs?

Answer: Adrenaline has α- and β-agonist effects (Table 35.7). Isoprenaline is a non-selective β-agonist with prominent cardiac (β_1) effects. The major side effect of both is cardiac arrhythmias. The newer drugs are selective β_2 agonists.

A girl with cystic fibrosis not complying with treatment

Age: 14 years

LEENA PATEL

Presentation

The cystic fibrosis (CF) team at the regional hospital have known Amy and her mother since her diagnosis at 8 months of age. She had been investigated for CF when she presented with a mucousy cough and frequent, pale, bulky, offensive stools. She is now a bright and attractive 14 year old. During a routine monthly check-up at the CF clinic, Amy is initially seen on her own and reports that she has been very well. She tells everyone about her very active social life, her recent trip to France and the pop concert she went to on Friday. When asked about specific symptoms, she says that she occasionally coughs up green mucus but has not had any trouble with her tummy. She does her physiotherapy before school and in the evening. The dietician shows Amy her growth chart and points out that her weight has fallen away from her expected position (Figure 36.1). Amy mentions that mornings are one big rush and breakfast is just not possible.

Self-test 1: From this presentation, what issues need further exploration?

Answers:
- Symptoms other than a productive cough and objective measures of respiratory status
- Chest physiotherapy schedule and other physical activities in the context of Amy's routine and social pressures
- Factors that might contribute to poor weight gain

- Level of adherence for different treatments (the morning physiotherapy must be difficult to fit in if Amy is so rushed)

It is worth remembering that patients with chronic illnesses tend to underestimate their disease severity and overestimate their level of self-care. Amy's mother's opinion about her level of adherence may be informative.

Self-test 2: What factors might contribute to Amy's poor weight gain?

Answers:
- Malabsorption from pancreatic insufficiency (suggested by frequent, pale, bulky, offensive stools) and not taking adequate pancreatic enzymes
- Inadequate calorie intake because:
  - oversleeps or is too busy to eat
  - appetite is poor as a result of lung disease
  - anorexic
- Diabetes mellitus

Self-test 3: Can you identify some of the regular medications Amy might be on and how frequently she might need these?

Answer: Amy is most likely to be on pancreatic enzyme replacement with meals and snacks, multivitamins daily and a prophylactic antibiotic against *Staphylococcus aureus*. In addition, she may also be on a number of other medications depending on the severity of her lung disease and other problems such as diabetes mellitus (Table 36.1, p. 384).

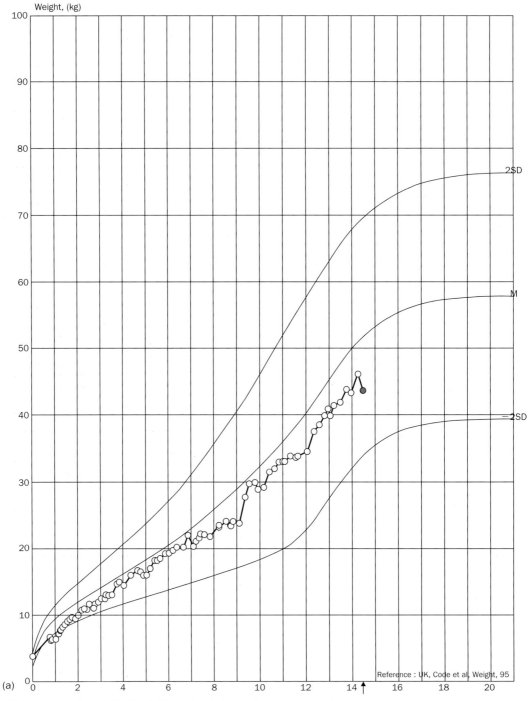

Figure 36.1 (a) Amy's weight chart. The red points are the most recent measurements.

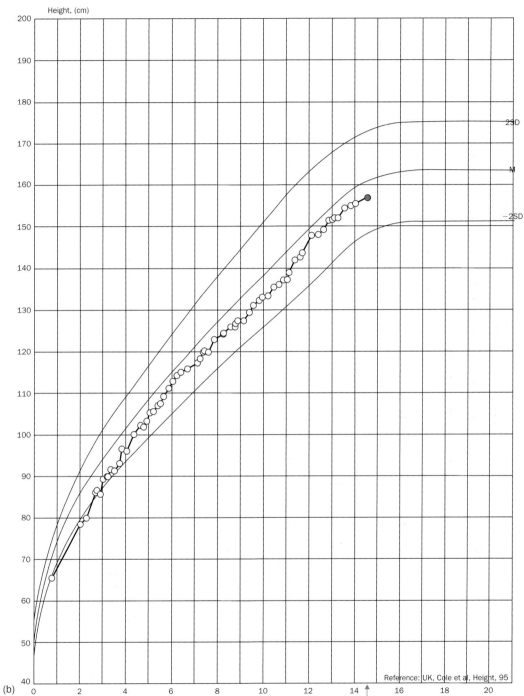

(b)

Figure 36.1 (*continued*) (b) Amy's height chart. The red points are the most recent measurements.

Table 36.1 Range of treatments that a child with cystic fibrosis may require regularly and proportion of patients reported to adhere to the treatment

Treatment	Percentage of patients reported to adhere to the treatment
Pancreatic enzyme replacement: oral capsules with meals and snacks containing fat and protein but not carbohydrate alone (e.g. an apple)	80–97
Adjuvants to pancreatic enzyme replacement: reducing gastric and duodenal pH with H_2-receptor blockers or proton pump inhibitors (once daily)	
Fat-soluble and water-soluble vitamins (up to three times a day)	45–90
Nutritional supplements: orally (one or more times a day) or as overnight gastrostomy feeds	30
Chest physiotherapy and airway clearance techniques (twice a day)	40–55
Bronchodilators: inhaled salbutamol or terbutaline (twice a day or more often)	
Anti-inflammatory: inhaled corticosteroids (twice a day)	
Mucolytic agents: nebulized DNAase (once daily)	
Prophylactic antibiotic against *Staphylococcus aureus*, e.g. oral flucloxacillin (four times a day)	70–95
Antibiotics for *Pseudomonas aeruginosa*, e.g. nebulized colistin or tobramycin (twice a day); intravenous ceftazidime or meropenem alone or in combination with tobramycin or colistin (three times a day for 2 weeks every 3 months or when exacerbation of symptoms)	
Diabetes mellitus: subcutaneous insulin (twice a day or more often); finger-prick blood glucose testing (at least once a day)	

Initial considerations and action

Patients with CF are recommended various treatments with the expectation that they will preserve health, slow disease progression and improve survival (Table 36.1). The improved survival over the past 50 years is attributed to the package of care, which includes (Figure 36.2):

- Enhanced airway clearance
- Prevention and aggressive treatment of infections
- Pancreatic enzyme therapy
- Better nutrition

  However, it must be pointed out that:

- The effectiveness of many treatments remains controversial

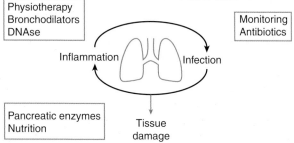

Figure 36.2 The major pathophysiological problem and treatments in cystic fibrosis.

- The treatments for cystic fibrosis are complex and time-consuming
- The minimum level of adherence required for a treatment to be clinically beneficial is not known but must be different for different treatments
- The extent to which patients adhere to treatments is influenced by many factors (Table 36.2) and, for younger children, this includes parents because they are primarily responsible for implementing the treatment

---

Self-test 4: Think of a time when you or someone close to you were recommended a treatment or change in life style. What factors contributed to adherence to the recommendation?

Answer: Check these with the factors listed in Table 36.2.

Defining compliance and adherence

Compliance is defined as the extent to which a person's behaviour coincides with medical advice. Many professionals prefer 'adherence' because it supports active participation by the patient in treatment decisions (Table 36.3). In practice, 'compliance' and 'adherence' tend to be used interchangeably.

Levels of adherence

The level of adherence for any treatment:

- Occurs along a continuum ranging from total participation with the treatment to total avoidance
- Is not static, changes over time and becomes particularly problematic during adolescence

Overall adherence rates in children with chronic diseases are no better than 30–70 per cent. Adherence in CF varies according to the treatment (see Table 36.1) and is better for those that immediately relieve symptoms (e.g. pancreatic enzymes) than treatments that offer longer-term benefits (e.g. chest physiotherapy). Not adhering to treatment may be a conscious decision (intentional non-adherence) or unintentional, e.g. because of a lack of understanding.

Individuals may be described according to their behaviour and honesty in reporting adherence as:

- Refusers – educated non-adherence
- Procrastinators – admit to some non-adherent behaviour
- Deniers – do not admit to non-adherence

Self-test 5: Michael is a 15 year old with CF. His father is a teacher and his mother a GP. Michael and his parents have a very good understanding about CF and the numerous treatments that he has to have. Does this mean that his level of adherence to the treatment is likely to be high?

Answer: Lack of knowledge is one factor that hinders adherence to treatment. But having knowledge does not necessarily imply a high level of adherence because many competing factors can influence Michael's decisions and behaviour. An individual might also make a conscious and well-reasoned decision not to take a treatment after weighing up the pros and cons of treatment (effectiveness, cost, inconvenience, discomfort) and quality-of-life issues. This is called educated (adaptive) non-adherence.

History

The purpose of the history and examination are to assess Amy's:

- State of health, especially in view of the respiratory symptoms and poor weight gain
- Physiotherapy, medicines and diet
- Level of adherence to the treatments
- Routine and social life

The CF team are already familiar with Amy's past and family history:

Amy has been relatively well until recently. *Pseudomonas aeruginosa* was first isolated from her sputum samples when she was 8 years old. Since then, Amy has had 2-week courses of intravenous antibiotics every 3 months. She came into hospital for the first few courses until her mother learnt to give them at home. Her mother is single and works part-time in a bakery, and her parents have helped her in

Table 36.2 Factors influencing adherence to treatments for cystic fibrosis (CF)

	Factors enhancing adherence	Barriers to adherence
Patient and family:		
Age	Good pattern of adherence established early on in life	Adolescence, mainly as a result of desire to be like peers
Knowledge and understanding	Good understanding of rationale for treatment and regimen	Inadequate knowledge about illness and treatment (e.g. fear of side effects), educated non-adherence
Perceptions and attitudes	Optimistic belief in treatment efficacy, personal control of illness	Underestimate illness severity, cultural stigma against accepting a chronic illness, denial, resentment, forgetful, tendency to consider short-term gains of not adhering
Health motivation	Motivation to achieve or maintain good health	Indifference to level of health, neglect
Health locus of control	Internal control orientation	External control orientation
Coping style and way thinking, feeling and acting	Hopefulness – optimistic, determined and positive	Resignation – avoidant, passive and helpless
Psychosocial context		Peer pressure to blend in with fads and fashions, struggle for control between patient and parent or other authority figure, competing life events (e.g. looking after unwell father)
Home environment	Organized supportive family or social network, nurturing parenting style, sensitivity to child's input	Chaotic family life, conflict between parents, non-CF crisis (e.g. mother starting work)
The disease:		
Duration of illness	Acute	Chronic
Stage of disease	Symptomatic	Asymptomatic
The treatment:		
Complexity of the regimen	Simplified regimen	Inconvenient, intrusive, time-consuming, embarrassing in public
Duration	Short term	Long term
Benefits and rewards	Immediate symptom relief (e.g. pancreatic enzymes, bronchodilators), greater sense of well-being	Little immediate benefit (e.g. chest physiotherapy, nebulized antibiotics)
Side effects	None or tolerable	Unpleasant

(continued)

Table 36.2 *(continued)*

	Factors enhancing adherence	Barriers to adherence
Requirements for lifestyle changes	Readily fits into daily routine	Involves major lifestyle changes, interferes with daily activities
Cost		Expensive
The health-care setting:		
Doctor/CF team–patient relationship	Constructive, trusting	
Patient's perception of the doctor/CF team	Friendly, warm, attentive	Indifferent, controlling, formal
Continuity of care	With same doctor or team	Different professionals on different occasions, conflict between professionals
Patient's encounter with professionals	Frequent contact	Brief and impersonal
Patient's satisfaction	High	Dissatisfaction

Table 36.3 Compliance versus adherence

	Compliance	Adherence
Patient's role in treatment planning	Passive and submissive recipient	Active and responsible participant
Role of health-care professional	Authoritarian, expects patient to obey	Supportive, permits patient autonomy
Health care	Paternalistic	Partnership between patient and provider

doing the best for Amy. Having received a lot of information from the CF team and the UK Cystic Fibrosis Trust over the years, Amy's mother has become an 'expert' on CF and Amy has been told more and more as she has got older.

Amy and her mother have a secure and friendly relationship with the various professionals in the CF team. Their approach is empathetic, non-threatening and non-judgemental, and this encourages openness with self-reporting. Seeing Amy on her own initially gives her space to express her own symptoms, thoughts and views. Amy is allowed to say when her mother should join in the consultation.

Health professionals are poor at judging adherence and few patients and parents will openly admit to non-adherence. Therefore some time is spent exploring the extent to which Amy adheres to different treatments.

The CF team are positive about any treatments Amy does rather than what she does not do. She may be encouraged to disclose by being told that:

- Total adherence is not expected
- Many people forget or can't fit in treatments for various reasons (Table 36.4)

The following are measures of adherence:

- Subjective measures: self-report, diary or chart, parent report
- Direct objective measures: consistency of lung function tests recorded at home and done in hospital, keeping appointments, drug concentration in blood or urine
- Indirect objective measures: capsule counts, prescription collection

Table 36.4   What to say to normalize non-adherence and ask about it

> We know that it can be difficult to do physiotherapy and stick to the diet and take so many medicines. Do you find any of the treatments difficult to fit in? When you are having a bad day, which treatments are you most likely to miss?
>
> Many people have trouble remembering to take their treatment. Do you ever forget? Have you ever intentionally not taken your medicines?

The history obtained from Amy and mother

Amy's mother thought that Amy had been coughing more and more, and bringing up a lot of mucus recently, possibly since the last clinic appointment, but Amy did not agree. Amy revealed that she finds the breathing exercises boring and only does a full session a few times a week when she feels that she needs it. Her mother added that this is whenever Amy has a lot of horrible green mucus because that always scares her. Her mother also said that Amy had too many parties and too many late nights. Amy said that she was fed up with her mother nagging and always telling her what to do. Amy names all her medicines, doses and the times that she takes them. She admitted not taking her pancreatic enzyme capsules when she is partying. She doesn't want people to think she's a 'druggie'. Mother chipped in that Amy had been out all day on Saturday and spent most of Sunday on the toilet. Her appetite is excellent, she does not complain of tiredness, excessive thirst and polyuria, and her periods are regular.

Self-test 6:

A **Why is the mucus that Amy coughs up greenish in colour?**

B **What is the relevance of regular periods?**

Answers:

A Because of the green pigments produced by *Pseudomonas aeruginosa*

B A teenager with CF might omit pancreatic enzymes to stay thin. This can be associated with amenorrhoea as in anorexia nervosa (see Chapter 38)

Interpretation of the history

Coughing is induced by increased mucus production associated with infection and inflammation (see Chapter 9). Mucus accumulating in the airways from lack of regular chest physiotherapy and suppressing a cough that might be embarrassing makes the matter worse. It is understandable that Amy finds physiotherapy boring. Doing physiotherapy and taking medicines compete with her other goals, such as fitting in with her peers and socializing, even though Amy knows that one consequence of not taking her pancreatic enzymes means suffering the unpleasant symptoms of malabsorption. Frequent episodes of malabsorption and worsening lung disease are likely to contribute to Amy's poor weight gain. She may not fully understand the positive association between weight (body mass index) and the state of her lungs. In the context of her previous good health, it is possible that she denies the significance of her symptoms to avoid facing the negative realities of the disease, and thus minimizes any psychological distress and maintains her self-esteem. Mother's authority is threatening to Amy's growing autonomy and she challenges her mother by disobeying.

Examination

Amy has an examination and the findings are compared with those from previous examinations:

General: not pale or cyanosed

Respiratory:

- Clubbing – but this is not new
- Intermittent cough during the consultation:
  - Amy tried to suppress it
  - sounded fruity
- No nasal discharge and no obvious nasal polyps
- No signs of respiratory distress
- Breath sounds are reduced in intensity all over
- Crackles are heard over both upper zones on the back: this contrasts with the examination 3 months ago when Amy had no abnormal signs in the chest

Abdomen:

- Not distended
- Liver and spleen are not palpable

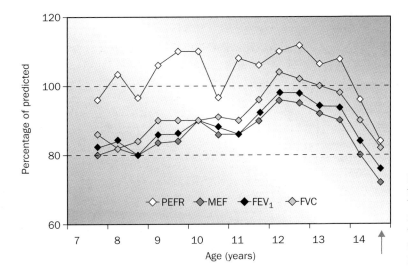

Figure 36.3 Chart showing Amy's lung function measured with a spirometer. The red arrow shows the most recent measurements. FEV$_1$, forced expiratory volume in 1 second; FVC, forced vital capacity; MEF, midexpiratory flow; PEF, peak expiratory flow.

Lung function assessment

Amy's lung function is also assessed using spirometry. This shows reduced:

- MEF$_{25-75}$ (midexpiratory flow between 25 and 75 per cent of expired vital capacity)
- FEV$_1$ (forced expiratory volume in 1 second)
- FVC (forced vital capacity)

They are lower than previous measurements (Figure 36.3).

The measurements provide information about the site of the disease and its severity. Initially in CF lung disease:

- MEF$_{25-75}$ is reduced because the smaller airways are involved
- Peak expiratory flow (PEF) is relatively normal because the large airways are normal (Figure 36.4)

With progressively worsening airflow obstruction through small airways and involvement of the larger airways, all spirometric measurements are reduced.

Self-test 7: What are the differences between a peak expiratory flow (PEF) meter and a spirometer and the measurements recorded by each?

Answer:

Peak expiratory flowmeter	Spirometer
Cheap, simple and easy to use	Battery operated and vary in cost
Tells us about what happens in early expiration, measures airflow obstruction in the larger airways and is useful in asthma	Also tells us about what happens in mid- and end-expiration, measures lung volumes–FVC and FEV$_1$ and airflow through smaller airways, and useful in cystic fibrosis and restrictive disorders

---

Interpretation of the examination

- Clubbing of the fingers and toes is associated with chronic lung disease in CF
- Crackles indicate retained secretions
- Breath sounds are of reduced intensity all over when there is extensive airway narrowing, and collapsed or damaged alveoli
- Productive cough with green mucus, which has been getting worse over 3 months, the new chest signs and the deterioration in lung function are features of progressing lung disease

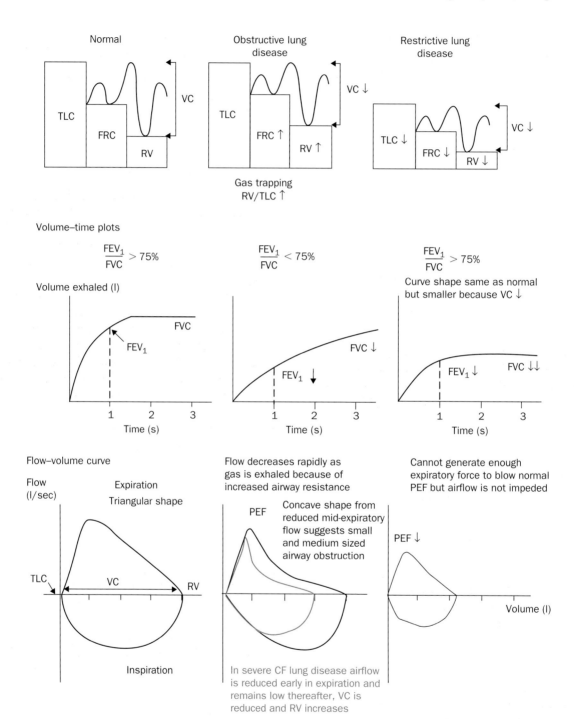

Figure 36.4   Differences in lung function between obstructive and restrictive lung disease. The usefulness of volume–time plots and flow–volume curves is illustrated. FEV$_1$, forced expiratory volume in 1 second; FRC, functional residual capacity; FVC, forced vital capacity; PEF, peak expiratory flow; RV, residual volume; TLC, total lung capacity; VC, vital capacity.

Not uncommonly, this is associated with poor weight gain or weight loss. The latter also occurs with diabetes mellitus which can contribute to worsening lung disease. However, Amy does not have any other symptoms of diabetes mellitus (see Chapter 34)

Her poor adherence to chest physiotherapy and medicines is likely to have influenced the recent deterioration in her lungs and nutritional state.

Self-test 8: Clubbing of the digits is a well-recognized feature in the following:

A Otherwise healthy children
B Congenital heart defects with left-to-right shunt
C Infective endocarditis
D Inflammatory bowel disease
E Coeliac disease

Answer: A, C and D are true. Clubbing is seen in cyanotic heart defects but not defects with left-to-right shunts (patent ductus arteriosus [PDA], ventricular septal defect [VSD], atrial septal defect [ASD]), which are acyanotic.

Crises in cystic fibrosis

Adjusting to CF also means adapting to periods of crises such as the following:

- The initial diagnosis
- First isolation of *Ps. aeruginosa*
- New treatments added to daily regimen
- First hospital admission with lung disease
- Awareness of disease progression
- Starting primary school
- Moving to secondary school
- Adolescence
- A complication such as diabetes mellitus or liver disease
- Learning about the death of someone with CF
- Boys finding out about infertility
- Girls finding out about the risk of passing CF on to children
- Transition from paediatric to adult care
- Perceived proximity to death

Investigations and results

Healthy airways are sterile below the first bronchial division. This is not so in children with CF and the common bacterial pathogens are:

- *Staphylococcus aureus*
- *Haemophilus influenzae*
- *Pseudomonas aeruginosa*

The organisms are identified from bacterial culture of cough swab samples from young children and sputum samples from older children. Infection of the smaller airways with *Ps. aeruginosa* is inevitable, is virtually impossible to eradicate and is the main cause of progressive lung disease.

The results of sputum culture from Amy's samples over the preceding 3 months are reviewed (Figure 36.5). *Ps. aeruginosa* has been isolated intermittently. This has been the pattern for Amy since the organism was first isolated and the CF team are aware that it is not a new finding. Amy's chest radiograph compared with the one last year shows new changes (Figure 36.6).

Self-test 9: The following antibiotics are effective against *Ps. aeruginosa*:

A Penicillin
B Cefotaxime
C Ceftazidime
D Meropenem
E Colistin

Answer: True: C, D and E, and also tobramycin, gentamicin, piperacillin and ciprofloxacillin.

Diagnosis

Amy has cystic fibrosis lung disease with recent deterioration.

She is only partially adherent with chest physiotherapy and pancreatic enzyme treatment. This is influenced by a number of factors:

- Busy social activities compete with treatment in terms of both motivation and time

CF Clinic List		AMY CROW							
Hospital Number:	581647	Date of Birth: 01/Jan/1988							
				MER	CAZ	PIP	CMN	TOB	CIP
Lab Number:	994176								
Cultures in progress									
Dated:	5/Jun/02	Received:	6/Jun/02						
				MER	CAZ	PIP	CMN	TOB	CIP
Lab Number:	991345								
COLIFORM BACILLI			++						
Dated:	17/May/02	Received:	20/May/02						
				MER	CAZ	PIP	CMN	TOB	CIP
Lab Number:	988633								
MUCOID PSEUDOMONAS AERUGINOSA			+++	S	S	S	S	S	R
SMOOTH PSEUDOMONAS AERUGINOSA			+	S	S	S	S	S	S
Dated:	4/May/02	Received:	6/May/02						
				MER	CAZ	PIP	CMN	TOB	CIP
Lab Number:	986160								
MUCOID PSEUDOMONAS AERUGINOSA			+++	S	S	S	S	S	R
Dated:	19/Apr/02	Received:	23/Apr/02						
				MER	CAZ	PIP	CMN	TOB	CIP
Lab Number:	983420								
MIXED COLIFORMS			+++						
Dated:	3/Apr/02	Received:	4/Apr/02						
				MER	CAZ	PIP	CMN	TOB	CIP
Lab Number:	983112								
YEASTS			+						
MIXED COLIFORMS			+++						
Dated:	20/Mar/02	Received:	23/Mar/02						
				MER	CAZ	PIP	CMN	TOB	CIP
Lab Number:	982975								
MUCOID PSEUDOMONAS AERUGINOSA			++	S	S	S	S	S	S
S-R PSEUDOMONAS AERUGINOSA			++	S	S	S	S	S	S
Dated:	8/Mar/02	Received:	10/Mar/02						

Figure 36.5 Amy's sputum microbiology results from all samples over the previous 3 months.

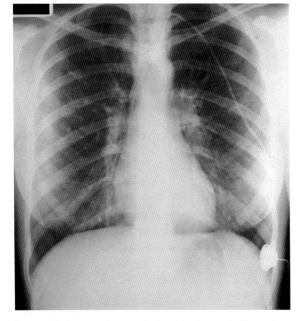

Figure 36.6 Amy's recent chest radiograph. There is widespread lung disease, bronchial wall thickening and diffuse shadowing. There is a totally implantable venous access device on the left with the tip in the superior vena cava.

- Desire to 'fit in' with peers and not be different
- Failure to appreciate significance of symptoms or denial
- Adolescent rebellion against mother's authority

Outcomes of poor adherence to treatment of cystic fibrosis

- Deterioration in lung disease, increased respiratory exacerbations
- Malabsorption symptoms
- Weight loss
- Increased hospitalization
- Time off school and work
- Worry about health, low morale
- Parental stress and conflict
- Wasted resources, e.g.
  - professionals' time is wasted in attempts to investigate symptoms and try new treatments
  - expensive treatment such as DNAase is used inappropriately
  - expensive tests are undertaken
  - unnecessary referrals are made

Management and follow-up

Non-adherence is not merely Amy's problem but also a problem for the CF team. It is important for professionals to:

- Address their own feelings and attitudes to non-adherence
- Optimize the way in which it is managed
- Enhance a multidisciplinary team approach
- Involve a clinical psychologist

How to communicate with patients or parents about specific issues

- Introduction: explain oneself, one's role, and invite patient or parent to share concerns
- Conduct of the interview:
  - courtesy, professionalism, appropriate non-verbal signals
  - engage patient/parents and develop a relationship
  - listen rather than talk
  - discuss rather than dictate or accuse
- Giving information about specific issues:
  - assess how much patient/parent already knows
  - tailor appropriately according to age of patient, family context, existing knowledge, stage of illness and goals
  - clear, unambiguous, non-technical, non-patronizing language, short sentences, avoid jargon
  - progress gradually from simple to complex
  - repeat information for reinforcement
  - use educational aids/models (e.g. bronchial tree and lungs, videos)
  - provide written information with diagrams
- Elicit further preoccupations, questions, anxieties, expectations
- Encourage discussion, questions, interruptions and requests for information from the patient/parent
- Check understanding:
  - check that information given is understood
  - identify and correct any misunderstandings or misconceptions
- Concluding: round off the interview, guidance towards seeking further help and information

Identify barriers to adherence and possible ways to overcome them

Through discussions, the CF team help Amy to identify obstacles to adherence and to come up with workable solutions. On social outings, Amy does not want people to know that she has CF. She wishes to try her mother's suggestion – excusing herself on the pretext that she needs 'the ladies' or to make a phone call, and then taking her pancreatic enzymes when she is away from public view. This measure is appropriate in the short term while Amy identifies a long-term strategy that will allow her to be open and honest about her condition and with which she feels comfortable.

Explore emotions, perceptions and beliefs

Changing the way a person follows medical advice requires changing their feelings (e.g. sadness, anger, fear, frustration, resentment), beliefs (e.g. 'the treatment is useless') and ways of coping (e.g. 'There's no cure and nothing really helps, I'm going to die anyway'). Open communication between Amy, her mother and the CF team is encouraged so that emotions and feelings might be expressed. Amy must not be criticized or made to feel guilty for her thoughts and actions. Her mother also needs advice and support about managing Amy's poor adherence and her own anxieties.

Education to help Amy understand what is to be done and why

Amy's mother has learnt and told Amy more and more about CF as she has got older. Both have had ongoing assessments of their understanding about different aspects of CF and have been updated regularly. Like many patients, Amy may not volunteer that she does not understand and may not ask questions. The CF team therefore reassess her understanding, especially about the rationale and benefits of regular chest physiotherapy ('What do you think is happening in your lungs?' 'What do you think will help?'), and the relationship between the state of her lungs and her nutrition ('Can you think of how your weight might affect your lungs?'). Although being honest about the severity of her lung disease and possible consequences of adherence and non-adherence, the CF team want to avoid frightening Amy.

Involve patients in their treatment

Self-management is beneficial in various ways (Table 36.5):

- Better understanding of the disease and treatment
- Feel in control, greater sense of competence
- Can see change in symptoms with treatment
- Better adherence

From being dependent as a child, Amy's involvement has gradually increased as she progresses to becoming an independent adult. She is encouraged to monitor and judge her symptoms, record sputum volume and lung function, and communicate with the CF team about treatment.

Tailor treatment and accept compromise

The CF team negotiate and compromise with Amy about the level of treatment likely to be clinically beneficial as well as manageable. While doing this, they bear in mind the following:

- Be sensitive to needs and choices of patients and families and tailor treatment to daily lifestyle and routine
- Establish realistic goals and make realistic treatment plans
- Simplify treatment and withdraw treatments if possible, offer choices (e.g. intermittent rather than continuous treatment), treatment holidays, alternative treatment methods (e.g. a chest physiotherapy technique that is less onerous)
- Coordinate and agree between professionals
- Introduce changes gradually with clear verbal and written explanations
- Point out which treatments are most important and why, so that, if a treatment must be missed, patients can make informed decisions

Table 36.5   Involving parents and patients with CF in their health care

● **Parents:**	– begin teaching self-management skills
– educate parents about CF	– point out connections between child's behaviour and measures of health
– prepare parents for increasing child's involvement over time	– ask if child has any questions
– help them and their child negotiate and renegotiate over time their separate and shared responsibilities	● **Adolescents:**
– role-play with children to help them respond positively when asked about their treatment or condition in public	– spend time alone with adolescent and give space to express
● **Preschool children:**	– explore what having CF means to the adolescent and the anxieties
– talk with child and listen	– develop shared treatment plan incorporating adolescent's goals and concerns
– explain illness and rationale for treatment	– clearly explain what needs to be done and the expected outcomes
– help child learn names of medicines and what each is for	– expect periods of non-adherence and explore reasons for them
– ask if child has any questions	– praise improvements in adherence
● **School-age children:**	● **Adult patient:**
– talk with child and listen	– treat as an equal partner
– reinforce understanding of illness and rationale for treatment	– recognize competing pressures of adulthood
– explain different treatments and reasons for any changes	– ensure that understanding of illness and treatments is accurate
– involve child in treatment planning	– respect their decisions

- Point out advantages of adhering and disadvantages of not adhering to treatment using visual displays of changes in self-monitoring diary, growth chart, lung function, chest radiograph and sputum microbiology
- Discuss any reservations that the patient might have about treatment
- Ensure frequent follow-up because absence of supervision results in relapse with non-adherence

Cues or reminders

It is human to forget and cues or reminders are helpful:

- Routinize treatments – do them at consistent times of the day or with daily routine activities
- Use a chart or calendar in the kitchen

Amy's current lifestyle is very erratic. As it may take time to establish a routine and she does not like her mother reminding her, Amy chooses to use a diary.

Positive feedback and motivation

The CF team give Amy confidence, hope and encouragement, and make her feel that what she does makes a difference. Mother is asked to give her positive feedback and remembers the time when Amy was at junior school – she earned stickers when she was good with her physiotherapy and exchanged them for horse riding lessons.

Ignoring minor negative reactions

Children often complain about their treatments and especially physiotherapy. Amy's mother is advised to acknowledge sympathetically (e.g. 'I know physio is hard but it does make you cough less afterwards') but not turn it into a big argument and to withdraw from arguments if they do ensue.

Behaviour management and the need for discipline

Discipline can be defined as setting rules and enforcing them in a way that is least bothersome to the parent and child. It is important in the everyday life of all children, irrespective of whether they have a chronic illness, and helps them develop self-discipline. Mother used 'time out' when Amy was younger but now it

would be more appropriate to take away a privilege such as the use of a mobile phone (see below). To ensure that they have positive things in their relationship and their lives do not just revolve around CF, mother and Amy need to have quality time together doing things unrelated to CF (e.g. shopping or going to the cinema).

The 'time-out' procedure

'Time out' is an effective discipline procedure in children aged between 18 months and 10 years. The child is:

- Required to sit quietly in a dull place (e.g. bottom of the stairs) for a set period (5 minutes or less)
- Allowed to leave 'time out' and asked to do what was originally requested
- Given positive feedback when he or she complies

Background information

Cystic fibrosis (see Chapter 11)

Genetic aspects

Over 1000 mutations have been identified in the CF gene (Figure 36.7). The most common mutation is δF508. Inheritance is autosomal recessive. One in 25 white people is a carrier (has one copy of an abnormal gene) and one in 2500 has the disease (two copies of an abnormal gene).

Further sources of information

Book

Hill CM, Dodge JA. *Practical Guidelines for Cystic Fibrosis Care*. London: Churchill Communications Europe, 1998

Articles

Gask L, Usherwood T. The consultation. ABC of psychological medicine. *British Medical Journal* 2002; **324**: 1567–9

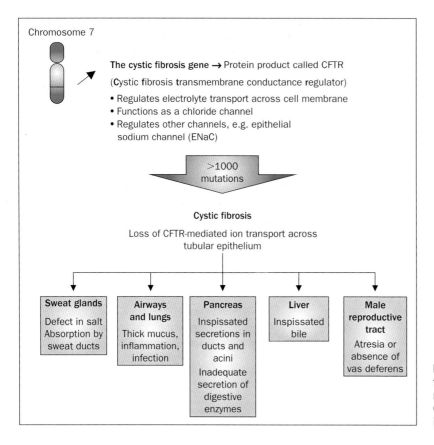

Figure 36.7 Defective cystic fibrosis gene (cystic fibrosis trans-membrane conductance regulator or CFTR) and multisystem involvement in CF.

Sockrider MM, Wolle JM. Helping patients better adhere to treatment regimens. Strategies for asthma, COPD, CF and tuberculosis. *Journal of Respiratory Diseases* 1996; **17**: 204–16

Website

www.cftrust.org.uk

The UK Cystic Fibrosis Trust website.

Self-test 10: Can you think of the professionals who make up a CF team?

Answers:

- Doctors including paediatrician, general practitioner, paediatric surgeon, ear, nose and throat (ENT) surgeon, microbiologist and radiologist
- Nurses, including clinical nurse specialists, community and hospital nurses
- Hospital and community physiotherapists
- Dietician
- Clinical psychologist
- Family counsellor
- Social worker
- Pharmacist

Self-test 11: Mohsin was born a few years after the death of his two siblings (at ages 10 and 12 years) who had cystic fibrosis. He too was found to have the condition soon after birth. Parents had found the physiotherapy routines and medications rather difficult for their first child, and treatment had become even more cumbersome when the second child was born 18 months later. They have refused all treatment for Mohsin because they believe that 'it does not work'. Should the parents' wishes be respected? Where do we draw the line between reasonable parental choices and child neglect?

Answer: The parents are not wilfully intending to neglect Mohsin and their decisions are based on their previous experiences. The CF team should respect their wishes and work with them towards a mutually agreeable goal.

Self-test 12: The following information is appropriate for most children with CF:

A Special schooling will be required

B Pancreatic enzymes are needed with any food they eat

C Extra salt is needed when away in a hot country

D Travel in an aeroplane is contraindicated

E They will be infertile

Answers: Only C is true. Remember that patients with CF lose more salt in their sweat – that is why they taste salty and it is the basis for the sweat test.

False:

A Children with CF do not require special schooling

B Only 85–90 per cent of CF patients have pancreatic insufficiency and require pancreatic enzymes with foods containing fat and significant amounts of protein, but not with foods that contain only carbohydrate (e.g. apple)

D Only those with advanced lung disease are at risk of becoming hypoxic in an aeroplane

E Only males with cystic fibrosis are infertile

Chronic disorder

Recurrent headache in a teenager

Age: 12 years

STEVEN RYAN

Presentation

A referral letter was received from a general practitioner:
Please see this 12-year-old girl who has been having serious problems with headaches over the last year or so. They are now starting to interfere with her school-work and her parents are very concerned about this. She also has asthma that is well controlled by an inhaled low-dose corticosteroid and she uses her reliever only before exercise. Her parents are worried about the possible causes of her headaches and the effect that they are having on her education. Examination of her cardiovascular system was normal and no abnormalities were found on neurological examination.

Self-test 1: What are the two most common specific headaches disorders seen in children and adolescents?

Answer: Migraine and tension-type headache.

Initial considerations and action

Chronic headaches are a common symptom in children and the vast majority of them do not indicate a serious underlying medical disorder. However, a small number do. The most worrying potential cause is a brain tumour. These most typically present with features of raised intracranial pressure. Therefore, the first task is to identify from the referral letter whether any features suggestive of such raised intracranial pressure are present.

Features in the history consistent with raised intracranial pressure:

- Waking during the night with headache
- Persistent vomiting
- History of several weeks of increasingly severe headaches
- Seizures
- Changed personality
- Deterioration in school performance
- History of abnormal neurological examination

If any of these criteria are present, then an urgent appointment should be offered.

As no such features are present in the referral letter, a routine appointment for 6 weeks' time is offered.

Self-test 2: Why is night-time headache seen in raised intracranial pressure?

Answer: As intracranial pressure (normally $<20\,cmH_2O$) is higher when lying down.

History

When Rebecca comes to outpatients with her mother and father the following history was obtained:

Apart from her well-controlled asthma, Rebecca has had no other significant health problems. Her headaches started in the autumn term of her first year at secondary school.

The headache is present virtually every day, although it varies in severity. It tends to come on around lunchtime and persists into the late evening. Its site is her forehead and vertex. Occasionally, it is present when she wakes up. The headache has slowly been getting worse and she has missed about a day a month from school with it over the last term. She occasionally feels nauseous with the headache, but has never vomited. She has never had any visual or sensory disturbance before or during the headache. Although she has time off school with the headache, she is able to get around the house.

Coughing and exercise do not make the headache worse. There is no obvious food or drink associated with the headaches. There is no history of nasal discharge or fever with the headaches.

Rebecca has used paracetamol to try to help her when she has a headache and, although it only provides partial relief, she is taking some virtually every day. At school she is said to be a conscientious student – a bit of a perfectionist in fact. Despite her headaches she continues to make good progress. Her father is a business consultant and spends a lot of time away from home and her mother has a part-time job in an office. She has had to take a couple of days off work to look after Rebecca. Rebecca's mother has occasional severe unilateral headaches followed by vomiting, after which she has to lie down in a darkened room for several hours.

It turns out that a cousin of Rebecca's was recently diagnosed with a brain tumour following a period of time with headaches, and the greatest concern of Rebecca's parents is that she might have the same problem.

Interpretation of the history

There are a number of important tasks in the history of a child with headaches. These are:

- Detecting features of raised intracranial pressure (see above)
- Characterizing the features of the headache to determine the headache syndrome
- Finding any factors that trigger headaches
- Building up a picture of how the child's and the family's lives are affected
- Taking a family history – an important feature of migraine

- Finding out which drugs have been used and in what dosages
- Mental state and psychological history

Meaning of the history in Rebecca

Raised pressure

There is no evidence from this history that Rebecca has raised intracranial pressure. She has none of the features listed above. The relatively long history, lack of vomiting, timing during the day, and lack of exacerbation by cough and exercise make raised intracranial pressure less likely – but it remains the parents' main concern

Headache syndrome

The two main types of headache in children are tension-type headache and migraine. Rebecca's headaches are most consistent with the former, although it is possible to have mixed headaches. Figure 37.1 illustrates the features that differentiate migraine from tension-type headache. Here the features of the headache are most

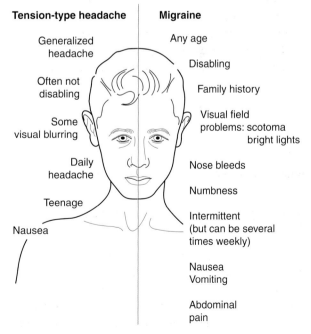

Figure 37.1 Differences between migraine and tension-type headaches.

consistent with tension-type headache, being daily in nature rather than episodic; they are not in the main disabling whereas migraine headaches are. Nor are there the classic features of vomiting or of visual or sensory aura. In adults, migraine headaches are typically unilateral but, in younger children especially, this is not the case.

Recurrent episodes of localized headache with fever and nasal discharge could indicate recurrent sinusitis, but Rebecca has no features of this.

Triggers

It is interesting that Rebecca's headaches started shortly after she started secondary school and this may have been an important trigger factor. Another possibility that has to be considered is analgesic headache. Regular medication with drugs such as paracetamol can cause a chronic daily headache, resulting in a vicious cycle of pain and analgesic intake.

Self-test 3: Which of the following are triggers for migraine in children?
A Citrus fruits
B Lack of sleep
C Hunger
D Exercise
E Bright sunlight

Answer: A–E are all true.

Disability

The headaches appear to be having an increasing effect on Rebecca's schooling. She is frequently having headaches at school, which will interfere with her learning ability, and she has missed a number of days at school. This has resulted in her mother having to take time off work. This could result in strain between her and her employer.

Family history

Rebecca's mother gives a history compatible with classic migraine without aura, but Rebecca shows no features of migraine – so far. Migraine is partially heritable and is typically transmitted through the mother.

Treatment

Rebecca has taken the most commonly used drug for children's headaches – paracetamol. The dose is not recorded. The typical dose used is around 15 mg/kg per day and paracetamol comes as tablets, soluble tablets, and infant and child suspensions. It is a safe and effective drug except in overdosage. It is most useful when used intermittently, but here may be contributing to the headaches.

Psychological factors

Here, the underlying concern about brain tumour may be very important and could well be adding to the anxiety about Rebecca's headaches, and this could exacerbate the headaches – if Rebecca is aware of the issue. The combination of a conscientious student and someone who is a perfectionist but is getting headaches during school time is recognized. Such children seem to pressurize themselves and may have high expectations.

Examination

Rebecca was examined. Here is a summary of the important findings:

- Height and weight on the 75th centile for age
- Slight frown and complaining of a headache at present
- Mild tenderness along the orbital ridge
- Nasal membranes and mouth and throat healthy
- Blood pressure is 108/76 mmHg and pulse rate 94/minute
- Pupils are reactive to light and equal with normal eye movements
- Optic fundi and retinas are normal (see Figure 25.1a, Chapter 25) and normal visual acuity
- Coordination (hand patting, finger–nose pointing, heel–toe walking forward and backwards)
- Balance normal
- All limb reflexes are present and symmetrical and both plantar reflexes are down-going

The purpose of the examination for most children and their parents is to provide reassurance that no significant underlying disorder is present and, in a small minority of children, to establish that such a disorder is present. It is especially important to exclude raised intracranial pressure.

Blood pressure should also be checked – although raised blood pressure is a very uncommon cause of childhood headaches. It should of course be checked using a correct-sized cuff (see Chapter 1). It is also possible to check the sinuses (by gentle percussion) for the tenderness that indicates active sinusitis, the temporomandibular joint and masseter muscle (both may be tender in tension-type headache), the teeth for evidence of nocturnal grinding (similarly), and the body of the occipitofrontalis muscle or its insertions (eyebrow ridge or occipital–nuchal crest may be tender in tension-type headache). Inspection of the nasal membranes is important to detect the inflamed swollen membranes of rhinitis, which may be accompanied by a purulent nasal discharge of associated sinusitis. Figure 37.2 shows the possible findings of the examination.

Interpretation of the examination

Rebecca is a healthy looking girl who is a normal weight for her height. The slight frown could well represent overactivity of the occipitofrontalis muscle – she has a headache at present and the tenderness at the orbital ridge confirms this. There is no evidence in the history of sinus disease. Importantly, there are no features in the examination consistent with significant intracranial pathology.

Features of raised intracranial pressure or space-occupying lesion on examination

- **Eyes:**
  Pupils of unequal size or reactivity
  Nystagmus
  Reduced visual acuity
  Reduced visual fields
  Papilloedema
- **Coordination and balance:**
  Unable to walk heel to toe
  Unable to pat hands in a coordinated fashion (dysdiadochokinesis)
  Fails finger–nose test

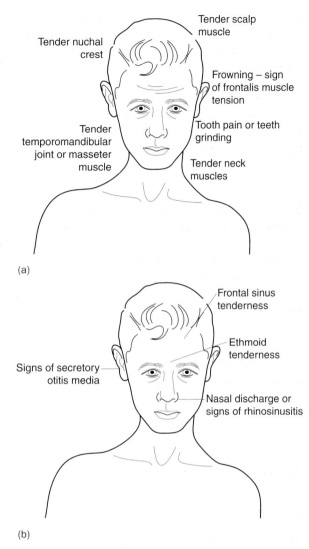

(a)

(b)

Figure 37.2 Possible examination findings in (a) tension-type headache and (b) sinus headache.

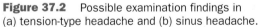

Cannot stand on one leg or falls over when standing with eyes closed

Differential diagnosis

The likely diagnosis here is tension-type headache (highly likely) and specifically chronic daily headache,

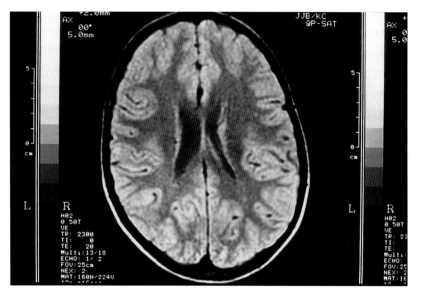

Figure 37.3   A healthy magnetic resonance scan.

although there remains a possibility of analgesic headache (quite likely). There is no evidence to support a diagnosis of raised intracranial pressure or space-occupying lesion (very unlikely).

Rebecca and her family are reassured, on the basis of the history and examination, that a brain tumour is unlikely, but despite this they remain concerned that this is still a possibility. It is also a possibility that the level of anxiety about this issue is contributing to the headache and may have precipitated the referral.

Investigations

For migraine and tension-type headaches, there are no specific diagnostic investigations. The most commonly ordered investigation is neuroimaging – either computed tomography (CT) or magnetic resonance imaging (MRI) to examine the anatomy of the brain. Even when ordered on highly selected groups of patients, only around 1–3 per cent will have such an abnormality. If sinusitis is suspected, scanning of the skull to examine the sinuses will probably give better information than plain radiographs of them.

On this occasion, because of the extreme anxiety, an MRI of Rebecca's head was requested. The image is shown in Figure 37.3 and is fortunately healthy.

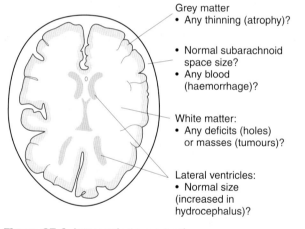

Grey matter
• Any thinning (atrophy)?

• Normal subarachnoid space size?
• Any blood (haemorrhage)?

White matter:
• Any deficits (holes) or masses (tumours)?

Lateral ventricles:
• Normal size (increased in hydrocephalus)?

Figure 37.4 Interpreting a magnetic resonance scan.

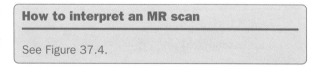

How to interpret an MR scan

See Figure 37.4.

Diagnosis

Following the MRI Rebecca is given a diagnosis of tension-type headache.

Treatment and follow-up plan

Rebecca's treatment plan comprises a number of elements:

- Reassured that the headaches do not have a serious basis
- Told to stop taking the analgesics on a regular basis
- Family are asked to consider what psychological factors might be at work
- Reassured that this type of headache is common
- Told that frequency and severity of headaches are very likely to reduce in time

First, she is reassured that the headaches do not have a serious basis. The hope is that this will reduce the component of anxiety caused by this worry, allowing her parents to deal with the headaches with less anxiety themselves.

Second, she is asked to stop taking the analgesics on a regular basis and in fact to take a holiday from them for several weeks, noting that the headaches may become temporarily worse.

Third, the family are asked to consider what psychological factors might be at work and to note that the headaches started shortly after Rebecca started her secondary school. Despite her good progress she is a perfectionist. Does she worry about things unnecessarily? Are there any particular concerns? They are asked to reflect on their lifestyle as a family. Do they get enough time for rest and relaxation?

Fourth, Rebecca is reassured that this type of headache is common and that both the frequency and severity of headaches are very likely to reduce in time.

Evidence-based medicine

Self-test 4: Which is the best initial source for evidence to answer this question? In a 12-year-old girl with tension-type headache which interventions are most helpful in reducing headache frequency and severity?

A Cochrane controlled trial register
B Cochrane database of systematic reviews
C Cochrane controlled trials register
D Search Medline for articles on headache in children
E Search through the indices of peer-reviewed paediatric journals

Answer: B

Ibuprofen, paracetamol, nasal sumatriptan and dihydro-ergotamine have been shown to be useful in acute migraine attacks. Flunarizine and possibly propranolol have been shown to be useful in prevention. A range of behavioural treatments such as progressive muscle relaxation and thermal biofeedback have been shown to be helpful in both migraine and tension-type headache.

Two months later Rebecca returns to the clinic with her mother. The headaches are considerably better since she stopped taking the regular paracetamol. At the parents' evening at Rebecca's school, her parents had a chance to discuss the situation with her form teacher who said that Rebecca had initially found the secondary school situation quite challenging, but was now making friends and good progress. She seemed much more relaxed. Rebecca was discharged from further follow-up.

Background information

Epidemiology

By the age of 11, three-quarters of all children will have had headaches. Between the ages of 5 and 15 years, about 1 in 10 children will have had a headache in the previous year. The most common headache type in children is migraine, and some surveys have suggested that as many as 9 of 10 children with headaches have migraine. As children get older, tension headaches become more predominant and more common in females. Children with chronic headaches lose an average of 3 days a year from school. There is also a sharp rise in the prevalence of migraine, which peaks around 15 years of age. Many children who subsequently develop migraine have suffered from recurrent abdominal pain, travel sickness and episodic night-time limb pain (growing pains).

Table 37.1 Drugs that modify the action of serotonin (5HT) receptors

Drug	Action	Comments
Pizotifen	5HT-receptor antagonist	Preventive treatment
		Site effects: sleepiness, weight gain
Sumatriptan	$5HT_{1A}$, $5HT_{1B}$, $5HT_{1D}$, $5HT_{1F}$ agonist	Acute treatment
		Highly effective in adults – nasal administration effective in children
Ergot alkaloids	$5HT_1$, $5HT_2$ agonist	Acute treatment, side effects caused by dopamine D_2-receptor and $5HT_2$ agonism – vomiting, diarrhoea and coronary vasospasm
		Not used in children

Aetiology

Although the fundamental aetiology of headaches is for the most part poorly understood, the role of triggers is much better worked out. Interestingly the classic food triggers described in adults (chocolate and cheese) are much less important in children, although one trigger also overlooked is citrus fruit. Other triggers include sudden vigorous exercise, bright light, lack of sleep and hunger. Psychological factors can be very important in both tension-type headaches and migraine.

Pathophysiology

The pathophysiology of migraine is complex. The simple model is that there is initially vasoconstriction causing an aura and then subsequent vasodilatation, which causes the headache. A more complex model is now proposed involving a migraine generator in the brain stem, a cortical spreading depression, the trigeminal system and release of vasoactive neuropeptides in blood vessel walls. Some rare forms, such as familial hemiplegic migraine, are associated with gene mutations on chromosome 19, some of which code for calcium channel proteins.

Hence, calcium channel blockers, such as flunarizine, have been used for treating and preventing migraine attacks.

Despite the complexity of migraine pathophysiology disturbances of serotonin (5-hydroxytryptamine or 5HT) metabolism are thought to be an important component of migraine susceptibility and of migraine episodes. Injection of serotonin has been demonstrated to abort some migraine attacks but at the cost of major side effects. Various drugs modify the action of 5HT receptors (Table 37.1).

Further sources of information

Articles

Annequin D, Tournaire B, Massiou H. Migraine and headaches in childhood and adolescence. *Pediatric Clinics of North America* 2000; **47**: 617–31

Ferrari MD. Migraine. *The Lancet* 1998; **351**: 1043–51

Websites

www.ama-assn.org/special/migraine/search/search.htm

www.aafp.org/afp/20020215.625.html

Self-test 5: Six-year-old James presented to outpatients, referred by his GP. He had a 6-week

history of increasingly severe headaches and these were waking him at night. He had started vomiting, especially in the mornings. He was somewhat better at the end of the day. When he was examined there was a degree of horizontal nystagmus.

A What are the most important features in this history?

B What could the nystagmus mean?

C What might you find if you examined his fundi?

D What investigation would you organize?

Answer:

A A short history, waking at night and morning vomiting are all consistent with raised intracranial pressure

B The nystagmus could indicate a cerebellar lesion

C Papilloedema

D An urgent CT or MRI of his head

Presentation

Referral letter from GP:
Please see Fiona aged 14 years whose parents are extremely concerned that she has lost approximately a stone in weight. Fiona started her periods at 11 and was having fairly regular periods until 6 months ago – she hasn't had one since. Her parents have tried to persuade her to eat more, but Fiona denies that there is a problem. Fiona is a high achiever and is continuing to do well at school.

Initial considerations and action

The information in the referral letter is limited, but there must be significant concern by the GP and parents to make a referral. Pathological causes of weight loss include anorexia nervosa, depression and a wide range of medical conditions.

Fiona's parents may be overanxious. It's not stated what Fiona's weight was before the weight loss – she may have been overweight. Dieting to achieve the ideal body shape is a very common occurrence in adolescence. Most fail to lose weight and give up, some achieve their goal and stop dieting, but approximately 1 per cent of teenagers develop anorexia nervosa.

Self-test 1: What is the significance of the amenorrhoea?

Answer: Periods may be irregular at menarche and it is not unusual for girls to have one or two periods and then quite a gap until the next. However, once a regular

pattern is established this is much less likely. Pregnancy always needs to be considered. Women who exercise intensively may have amenorrhoea and it is also an indicator of significant weight loss.

The amenorrhoea is a worrying feature and is indicative of significant weight loss (note that pregnancy should always be considered).

The paediatrician arranges to see Fiona and her parents in the outpatient clinic and needs to consider:

- Whether features of anorexia nervosa are present
- Physical causes causing weight loss and poor appetite
- Psychiatric conditions associated with weight loss and poor appetite

Warning signs of anorexia nervosa

- Deliberate self-starvation with weight loss
- Fear of gaining weight
- Refusal to eat/avoidance of 'fattening' foods
- Denial of hunger
- Use of laxatives or purgatives
- Self-induced vomiting
- Constant exercising
- Greater amounts of hair on the body or face (lanugo hair)
- Sensitivity to cold
- Absent or irregular periods
- Loss of scalp hair
- A self-perception of being fat when the person is really too thin (distorted body image)

Medical illnesses with significant weight loss

- Tuberculosis (TB)
- Acquired immune deficiency disease (AIDS)

- Anterior pituitary insufficiency
- Addison's disease
- Hyperthyroidism
- Diabetes mellitus
- Inflammatory bowel disease
- Hypothalamic tumours
- Malignancy

Features of depression in adolescents

- Apathy, boredom, lack of interest in usual activities, lack of energy
- Fall-off in school performance and loss of concentration
- Preoccupation with minor ailments
- Irritable mood, feelings of sadness and hopelessness
- Loss of appetite and weight, or comfort eating and excess weight gain
- Sleep disturbance leading to tiredness
- Loss of libido
- Slowing of thought and movement
- Suicidal thoughts

History

Fiona attends the outpatient clinic with her mother and father.

A year ago, Fiona's cousin had asked her to be a bridesmaid and as she was a bit plump she decided to lose some weight. Fiona's mum also wanted to lose weight and they decided to go to a slimming club together. Both mother and daughter started on a healthy eating plan. The rest of the family were very supportive and, when Fiona went for the first fitting of the bridesmaid dress, her cousin was impressed by her weight loss. However, as the wedding approached, Fiona became more and more concerned that she would look fat on the photographs. She stopped going to the slimming club and took up jogging. At this stage her parents became concerned that the exercising and dieting had taken over her life and that she was now too thin. She denied that she was dieting. She explained that she was eating sensibly, which was why she had become a vegetarian. Her parents knew she was misleading them about how much she was eating and that she was throwing food away.

Fiona acknowledged that she sometimes did this if her mother had used animal fat in cooking. She hadn't wanted to say anything in case it hurt her mother's feelings.

Fiona is a bright girl who has always been a high achiever in school, which she enjoys. She is conscientious, organized and very methodical. Fiona has always been considerate of others and up until now hadn't caused her parents any concern. She doesn't have a boyfriend.

Fiona is the eldest of three children. She has a brother aged 10 years and a sister aged 7.

Fiona described herself as being in good health and usually having lots of energy. She started her periods at 11 years and had a regular 30-day cycle until 8–10 months ago. She hasn't had a period since. Review of systems didn't reveal any additional symptoms. Fiona didn't see herself as being too thin and gets very irritated when people comment on this. However, she had been feeling more tired recently and was concerned about how this might interfere with her exercise programme and homework. She sleeps well. On specific questioning, Fiona denied making herself sick, using laxatives or diuretics.

Self-test 2: Which of the warning signs for anorexia nervosa is most helpful in distinguishing it from other conditions?

Answer: Distorted body image.

Meaning of the history

Anorexia nervosa

Fiona's parents describe a typical picture of anorexia nervosa – individuals starve themselves, avoid high-calorie foods and exercise constantly. They feel hungry, although they deny this. Fiona's distorted body image is an important factor. The features of bulimia – binge eating, self-induced vomiting, and use of laxatives and diuretics to control weight gain – are also commonly seen in anorexia nervosa. Fiona has denied this, but self-reporting of eating patterns and other behaviours has to be interpreted with caution. Independent observation is important. Many adolescent girls go through a phase of vegetarianism and this is common in young people with anorexia nervosa.

Criteria for diagnosis of anorexia nervosa
- Determined food avoidance
- Weight loss in the absence of physical or other mental illness
- Any two or more of the following:
  – self-induced vomiting
  – marked fear of weight gain
  – distorted body image
  – preoccupation with body weight
  – preoccupation with energy intake
  – extensive exercising
  – laxative abuse
  – amenorrhoea

How to detect tricks to keep weight down

- Style of clothes – baggy clothes worn to hide emaciation
- Excessive exercise, often secretive, constantly moving to use up as much energy as possible
- Regular trips to the bathroom after meals: is this to induce vomiting after eating?
- Use of laxatives and diuretics
- How much food is actually being eaten and what is its calorie and fat content?
  – becoming vegetarian to justify a change in eating habits
  – hiding food/throwing food out
  – filling the plate with vegetables/lettuce
  – eating slowly
  – insisting on 'healthy' cooking, i.e. no frying, use of cooking oils, only boiling or steaming
  – offering to cook the family meals to take control over calories served
  – returning home late from friends saying they've already eaten

Self-test 3: Which groups of young people are prone to develop anorexia nervosa?

Answer: Gymnasts, ballet dancers, models.

Physical causes for weight loss and poor appetite

A careful history and examination should exclude other conditions that may present with anorexia and weight loss; young people with chronic illness don't feel like eating and have other symptoms. Some of the symptoms of juvenile hypothyroidism are similar to those seen in anorexia nervosa; however, it is usually associated with a goitre and results in weight gain rather than weight loss. Fiona reports that she is well and that she has a normal appetite.

Features of hypothyroidism in young people
- Cold intolerance
- Dry skin and cold extremities
- Bradycardia
- Thin dry hair
- Puffy eyes
- Goitre
- Constipation
- Slow to relax reflexes
- Short stature
- Delayed puberty
- Obesity
- Deterioration in schoolwork
- Learning difficulties

Psychiatric conditions

Psychiatric states that may be confused with anorexia nervosa include depressive disorders, obsessive–compulsive disorder (OCD) and less commonly drug misuse. Many girls with anorexia nervosa suffer low mood and a significant number are seriously depressed and it may be difficult to know if the depression is primary with secondary loss of appetite and weight, or vice versa. The presence of other symptomatology and attitudes to bodily appearance will usually clarify the diagnosis. Fiona doesn't have features of depression.

Signs of drug misuse
- Unexplained absences from home or school
- Loss of interest in schoolwork
- Intoxication
- Change in behaviour
- Mixing with known users
- High rates of spending money and stealing money

Obsessional disorders in childhood
Definitions
- **Obsession:** a recurrent intrusive thought that is recognized to be irrational but cannot be ignored

- **Compulsion:** a behaviour carried out (usually repeatedly) to reduce the anxiety associated with the obsessional idea

Clinical course
- Usually begins in middle childhood, often with fluctuating course
- Common themes of obsessional ideas:
  - cleanliness
  - washing/dressing
  - contact/contamination with disease or illness
  - foreboding and sense of doom
- Mood disturbance, usually depressive
- Family members involved in rituals

Treatment
- Medical treatment of any mood disturbance
- Identify and manage any precipitating stress
- Enlist help of family and school
- Behavioural techniques

Prevalence
- Rare – prevalence of 0.3 per cent

Self-test 4: Which of the following symptoms are seen in depression?

A Loss of appetite

B Sleep disturbance

C Over-eating

D Increase in energy levels

E Fear of weight gain

Answer: A, B, C.

Examination

Fiona is examined.

General appearance

- Bright alert appearance
- Fine downy (lanugo) hair over face, trunk and limbs
- Dry skin and hair
- Normal teeth, Russell's sign negative (callus on middle fingers caused by self-induced vomiting)

Growth

- Height 160 cm (50th centile)
- Weight 40 kg (2nd–9th centile)
- Bones protruding through skin

Cardiovascular system

- Blood pressure 90/60 mmHg
- Pulse 60/minute
- Adequate peripheral circulation, but hands and feet somewhat cold

Respiratory system

- Normal

Abdomen and genitalia

- Pubertal developmental – breast and pubic hair development both Tanner stage 4
- Abdomen – normal

Neurological examination

- Normal, including no deficit of visual fields and normal fundal examination

---

Self-test 5: Why is it important to examine the teeth?

Answer: As an indication of possible bulimia. The teeth may be eroded by gastric acid caused by recurrent vomiting.

The purpose of the examination is to assess the nutritional status and medical well-being. Parts of the body may be covered in lanugo hair and the skin may be coarse and rough. The body may develop a low metabolic rate as a result of starvation with slow-to-relax tendon reflexes, reduced peripheral circulation, low blood pressure and bradycardia. Low plasma proteins can lead to ankle oedema. In very severe cases, the young person can be tipped into cardiac failure.

Self-test 6: Why have the visual fields specifically been recorded in the examination?

Answer: Panhypopituitarism caused by expanding tumours in the pituitary region can result in visual field

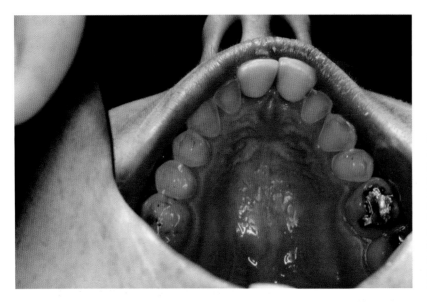

Figure 38.1 Upper teeth in an 18-year-old bulimic patient. The enamel has been eroded by gastric acid exposing the underlying dentine, which is yellow. The remaining white enamel can be seen on the buccal aspects of the teeth. This can be sensitive and disfiguring, and functional problems can also occur. (Photograph courtesy of A Milosevic, Liverpool University Medical School.)

defects which result from pressure on the optic chiasma. Hypopituitarism may present with weight loss, growth failure and failure to develop, or regression in sexual maturation with amenorrhoea.

It is important to examine the teeth to detect changes caused by recurrent vomiting – dentists are adept at picking up eating disorders (Figure 38.1). The patient may be eating adequate amounts, but relies on vomiting to control the weight.

Interpretation of the examination

The history and findings on examination are typical of anorexia nervosa. Fiona is significantly underweight – 80 per cent of the expected weight for her height. There is no evidence of cardiac failure or depression.

Investigations

Investigations will depend on the severity of symptoms and clinical indicators of possible medical conditions. The following investigations are carried out on Fiona:

- **Full blood count (FBC):** normal
- **Thyroid function tests (TFTs):** normal
- **Urea and electrolytes (U&As):** normal
- **pH:** normal
- **Plasma proteins:** normal
- **Blood luteinizing hormone (LH) and follicle-stimulating hormone (FSH):** low
- **Urine LH and FSH:** low
- **Cortisol:** high

Low triiodothyronine (T_3) is not uncommon in anorexic patients and may give rise to false suspicions of hypothyroidism. Use of laxatives, diuretics and vomiting can result in metabolic abnormalities such as hypokalaemia and alkalosis. Low FSH and LH result in amenorrhoea. Mild anaemia may be present with low iron stores.

Diagnosis

Anorexia nervosa

Treatment and follow-up plan

Anorexia nervosa is a serious and potentially life-threatening condition. A comprehensive approach to management is necessary, paying attention to physical, social and psychological factors. This includes the role of the family, school and peers, as well as physical aspects. Access to a multiagency team is essential. The paediatrician discusses Fiona urgently with the Child and Adolescent Mental Health Team and arranges to work jointly with them to advise on medical issues.

Treatment aims

- Engagement in the therapeutic process for Fiona and her family
- Recognition/acknowledgement of the problem – motivational interviewing
- Alteration of eating habits to ensure restoration of weight loss and correction of nutritional deficiency
- Treatment of individual and family psychopathology:
  - individual or cognitive – behavioural therapy
  - family therapy
  - drug treatment for any associated conditions, e.g. depression or OCD
  - follow-up contact to monitor weight and general progress

Recognition of the problem and engagement

Treatment of anorexia nervosa is difficult, because people with anorexia believe that there is nothing wrong with them. The first crucial steps are recognition of the problem and engagement of the young person and family in the therapeutic process. This may need several extended interviews with the parents and young person. The seriousness of the condition, the eating habits of the individual (fear of fatness, dieting, binge eating, over-exercising, avoidance of food etc.) must be discussed openly in order to establish a therapeutic alliance. Only when this has occurred is it possible to commence a specific treatment programme.

Motivational interviewing

The psychiatrist explains the condition to Fiona and her parents and explores Fiona's motivation for change. Fiona admitted to some tiredness, which could be used as a motivator to improve her eating because she feels it could interfere with her schoolwork. An explanation that her tiredness is the result of undernutrition and advice from

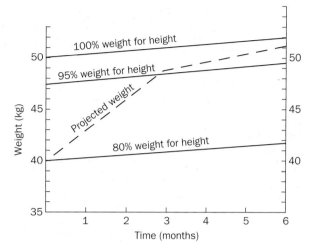

Figure 38.2 Growth chart over a 6-month period, showing target weight range of 95–100 per cent expected weight for height, starting weight of 80 per cent expected for height and projected weight with a gain of 2.5 kg/month.

the dietician on healthy eating may be a useful start. Fiona's morbid fear of becoming fat is acknowledged, with continual reassurances that the aim of treatment is not to make her fat but healthy.

Alteration of eating habits

Management focuses on improving the patient's well-being by improving her eating. Weight is monitored, but being mindful that weight gain is what the patient will be most fearful of. A target weight needs to be set (weight appropriate for height). It is helpful to have a weight range to work to rather than a specific weight. Menstruation is unlikely to occur at less than 94 per cent height for weight. It is wise therefore to set a target range of 95–100 per cent. (No individual with anorexia nervosa will want to be of average weight.)

The paediatrician uses the growth chart to agree a target weight with Fiona and plots on a graph the anticipated weights on a monthly basis. Weight gain is expected at 2–2.5 kg per month (Figure 38.2). The dietician provides dietary advice so that Fiona has an appropriate daily calorie intake to ensure its attainment. Fiona's weight is 40 kg, which is 80 per cent of the weight expected for her height. In 3 months she should have reached the target weight range.

Most cases are now managed by frequent outpatient visits. Hospital admission to a paediatric or psychiatric unit would be indicated if there was evidence of:

- Dehydration and metabolic disturbance
- Signs of circulatory failure such as low blood pressure, slow pulse, poor peripheral circulation
- Persistent vomiting or haematemesis
- Significantly worsening weight loss or weight less than 80 per cent for height
- Severe depression with risk of suicide.

In hospital, nursing care and support are important aspects of management. Nursing staff have to be vigilant about food hoarding and vomiting. Management usually involves graded privileges dependent on satisfactory weight gain. It may involve supervising family meals at home during weekend leave.

Individual and family therapy

Establishment of a trusting relationship between the young person and individual therapist is important at the outset. Acceptance of the problem and willingness to discuss attitudes and ideas about body image, growth and development, family and peer relationships are necessary, not only to modify eating habits, but also to change family and interpersonal relationships. Once acceptable weight gain has been achieved, individual psychotherapeutic approaches become more worth while. The young person can be helped to achieve more autonomy in decision-making and feel more in control of her life generally. The patient and her family can be counselled in more constructive ways of handling conflict and relationships.

The presence of siblings at the sessions can be very helpful. It is crucial to get family and friends to support the management.

Liaison with school is essential – eating disorders affect the young person's education. They may deny that they are physically too weak to cope with the demands of the normal school day. Their pursuit of perfectionism may drive them to achieve while remaining dissatisfied with the results. Obsessional traits may result in compulsive work habits, and their difficulties in personal relationships can interfere with appropriate peer and teacher interaction.

Medication

Medication has only a small part to play in management. Severe anxiety and tension may merit the use of an anxiolytic. Antidepressants may be used if depression is a prominent component. Choice of antidepressant is usually a selective serotonin reuptake inhibitor that is also of use for symptoms of OCD.

Follow-up

Weight gain is usually the easy part and Fiona reaches her target weight without much difficulty. More difficult is the restructuring of the young person's and the family's attitude to food and their pattern of interaction. Regular supervision, support and contact with the therapist are set up to maintain progress. Often a compromise has to be made between an ideal resolution of the problem and a realistic appraisal of the family and the child's capacity to change. Fiona and her family attend the sessions regularly. Communication improves and the family feel that they can be discharged.

Background knowledge

Anorexia nervosa

Epidemiology

The age of onset may be anything from 6 to 60 years, but most begin in the teenage years with a prevalence of about 1 per cent of teenagers. The incidence rate has been increasing, although severe forms are still relatively uncommon. The peak age of onset is 14 years and girls outnumber boys by 20 to 1.

Aetiology

Family factors
Characteristic patterns of family functioning have been described, although these are not universal:

- Enmeshment or over-involvement
- Over-protectiveness
- Rigidity
- Poor conflict resolution

Restricting their eating gives the young person a feeling of control over his or her life and body.

Genetic factors

Evidence from twin and family studies suggest that there may be a genetically determined element.

Individual factors

Affected individuals are usually hard-working and quiet with obsessive and perfectionist traits. There may be a desire not to enter the adult world of womanhood with its implications for independence, sexuality and motherhood. Sexual abuse needs to be considered.

Societal factors

Such attitudes to female appearance are probably relevant. Extremely thin models and pop stars have become celebrities and role models for young girls.

Pathophysiology

Starvation and malnutrition significantly affect a broad spectrum of physiological parameters. The endocrine changes are secondary to the condition, but once established inhibit recovery and are a significant factor in the maintenance of the condition. Psychological improvement can occur quite rapidly once the physical changes of malnutrition are reversed.

Prognosis

- About a third make a full recovery with a normal attitude to bodily appearance and their adolescent development
- A third retain a reasonable body weight but remain preoccupied with their appearance and have minor psychosexual problems
- A third develop a chronic relapsing course. Those who have developed the condition before puberty may remain short in stature and never menstruate. Personality problems remain severe in this group, suicidal attempts are common and 5 per cent die by suicide, malnutrition or infection

Further sources of information

Books

Rutter M, Taylor E, Hersov L (ed.) *Child and Adolescent Psychiatry, Modern Approaches*, 3rd edn. London: Blackwell Science, 1994

Lask B, Bryant-Waugh R (ed.) *Childhood Onset Anorexia Nervosa and Related Eating Disorders*. Hove: Lawrence Erlbaum Associates Ltd, 1993

Article

Milosevic A. Eating disorders – a dentist's perspective. *European Eating Disorders Review* 1999; **7**: 103–10

Self-test 7: John, aged 13 years, presents with a 3-month history of loss of appetite and some weight loss and constipation. He is finding it increasingly difficult to get up in the mornings and consequently is late for school. His schoolwork is deteriorating, and he is complaining of feeling cold and tired all the time.

A Which medical condition needs to be considered?

B Which additional points in the history would help determine whether or not John has anorexia nervosa?

C Which additional points in the history would suggest OCD?

D What is the likely diagnosis?

Answer:

A Hypothyroidism

B Distorted body image, fear of gaining weight

C Obsessive–compulsive behaviours that are interfering with normal functioning

D Depression

Chronic disorder

A tired teenager

Age: 15 years

STEVEN RYAN

Presentation

Fifteen-year-old Camilla was returning for a follow-up clinic appointment at the hospital; she had been 6 weeks earlier, having been referred by her general practitioner. The doctor who had seen her in the first hospital clinic had written this at the end of the case notes:

- Tired teenager
- Possible chronic fatigue syndrome
- For investigations to exclude an underlying disease
- To keep symptom diary

Camilla returned to the clinic today for her test results and to share the contents of her diary. Both her parents accompanied her, as they did at the initial visit. Camilla walked into the room in a laboured way and sat down, exhaling loudly as if she was exhausted.

Self-test 1: What is the minimum duration of symptoms before chronic fatigue syndrome can be diagnosed?

A 1 week
B 6 weeks
C 3 months
D 6 months
E 1 year

Answer: D.

Initial considerations and action

Tiredness is a common symptom in adults and is also seen in teenage years. It is an uncommon symptom in younger children. It has a very large range of potential causes including definitive organic disorders, such as hypothyroidism, and much less well-defined disorders, such as chronic fatigue syndrome (myalgic encephalomyelitis [ME]). Obviously mental health problems are highly associated with this symptom but it is important to note that association does not necessarily mean causation. A young person might become depressed by chronic fatigue – whatever its cause. The groups of causes that need to be considered are:

- Tiredness is a common 'normal' symptom in teenagers – lifestyle factors may be important (Figure 39.1)
- Chronic viral infection, e.g. Epstein–Barr virus
- Chronic fatigue syndrome (also known as ME)
- Haematological, e.g. iron deficiency anaemia
- Endocrine, e.g. hypothyroidism
- Psychological, e.g. depression, anxiety
- Malignancies, e.g. lymphoma
- Cardiorespiratory insufficiency
- Gastrointestinal, e.g. coeliac disease
- Renal, e.g. chronic renal failure
- Musculoskeletal, e.g. myopathy

Self-test 2: In hypothyroidism which three of the following symptoms are more likely?

A Intolerance of cold
B Palpitations
C Weight loss
D Gruff voice
E Hair loss

Answer: A, D, E.

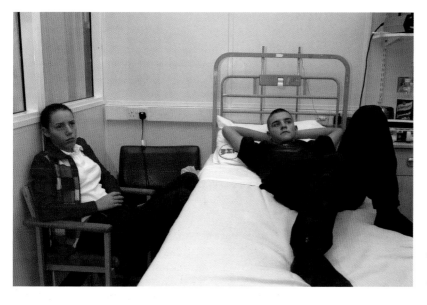

Figure 39.1 A teenager may report lethargy and excessive somnolence without organic disease. In fact parents are more likely to comment on it!

History

The purpose of the history is:

- To help make the diagnosis
- To quantify the degree of disability and lifestyle disruption, and especially to quantify the effect on schooling

Camilla was initially allowed to talk about her problem without interruption and the following details had emerged:

She had been well until 6 months ago – the previous summer – around the time of her annual exams. She did not remember a specific illness but gradually became less energetic. It was more difficult to wake up in the morning and her sleep was less restful. Her exercise tolerance had decreased and she had given up sports at school (though she did not like sports much in any event). The symptoms had got worse over a month or two and then had remained pretty static, although she had good days and bad days. The mornings were particularly difficult. She had missed several weeks at school and sometimes did not get to school until the afternoon.

From time to time she had a variety of other symptoms, including swollen glands, sore throats, vertigo and headaches.

She had an unremarkable past medical history other than an appendectomy 3 years earlier.

She had been prescribed two courses of antibiotics during her illness – for sore throats – but these had made little difference to the symptoms.

Camilla and her mother described the family history:

- **Mother:** 38 years old – coeliac disease (presented with diarrhoea in infancy) on gluten-free diet
- **Father:** 40 years old – fit and well
- **Brother:** 11 years old – mild asthma

Subsequently a more directed history was undertaken to consider the possible diagnoses above.

- **Chronic viral infection:**
  - no contact history
  - minor lymphadenopathy
  - some puffiness around eyes

Self-test 3: Give three causes of puffiness around the eyes.

Answers: Nephrotic syndrome (or other cause of reduced serum albumin), nephritic syndrome (mild), glandular fever, allergy.

- **Chronic fatigue syndrome:** (also known as ME):
  - a diagnosis of exclusion
- **Anaemia:**
  - no history of preschool anaemia
  - currently rather poor diet and Camilla was a vegetarian
  - not taking any nutritional supplements
  - menstrual periods were regular and light
- **Endocrine:**
  - hypothyroidism:
    no constipation
    hair and skin in good condition
    no change in voice
    good tolerance of cold, preferring this to warmth
  - hypoadrenalism (Addison's disease):
    no loss of weight or wasting
    some abdominal pain
    some anorexia
    no craving for salt
- **Psychological:**
  - no unrealistic worries
  - no obsessions or compulsions
  - 'fed up' with being ill
  - episodes of crying
  - no suicidal ideas
  - some sleep disturbance
  - no history of depression in either parent
- **Malignancies:**
  - lymph glands mildly enlarged from time to time
  - fever from time to time but no night sweats
  - no cough
- **Cardiorespiratory insufficiency:**
  - no cough, breathlessness or wheeze
  - no chest pain, palpitations or fainting
- **Gastrointestinal:**
  - intermittent, colicky, mild-to-moderate, central abdominal pain
  - occasional loose motions
  - no vomiting, though sometimes nauseous
- **Renal:**
  - no history of urinary tract symptoms or infection
  - no family history of chronic renal disease
- **Musculoskeletal:**
  - generally fatigued but no specific muscle weakness or pain
  - no joint swelling, pain or stiffness

Meaning of the history

Camilla gives a clear history of prolonged fatigue with a number of non-specific associated symptoms. The level of disability seems beyond that which would occur in otherwise healthy teenagers. Chronic viral infection or chronic fatigue syndrome remains a strong possibility. Camilla's mental state seems reasonable – she does not seem to be clinically depressed, but the illness is taking its toll. No strong candidates emerge from the other potential diagnoses.

Examination

The aim of the examination is primarily to search for clues to possible diagnoses. It is also important that, even if the examination is unlikely to be positive, it is carried out thoroughly because it is important that the family see that their concerns are taken seriously. Camilla is examined and these are the findings.

General examination

- **Skin:** warm, healthy, no pigmentation or depigmentation
- **Nails:** no pallor or clubbing
- **Conjunctiva:** no clinical anaemia
- **Hair:** good condition – no recent loss
- **Neck:**
  - small, smooth, mobile, lymph nodes in anterior and posterior triangles bilaterally
  - tonsillar glands larger (1.5 cm) but also smooth and firm and non-tender
  - no other lymphadenopathy anywhere
  - no goitre
- Height/weight within normal limits (body mass index 22 kg/m^2)

Ears, nose and throat

- Ear drums grey and healthy with good light reflex
- Nasal membranes healthy
- Moderately enlarged tonsils with scarring and pitting
- Petechiae observed on posterior palate

Cardiovascular system

- Heart rate 78/minute
- Blood pressure 108/68 mmHg
- Normal cardiac examination

Respiratory system

- Normal

Abdomen

- Normal

Central nervous system

- No abnormality was detected
- No loss of power identified (all major muscle groups score 5/5 on MRC grading)
- Limb tendon reflexes all present and appropriate
- Plantar reflexes down-going

> ### How to test muscle strength using the MRC grading system for muscle power
>
> Table 39.1 shows the Medical Research Council's (MRC's) scheme for measuring and recording muscle power. For each joint and each specific movement involved, the power is recorded on the scale in the table. The score can be used for diagnostic purposes but also for monitoring conditions and their treatment.

Locomotor system

- Full range of non-painful joint movements throughout the body
- No swelling of joints

This examination is reassuring and helps to exclude a number of possible diagnoses:

- **Anaemia:** there are no features consistent with anaemia
- **Malignancy:** the lymphadenopathy seen here is common. The features that go against malignancy are the smooth, small and mobile nature of the lymph glands. The tonsillar (or jugulo-digastric glands) are commonly enlarged in healthy children

Table 39.1 Grading for muscle power of the Medical Research Council (MRC)

Muscle response	Score
No movement	0
Muscle belly moves but the joint does not move	1
Joint moves with gravity eliminated	2
Joint moves against gravity	3
Joint moves against gravity and some resistance	4
Full strength	5

- **Hypothyroidism:** the healthy skin and hair, warm peripheries, lack of goitre and normal reflexes (slow relaxation in hypothyroidism) make a thyroid disorder less likely
- **Addison's disease:** sometimes difficult to exclude on examination, but skin pigmentation and low blood pressure might be seen

The moderately enlarged tonsils are non-specific but palatal petechiae are sometimes seen in Epstein–Barr virus infection (Figures 39.2 and 39.3).

Investigations

The doctor now reviewed the investigations with Camilla and her mother.

Haematology

See Table 39.2.

- **Film:** shows atypical lymphocytes
- **Anti-endomysial antibodies for coeliac disease:** negative

Biochemistry

See Table 39.3, p. 419.

Thyroid function tests

See Table 39.4, p. 419.

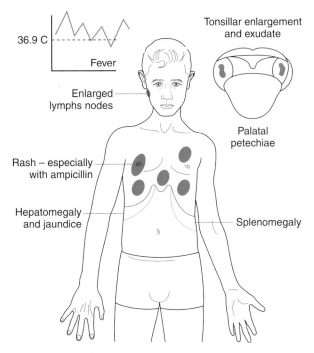

Figure 39.2 Findings that can be seen in Epstein–Barr virus infection (glandular fever/infectious mononucleosis).

Viral serology

- **Epstein–Barr virus (EBV):**
  - anti-EBNA-1 IgG: positive (EBNA is Epstein–Barr nuclear antibody)
  - EBV anti-capsid antigen IgM: negative
  - heterophile antibody: negative
- **Cytomegalovirus (CMV):** no antibodies detected

Meaning of the investigation results

Importantly, these investigations have not only provided the likely diagnosis, but also excluded a number of other diagnoses. There is no anaemia, renal function is normal and there is no evidence of an endocrine disorder. There is strong evidence to support the presence of Epstein–Barr virus infection. The C-reactive protein level is increased moderately and this is in keeping with a viral infection. The anti-capsid IgM (immunoglobuin M) antibody is elevated early in the infection but then declines. The appearance of nuclear antigen-1 antibody appears later in the 'convalescent' phase but then persists.

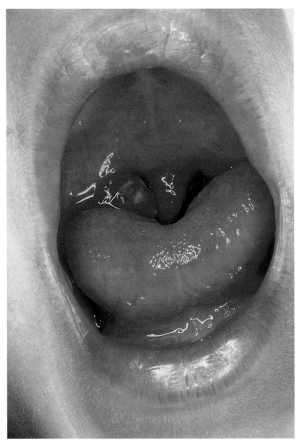

Figure 39.3 Tonsillitis in glandular fever

Table 39.2 Haematology results of investigations for Camilla

Parameter	Value	Expected range
Haemoglobin (g/dL)	12.9	11.5–15.8
White cell count ($\times 10^9$/L)	13.74	4.9–13.7
Platelet count ($\times 10^9$/L)	293	150–400
Neutrophil count ($\times 10^9$/L)	4.29	1.6–9.0
Lymphocyte count ($\times 10^9$/L)	13.78	2.2–9.8

Heterophile antibodies represent a non-specific test for IgM antibody, which agglutinates sheep red cells. This is the basis of the glandular fever screening test (Monospot). Although positive in many during the

Table 39.3 Biochemistry results for Camilla

Parameter	Value	Normal range
Creatinine (μmol/L)	43	30–62
Urea (mmol/L)	4.8	2.3–6.4
Sodium (mmol/L)	136	135–145
Potassium (mmol/L)	4.4	3.5–5.5
Glucose (random) (mmol/L)	6.6	>2.8
Total bilirubin (μmol/L)	14	0–15
Alkaline phosphatase (IU/L)	480	177–1036
Alanine aminotransferase (IU/L)	18	8–36
Aspartate transaminase (IU/L)	24	12–41
C-reactive protein (mg/L)	24	0–8

IU, international unit.

Table 39.4 Thyroid function test results for Camilla

Parameter	Value	Expected range
Thyroxine (nmol/L)	94	76–155
TSH (mU/L)	0.70	0.3–3.8
Cortisol (9am) (nmol/L)	191	140–500

TSH, thyroid-stimulating hormone.

early illness, it is invariably negative subsequently. Atypical lymphocytes are another non-specific marker of viral infection.

Diagnosis

Epstein–Barr virus infection (glandular fever, infectious mononucleosis).

Management and prognosis

The patient was reassured that her symptoms were related to virus infection and that in time her symptoms were very likely to abate and she would recover full health. She was informed that there was small likelihood of a more persistent postviral fatigue syndrome.

No specific treatment is routinely used for this illness and treatment is supportive. Camilla's school were informed about the illness (with her permission) – specifically they were told that the symptoms might persist for up to a year, that the symptoms were quite variable, and that a flexible approach to education would be required until Camilla had recovered.

Subsequently, Camilla did make a good recovery and was able to return to school full-time 3 months later.

Background information

Epstein–Barr virus

Epstein–Barr virus is a member of the herpes virus family and most people become infected with EBV at some time during their lives (usually by 40 years of age), although many infections are asymptomatic. Infants become susceptible when maternal antibody protection (present at birth) is lost. Many children become infected, usually without symptoms or with symptoms that are indistinguishable from the other mild illnesses of childhood. Symptoms seem more likely to occur in adolescence when 'infectious mononucleosis or glandular fever' is quite likely. It is known as the 'kissing' disease because it is felt that close social contact may help its transmission.

Typically patients have recovered within 2 months but the virus remains and symptoms regularly continue for up to a year. As with other herpes viruses it remains latent in a few cells in the throat and blood for the rest of life. From time to time, the virus can reactivate (asymptomatically) and is commonly found in the saliva of infected people. This reactivation usually occurs without symptoms of illness. A late event in a very few carriers of this virus is the emergence of Burkitt's lymphoma (especially in Africa). EBV plays a key role in these malignancies, but is probably not the sole cause of the disease.

Chronic fatigue syndrome

Feeling tired is a common symptom – especially in adulthood, so what makes chronic fatigue syndrome different? It is defined as 'severe disabling fatigue that lasts at least 6 months, made worse by minimal physical or mental exertion, and for which there is no adequate medical explanation'.

Features of chronic fatigue syndrome

- Fatigue (severe tiredness) is the main symptom, present for at least 6 months
- Fatigue is severe, disabling, and affects physical and mental function
- Other symptoms are often seen:
  - muscle aches, especially after physical exertion
  - mood swings
  - sleep disturbance
  - poor appetite
  - sore throats
  - fever
  - faintness or dizziness
- No other cause found

A large number of theories about the cause for the condition have been postulated, and causes and treatments drift into and out of fashion. A large body of medical opinion remains sceptical about the condition and somewhat derogatory terms have been used to describe it, 'yuppie flu' being one of them. In all reality we are not dealing with a single disorder here, but a complex disorder with a range of initiating and maintaining factors both physical and psychological. Important principles of management include:

- Acknowledging the physical and psychological nature of the disease
- Graded introduction of physical exercise can be useful
- Cognitive–behavioural therapy can be useful
- Negative processes, such as blaming the patient for the illness or accusing him or her of malingering or of having nothing wrong, are usually unhelpful
- Avoiding expensive and experimental remedies

Further sources of information

Article

Hickey SM, Strasburger VC. What every pediatrician should know about infectious mononucleosis in adolescents. *Pediatric Clinics of North America* 1997; **44**: 1541–56

Websites

www.hwl.co.nz/laboratory/News/epstein_barr_virus_serology.htm

Epstein–Barr virus serology.

www.cdc.gov/ncidod/diseases/ebv.htm

Background on Epstein–Barr virus.

www.science.org.au/nova/026/026key.htm

Self-test 4: A 14-year-old girl presents with tiredness. She says she hates the cold and she is fed up because her hair is in poor condition. She has also put on a lot of weight recently. She has a blood test, which shows the following thyroid function tests:

Thyroxine (nmol/L)	54 (normal range 76–155)
Thyroid-stimulating hormone or TSH (mU/L)	28 (normal range 0.3–3.8)

A What is the underlying problem?
B Why is the TSH level raised?
C What would you find if you tested the deep tendon reflexes of her knee?
D What treatment is required?
E For how long?

Answers:
A Primary hypothyroidism (failure of the thyroid gland)
B As the pituitary is trying to stimulate a failing gland
C A slow relaxation phase
D Thyroxine replacement
E For life

A girl with recurrent fainting attacks

Age: 15 years

STEVEN RYAN

Presenting complaint

A hospital paediatrician receives the following referral letter from a general practitioner:

> Please would you see Rebecca aged 15 – she has collapsed to the ground on a number of occasions, at school and at home. In between attacks she is healthy. She has an uncle with epilepsy and the family are worried that she too may have epilepsy, and would like a brain scan and an EEG to be performed. I examined her and could find no abnormality.

Initial considerations and action

The key differential diagnosis here is shown in Table 40.1.

The history, examination and investigations will be aimed at deciding which system is involved and then at

Table 40.1 Examples of underlying disorders in the differential diagnosis

Underlying disorder type	Example
Cardiovascular	Syncopal episodes
Neurological disorder	Epilepsy
Psychological disorder	Factitious seizure
Metabolic	Hypoglycaemia

trying to determine the specific disorder. It is important to differentiate common non-serious disorders (e.g. simple faints in teenagers) from serious disorders (e.g. underlying cardiac arrhythmias). The most important tool in determining this is the history. Some causes of acute collapse can be discounted because they are unlikely to be recurrent (see Chapter 22).

Self-test 1: For each of the five statements below say whether an epileptic seizure or a syncopal episode (faint) is more likely.

A Patient has no memory of episode

B Patient remembers tunnel vision and then eyesight blacking out

C Episodes occur on rising to a standing position first thing in the morning

D Patient had tremulous jerking for several seconds

E Episode occurred while patient was lying down

Answer: A: fit; B: faint; C: faint; D: faint; E: fit.

History

First of all the history of the individual episodes is reviewed. Unless there have been very large numbers of episodes or all episodes have been identical, it is best to record the information in a systematic way. Rebecca's mother has kept a diary of the events (Figure 40.1).

No.	Where and when	Situation	Description of attack	Other comments
1	School – assembly 09:15	Standing	Felt hot, weak, room span, fell	Missed breakfast
2	Home 21:00	Getting out from bath	Vision quickly became black, fell – hitting head on side of bath	
3	School 12:15 (pre-lunch)	Coryza 2 days, feverish	Felt hot, light-headed, vision blacked out, fell	Took 2 days to recover from cold
4	School 15:30 (lessons just finished)	Cut knee on way out of school	Went pale, felt nauseous, fell to ground outside school	Never liked the sight of blood. Headache afterwards (did not hit head)

Figure 40.1 A diary of symptoms.

A further history is obtained:

Features consistent with epilepsy

- None of the following:
  - urinary incontinence
  - frothing of saliva
  - tongue biting
  - no memory of episode
- Shaking:
  - a few brief jerks of Rebecca's limbs were noted on occasion

Past medical history

- Three febrile convulsions between ages 1 month and 4 years
- Always been a thin child
- Otherwise well
- She regularly misses meals and particularly breakfast

Family history

- The mother's brother has primary generalized epilepsy, well controlled on sodium valproate
- His fits started at a similar age to those in Rebecca
- The family are very concerned that Rebecca might have epilepsy
- There is no family history of heart disease, arrhythmia, sudden collapse or death

- No history of hearing loss within the family
- None of the attacks has occurred during exercise or immediately related to a sudden stimulus
- Rebecca is mentally well and the family are settled with no recent significant life events. She is also happy at school. She has seen her uncle have a fit – which she found very distressing

We are now in a position to consider the initial differential diagnosis.

Cardiovascular

- This seems the most likely cause – feeling unwell before falling is consistent with reduced blood flow in the brain
- This is also supported by the pallor that was observed
- Standing still for long periods, getting out of a hot bath, an emotional shock, underlying viral illness and hunger are all in keeping with syncope (simple fainting)
- Episodes occurring during exercise, and especially during swimming and immediately at the time of a shock or loud noise, are indicative of an underlying serious arrhythmia (e.g. prolonged QT syndrome), which needs to be dealt with early
- Prolonged QT syndrome may also be associated with a family history of sudden death in young people and with hearing loss; both these situations indicate that

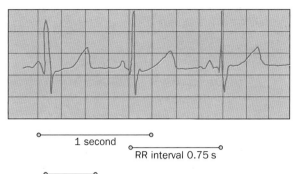

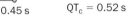

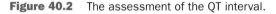

Figure 40.2 The assessment of the QT interval.

prolonged QT syndrome can be genetically determined (Figure 40.2 shows assessment of QT interval)

● The subsequent headache after one of the episodes is frequently seen and may represent an adrenaline (epinephrine) effect

Neurological disorder

● Although a few brief jerks were observed on one occasion, no sustained clonic jerking has occurred
● The patient remembering the attack in which consciousness is lost is a key point – this makes primary generalized epilepsy unlikely

Psychological disorder

● Factitious seizure seems unlikely because the attacks tend to be theatrical, evolving and prolonged
● Rebecca's attacks have not been like her uncle's and factitious attacks may mirror those observed elsewhere
● There is no history of family or personal psychological problems
● There is no history of hyperventilation or anxiety attacks

Metabolic

● Hypoglycaemia may have provoked at least one attack and is a known factor in syncopal episodes
● The onset of episodes is rather quick for hypoglycaemia

The history points towards syncopal episodes and the examination must make this a priority. However, the family's initial concern is the neurological disorder epilepsy and a thorough examination of the central nervous system will help to provide reassurance.

Self-test 2: Describe the usual neurological findings in a child with primary generalized epilepsy.

Answer: Such children are normally healthy on routine physical examination.

Examination

Cardiovascular system

● Pulse rate: 80/minute – regular – normal volume and character
● Blood pressure:
  – right arm lying down 110/72
  – right arm immediately on standing 94/64
● Precordium: apex undisplaced, no thrills, no heaves
● Auscultation: normal heart sounds heard, no additional sounds or murmurs

Self-test 3: Why is blood pressure taken lying down and standing up in this case?

Answer: To determine whether any postural hypotension is present. This sometimes accompanies a tendency to syncope.

How to take blood pressure in a child

● Make sure you use the right size cuff (Figure 40.3). Its length when on the upper arm should be two-thirds of the shoulder – elbow distance
● It is important that the arrow indicating the relative position to the brachial artery should be in the right position

- The cuff should be inflated until the radial artery (or brachial artery in younger children) can no longer be palpated
- The cuff is then slowly deflated. Systolic pressure is indicated when the artery is initially auscultated and diastolic pressure when the sound stops

Nervous system

- A thorough examination of the CNS revealed no abnormality

Growth

- Height: 171 cm (90th centile)
- Weight: 59 kg (just over 50th centile)
- Weight for height: 88 per cent

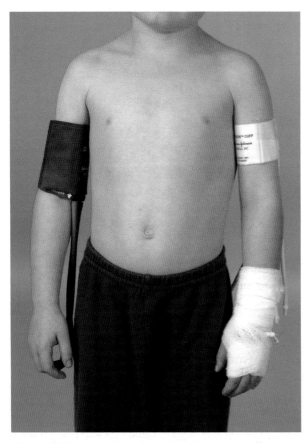

Figure 40.3 An appropriate blood pressure cuff on the left and one that is too small on the right.

No significant pathology has been detected but, interestingly, there has been a fall in blood pressure (BP) when Rebecca stands up. The definition of orthostatic or postural hypotension is a reduction in systolic BP of at least 20 mmHg or a reduction in diastolic BP of at least 10 mmHg. Although not meeting this definition, the finding is consistent with a diagnosis of 'neurocardiogenic' or 'vasovagal' syncope. Underweight, tall (but otherwise well) children do seem to be at particular risk of this disorder, and Rebecca fits this profile well.

Investigations

The family was initially keen to exclude the diagnosis of epilepsy with a brain scan and an electroencephalogram (EEG). They are told that epilepsy is a clinical diagnosis based on the history of the events. It is clear from Rebecca's history that the episodes are not epileptic and a cardiovascular cause is more likely. Any investigations should be aimed at that system. As a result of the thorough examination, acknowledgement of their concerns and clear explanation, the families are happy to pursue investigation of the cardiovascular system.

An electrocardiogram (ECG) is undertaken. It is reported as shown in Table 40.2. Comment based on this ECG: 'This ECG seems to be healthy and in particular the QT interval is within normal limits.'

For this patient this degree of investigation is adequate given the limited number of attacks, although other investigations can be done:

- **Exercise ECG:** if exercise-induced symptoms, prolonged QT suspected
- **Echocardiogram:** exercise-induced symptoms or family history of collapse
- **Tilt-test (see below):** very troublesome fainting, treatment considered, true abnormality of autonomic nervous system suspected

Diagnosis

Neurocardiogenic syncope (vasovagal episodes – simple faints).

Table 40.2   Rebecca's ECG

Component	Feature	Assessment	Expected values
P waves	Rate (/min)	78	60–120
	Rhythm (regular/irregular)	Regular sinus rhythm	
	Axis (°)	+60	0 to +90
	Size (mm)	1.5	<2.5
	Duration (ms)	80	<120
	Association with QRS complex	1:1	1:1
PR interval duration (lead II) (ms) (from start of P wave to start of QRS complex)		120	90–175
QRS complex	Duration (ms)	50	34–88
	Axis (°)	+60	+10 to +130
	Configuration	Normal	
ST segment depression or elevation		Neither	Neither
T wave	Inversion present	No	No
	Size	Normal	Normal
QT interval duration (corrected for heart rate QT$_c$) (ms)		380	<440

Management and prognosis

Rebecca was reassured that she did not have a serious health problem and would not die. Nor did she have epilepsy. The nature of the episodes (why and how they occur) was discussed with her. In particular, the provoking factors in Table 40.3 were discussed along with possible solutions.

Rebecca was also given advice on what to do if she felt she was going to faint and it was suggested that, if the first manoeuvre was unsuccessful, she could move to the next:

1 Sit down
2 Sit down with head between legs
3 Lie down
4 Lie down with legs up

Rebecca was also asked to keep a diary and return for review in 3 months. During that time she had one further

Table 40.3   Provoking factors

Factor	Possible solution
Being tall	None!
Being thin	Discuss improved diet
Standing still	Move!
Missing meals	Do not miss meals
Intercurrent infections	Be prepared for possible episodes
Standing up	Take care, rise slowly, sit back down quickly – especially rising from a hot bath
Emotional shock/pain	Avoid!
Hot, stuffy environments	Seek cool environment – cool drink

episode during morning assembly at school. She lay down on the floor and, although she felt unwell, she did not lose consciousness. Once they understood the problem, her teachers were helpful in preventing attacks occurring. Over the following year the episodes stopped.

Background information

ECG in children

This procedure is essentially performed in the same way as in adults with the leads positioned in the same way (Figure 40.4). The P wave represents atrial depolarization and the PR interval the conduction from the atrioventricular node into the bundle of His and ventricular conducting system. The QRS complex then begins with the onset ventricular depolarization and the T wave is ventricular repolarization (Table 40.4).

The direction in which polarization of the atria and ventricles occurs is called the axis and is determined using the limb leads in the coronal plane.

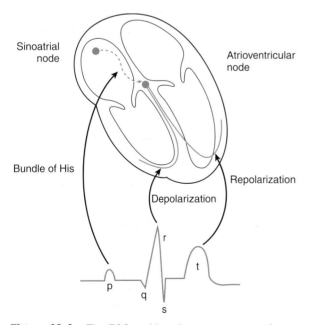

Figure 40.4 The ECG and how its components relate to conduction within the heart.

The physiology of fainting and not fainting

Not fainting

When a typical teenager stands, about a pint of blood is forced downward by gravity to the lower abdomen and into the legs. Within a few seconds, there is decreased in venous return to the right side of the heart. The pressure receptors in the heart, lungs, carotid sinus and aortic arch are activated and provoke an increase in the sympathetic system input to the cardiovascular system. By vasoconstriction of blood vessels in the above areas and through increased cardiac output, a healthy teenager is able to stabilize and normalize cardiac output within a minute. This neurally mediated mechanism is the way by which hominids can adapt to having an upright posture.

Fainting

This is vasovagal or neurocardiogenic syncope usually (but not always) on standing. Venous pooling in the lower body begins but the body's autoregulatory response fails, cardiac output is diminished, brain blood flow falls below a critical level and syncope occurs. The body's response of then falling over is a final regulatory mechanism that restores brain blood flow. The restriction in blood flow does not cause permanent brain injury. The failure is related to an inappropriate response of the autonomic nervous system, which, for example, may result in a paradoxical bradycardia and peripheral vascular dilatation, which worsens cardiac output. The bradycardia is often related to forceful contractions and the patient may report a pounding heart beat before collapse. These mechanisms can be elucidated using the tilt-table test. The patient is placed horizontally on a flat table and strapped down. Blood pressure and heart rate are monitored. The table is then tilted to a more vertical position and in many patients this provokes some of the symptoms as well as hypotension and bradycardia. This can be used to diagnose the condition if there is uncertainty.

Treating fainting
Usually no specific treatment is indicated or used but in problematic or frequent attacks increased salt intake, fludrocortisone treatment, β blockade and even more rarely electrical heart pacing may be used.

Table 40.4   Components of the ECG, abnormalities and their meanings

Component	Feature	Abnormality	Meaning
P waves			
	Rate	Slow	Sinus bradycardia
		Fast	Sinus tachycardia
	Rhythm	Irregular	Atrial fibrillation
			Sick sinus syndrome
	Axis	Abnormal	Heart not in usual position
			Leads in wrong place
			Atrial position abnormal
	Size	Large	Right atrial hypertrophy
	Duration	Long	Left atrial hypertrophy
	Association with QRS complex	Absent	Heart block
PR interval duration (lead II) (from start of P wave to start of QRS complex)		Short	Short circuit to atrioventricular node, e.g. Wolff–Parkinson–White syndrome
		Long	First-degree heart block
QRS complex			
	Duration		
	Axis	Right deviation	Right ventricular hypertrophy
	Configuration	Q waves in right chest	Right ventricle enlargement
		Deep Q waves II, II, V4–6	Left ventricle enlargement
		Large R in V1	Right ventricular hypertrophy
		Large S in V6	Right ventricular hypertrophy
ST segment depression/elevation		Depression	Ischaemia
		Elevation	Pericarditis, infarction
T wave			
	Size		Enlarged and peaked in hyperkalaemia
			Small in hypothyroidism, hypokalaemia
	Inversion		Ischaemia, infarction and myocarditis
QT interval duration (corrected for heart rate QT_c)		Prolonged	Prolonged QT syndromes
			Hypocalcaemia
			Bundle-branch block
			Myocarditis

Table 40.5 Information for Self-test 4

No.	Where and when	Situation	Description of attack	Other comments
1	Home 07:00	Sitting in kitchen	Fell off chair, went totally rigid for 1 minute, shook all over 2 minutes Slept No memory of episode	Drowsy for several hours
2	School 08:30	At desk	Fell off chair, stiff then shaking, frothy secretions in mouth No memory of episode	Incontinent of urine

Further sources of information

Book

Archer N, Burch M. *Paediatric Cardiology. An Introduction*. London: Chapman and Hall Medical, 1998

Articles

Di Girolamo E, Di Iorio C, Leonzio L, Sabatini P, Barsotti A. Usefulness of a tilt training program for the prevention of refractory neurocardiogenic syncope in adolescents: A controlled study. *Circulation* 1999; **100**: 1798–801

Strieper MJ, Auld DO, Hulse E, Campbell RM. Evaluation of recurrent pediatric syncope: role of tilt table testing. *Pediatrics* 1994; **93**: 660–2

Websites

www.epilepsy.org.uk/info/ffftfrm.html

Fits, faints and funny turns from a neurological perspective.

www.childrenheartinstitute.org/educate/syncope/neurocar.htm

A good guide to the pathophysiology of syncope.

Self-test 4: Table 40.5 gives some of the information about a previously healthy 8-year-old boy who reports two episodes.

A What is the most likely system responsible for these episodes?
B What is the likely diagnosis?
C What test would be most useful?
D Would any treatment be reasonable and, if so, give an example?
E How should the boy change his lifestyle?

Answer:
A Nervous system
B Primary generalized epilepsy
C An electroencephalogram to determine the epilepsy syndrome and to help choose an appropriate treatment
D Sodium valproate, carbamazepine, lamotrigine
E Consider restricting climbing at any height, taking a bath with the door locked, cycling in busy streets or without a helmet, swimming without direct and continuous supervision

Index